Illustrated Pediatric Dentistry (Part 2)

Edited by

Satyawan Damle

Former Professor of Pediatric Dentistry,
Dean Nair Hospital Dental College,
Mumbai, India

Former Vice Chancellor,
Department of Pediatric Dentistry,
Maharishi Markandeshwar University,
Mullana, Ambala, India

Ritesh Kalaskar

Department of Pedodontic and Preventive Dentistry,
Government Dental College & Hospital, Nagpur,
India

&

Dhanashree Sakhare

Founder, Lavanika Dental Academy
Melbourne
Australia

Illustrated Pediatric Dentistry (Part 2)

Editors: Satyawan Damle, Ritesh Kalaskar and Dhanashree Sakhare

ISBN (Online): 978-981-5080-77-3

ISBN (Print): 978-981-5080-78-0

ISBN (Paperback): 978-981-5080-79-7

need for a court order if at any point you breach any terms of this License Agreement. In no event will any delay or failure by Bentham Science Publishers in enforcing your compliance with this License Agreement constitute a waiver of any of its rights.

3. You acknowledge that you have read this License Agreement, and agree to be bound by its terms and conditions. To the extent that any other terms and conditions presented on any website of Bentham Science Publishers conflict with, or are inconsistent with, the terms and conditions set out in this License Agreement, you acknowledge that the terms and conditions set out in this License Agreement shall prevail.

Bentham Science Publishers Pte. Ltd.
80 Robinson Road #02-00
Singapore 068898
Singapore
Email: subscriptions@benthamscience.net

BENTHAM SCIENCE

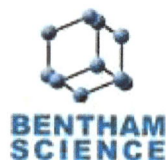

CONTENTS

FOREWORD 1

It is my great pleasure to pen down a foreword for this tremendous book on Pediatric Dentistry for a legend and doyen of the subject, a mentor and guide to the brightest of minds in the field of dentistry.

Rising from the fundamentals, comprehensive in-built, contemporary and authoritative in construct and approach, and hands-on to the core, *Illustrated Pediatric Dentistry* is a wonderful work engineered by some of the best-known academics in this noble realm. The chief author, *Professor Satyawan Damle*, is a colossus among giants, having been a celebrated teacher, distinguished leader, and dynamic policymaker at several dental institutions and universities, including the most prized, the University of Mumbai.

Prof. Satyawan Damle is the rare blend of a gifted clinician and a carved-out academic guru whose intellect has emerged with decades of practice. It is no secret that the degree of acquisition of knowledge by students is one of the measures of the effectiveness of a medical curriculum; and with Pediatric Dentistry being one of the crucial epicentres of growth, it has the potential to make momentous advancements in the evolutionary trajectory of oral and general health.

His co-editors *Ritesh Kalaskar & Dhanashree Sakhare* are examples of excellence in their arena. The work reflects their collective understanding of where pediatric dentistry stands today, what have been the treasures and well-kept secrets of the past, and where this tree of knowledge finds fruition today pawing way for the future.

Embedding best care practices of all times, *Illustrated Pediatric Dentistry* is a comprehensive yet concise work, which fulfils the essentials of the pediatric dentistry curriculum both for graduates and postgraduates across all universities.

Walking you through the nitty-gritties of preventive, curative and restorative childhood dentistry, be it the behavioral challenges, cariology, endodontics, traumatology, para-surgical themes such as the use of conscious sedation and general anaesthesia at that age, and the management of medically compromised children, the work is a tree of knowledge, nurtured with experiential learning, and carries wonderful blossoms of practical wisdom.

Let us savour and celebrate the chef-d'oeuvre. Indeed, Illustrated Pediatric Dentistry is a must-read and must-assimilate work for each one of us. Students, practitioners and teachers of Pediatric dentistry will cherish it as a treasured possession on their shelves. I congratulate Prof. Damle and Bentham Science, Singapore, for publishing this irreplaceable tome.

Prof. (Dr.) Mahesh Verma
Vice Chancellor
Guru Gobind Singh
Indraprastha University,
New Delhi,
India

FOREWORD 2

I am delighted to write this foreword for a Book of Illustrated Pediatric Dentistry edited by Professor Satyawan Damle and other academicians. Prof. Satyawan Damle is a well-known researcher and academician with over 44 years of clinical and teaching experience in Dentistry. Besides the several posts and hats he wore in the various roles he played for the profession, he is also a recipient of several awards and recognitions, including the Lifetime Achievement Awards, Outstanding Public Servant Awards, and Research Awards and Fellowships. He is an active member of the Indian Council of Medical Research. Despite his extraordinary achievements as a Pediatric dentist, researcher, and academician, Prof Satyawan Damle will always be known as the longest-serving chief editor of Indexed journals. For almost 35 years. He dedicated himself to overseeing the publication of the highest-quality peer-reviewed studies and opinion pieces on child dental health.

Prof. Damle is actively involved in writing several books on Pediatric Dentistry and Dentistry, which is the testimony of his in-depth knowledge of the subject. The Book of Illustrated Pediatric Dentistry is their new venture initiated by him. I am confident that this book will be accepted by students and faculty involved in teaching Pediatric Dentistry. His work as a teacher, researcher, innovator, visionary and extraordinary academician made him a legend. His role as a mentor and friend made him a role model to those of us who know him and worked with him. His legacy persists not only in academics but also as an able administrator, as he proved his mettle as the Dean of a dental school, Director of Medical Education, Joint Municipal.

Commissioner of Mumbai and, ultimately, the Vice Chancellor of a University. Prof. Damle has worked conscientiously and untiringly to present an unmatched educational endeavour. The topics in this book display a clear and succinct clinical expertise and the capability of imparting updated education and information to Oral Health Professionals. The entire volume of this book deals with ultramodern and current state-of-the-art techniques. I take this opportunity to congratulate Prof. Satyawan Damle and his team of contributors - Ritesh Kalaskar and Dhanashree Sakhare for publishing this Textbook for Bentham Science.

Dr. Ashok Dhoble
Secretary General
Indian Dental Association H.O.
Mumbai, Maharashtra 400025,
India

PREFACE

It is imperative to have an established approach to handling Children's oral diseases. **'Illustrated Pediatric Dentistry,'** is an unpretentious endeavour to integrate the latest developments and up-to-date reviews in the field of Pediatric dentistry by distinguished writers. The book intends to allow students to understand the conceptions of Pediatric dentistry and create a spur to discover the subject by advance reading. Several illustrations, descriptions and graphic drawings have been included to attract the students and make the subject simple to comprehend. A healthy mouth is a gateway to a healthy body and the best time to inculcate healthy habits is through childhood. Prevention of the initiation of oral diseases and training appropriate oral hygiene methods are commenced best throughout the formative years of the child. With a substantial percentage of the worldwide population being in the Pediatric age group, it is imperious to have a scientific approach in the behaviour management, prevention and treatment modalities in the dental office, as Pediatric dentistry is a fast-growing division of dental disciplines that lays the basis for the impending dental health of the populace.

The book has been divided into several sections. The sections on child psychology and the emotional development of children are important to learn the basics of various behaviour management strategies. The section on dental caries sensitizes the reader towards the most common dental disorder that is seen in children, and preventive procedures aimed towards lessening dental caries are the necessity of the hour. While an endeavour has been made to include the growth and development of the facial structures and dentition and along with their disturbances and the interceptive and preventive procedures to monitor the erupting teeth.

Pediatric Operative techniques, including endodontics and management of teeth with immature apices affected due to dental caries and traumatic injuries have been given prominence. Innovations in the field of Pediatric dentistry are transpiring amazingly fast, and it is crucial to stay up to date with the latest materials, equipment and techniques to deliver the highest quality of care to our little patients.

The new book cannot be successfully compiled without the collective contribution regarding meticulous reviews of the manuscript to keep pace with the latest innovative novelties. The credit for introducing a new textbook goes to the contributors for their engrossment, devotion and dedication in presenting a manuscript after applying prudent and well-adjudged scrutiny and analytical approach and have excelled in exploring the things to the ultimate.

Accumulation of information and its cogent management would not have been conceivable without the efforts of the contributors who have painstakingly submitted their manuscripts to shape this gargantuan task and to introduce this book in the service of Pediatric dentistry.

Satyawan Damle   **Ritesh Kalaskar**
Former Vice-Chancellor,   Department of Pedodontic and Preventive Dentistry
Maharishi Markandeshwar University,   Government Dental College & Hospital, Nagpur
Mullana (Ambala), India   India

Dhanashree Sakhare
Founder,
Lavanika Dental Academy,
Melbourne
Australia

ACKNOWLEDGEMENTS

We do not find such appropriate words to praise the unique nature of Dr. Mahesh Verma, Vice Chancellor of Guru Gobind Singh Indraprastha University, New Delhi, who himself being a great resolute and connoisseur of dentistry occupying an illustrious position with an eminent background in dentistry, has spared his valuable time from his busy schedule to inscribe the foreword for the textbook of "Illustrated Pediatric Dentistry". We take it as inventiveness and encouragement rather than a morale-boosting for us to uphold and keep up our determination to satisfy our hunger for academics for the advantage of budding dental professionals.

We also do not find such befitting words to laud the unique nature of Dr. Ashok Dhoble Hon, General Secretary, Indian Dental Association Head Office, who himself being a great advocate and connoisseur of dentistry occupying a distinguished position with an illustrious background in dentistry has spared his precious time from his busy schedule to write the foreword for the Textbook of Illustrated Pediatric Dentistry. I take it as an inspiration and encouragement rather than a morale-boosting for us to uphold and keep up our determination to satisfy our hunger for academics for the advantage of budding dental professionals.

We are also indebted and beholden to the contributors for their altruistic and substantial contribution to make this Textbook of Illustrated Pediatric Dentistry, a great academic endeavour. The contributors are highly competent and knowledgeable clinicians known for their aptitude and capability, which have successfully recognized the most complex and convoluted details of each topic, duly integrating and blending the latest advancements and innovations in Pediatric Dentistry. They are a terrific hard worker and legendary luminaries known for their admirable accomplishments and remarkable involvement in dental education. They have made lots of efforts to lead things to excellence. Credit goes to these patrons and benefactors for the benevolent bequest of their vast knowledge and experience for the betterment of dental education.

We would also like to thank Dr. Priyanka Bhaje, Dr. Parag Kasar, Dr. Sharath Chandra, Dr. Prachi Goyal and Dr. Vidya Iyer for their painstaking efforts and intransigent toil during the editing of this book. They displayed exceptional patients, forbearance, and commitment during the preparation of the book Our dream has come true due to the support of our past and present students. Credit also goes to our family members for their tolerance, Love, and affection.

We would like to appreciate the efforts of Mrs. Humaira Hashmi & Mrs. Fariya Zulfiqar of Bentham Science for giving us an opportunity to pen down our ideas and academic work to reality. We also convey our kind and sincere appreciation to Pascali Pascalis.

Representative of Porter Instrument Business Unit of Parker Hannifin Matrx by Parker and Parker-Porter Product for permitting us to use the company products in our book.

Lastly, we would like to state that fortune favours those who defy complexities and overcome them on their own. We also passionately believe that Man is the architect of his own destiny, and God is on the side of those who toil and perspire to make their providence.

We place our sincerest admiration and gratitude to all those who have delightfully contributed to this cause and for their wishes and devotions made for understanding our dream.

Satyawan Damle
Former Vice-Chancellor,
Maharishi Markandeshwar University,
Mullana (Ambala), India

Ritesh Kalaskar
Department of Pedodontic and Preventive Dentistry
Government Dental College & Hospital, Nagpur
India

&

Dhanashree Sakhare
Founder,
Lavanika Dental Academy,
Melbourne
Australia

List of Contributors

Aditi Pashine	Associate Dentist, MyDentist, Aberystwyth, UK
Aman Chowdhry	Professor, Faculty of Dentistry, Jamia Milia Islamia (A Central University), New Delhi, India
Armelia Sari Widyarman	Department of Oral Biology, Faculty of Dentistry, Universitas Trisakti, Jakarta, Indonesia Departmental Head of Microbiology, Faculty of Dentistry, Universitas Trisakti, Jakarta, Indonesia
Arun M Xavier	Department of Pediatric and Preventive Dentistry, Amrita School of Dentistry, Cochin, Kerala, India
Bhavna Dave	Department of Pediatric and Preventive Dentistry, K. M. Shah Dental College, and Hospital, Sumandeep Vidyapeeth Deemed to be University, Vadodara, Gujarat, India
Bhavna Gupta Saraf	Department of Pedodontics and Preventive Dentistry, Sudha Rustagi College of Dental Sciences and Research, Faridabad, Haryana, India
Deepika Bablani Popli	Department of Oral Pathology and Microbiology, Faculty of Dentistry, Jamia Millia Islamia, New Delhi, India
Dhanashree Sakhare	Founder Lavanika Dental Academy, Melbourne, Australia
Eko Fibryanto	Department of Conservative Dentistry, Faculty of Dentistry, Universitas Trisakti, Jakarta, Indonesia
Enrita Dian R.	Department of Pedodontic, Faculty of Dentistry, Universitas Trisakti, Jakarta, Indonesia
H. Sharath Chandra	SJM Dental College and Hospital, Chitradurga, Karnataka, India
Jay Gopal Ray	Dr. R Ahmed Dental College and Hospital, Kolkata, West Bengal, India
M. Vijay	Department of Orthodontics, CSI College of Dental Sciences and Research, Madurai, Tamil Nadu, India
M.H. Raghunath Reddy	Professor and Head, SJM Dental College and Hospital, Chitradurga, Karnataka, India
Monika Rathore	Department of Pedodontics and Preventive Dentistry, BBD College of Dental Sciences, BBD University, Lucknow, U.P, India
Neerja Singh	Department of Pedodontics and Preventive Dentistry, BBD College of Dental Sciences, BBD University, Lucknow, U.P, India
Parag Kasar	Chief Pediatric Dentist at Deep Dental Clinic, Nerul, Navi Mumbai, India
Prachi Goyal	Maharishi Markandeshwar College of Dental Sciences and Research, Ambala, India
Pratik Kariya	Department of Pediatric and Preventive Dentistry, K. M. Shah Dental College, and Hospital, Sumandeep Vidyapeeth Deemed to be University, Vadodara, Gujarat, India
Priyanka Bhaje	Rungata College of Dental Sciences and Research Center, Bhilai, Chhattisgarh, India

Raghavendra M. Shetty   Department of Clinical Sciences, College of Dentistry, Center of Medical and Bio-allied Health Sciences Research, Ajman University, Ajman, UAE

Satyawan Damle   Former Professor of Pediatric Dentistry, Dean Nair Hospital Dental College, Mumbai, India
Former Vice Chancellor, Department of Pediatric Dentistry, Maharishi Markandeshwar University, Mullana, Ambala, India

Shailaja Chatterjee   Department of Oral Pathology, Yamuna College of Dental Sciences and Research, Yamuna Nagar, Haryana, India

Shruti Balasubramanian   Department of Pediatric and Preventive Dentistry, Government Dental College and Hospital, Nagpur, India

Tri Erri Astoeti   Department of Dental Public Health and Preventive Dentistry, Faculty of Dentistry, Universitas Trisakti, Jakarta, Indonesia

Trisha Gadekar   Department of Pediatric Dentistry, Mamata Dental College, Khammam, Telangana, India

Vidya Iyer   Department of Orthodontics, CSI College of Dental Sciences and Research, Madurai, Tamil Nadu, India

CHAPTER 1

Swellings of Orofacial Structures in Children

Jay Gopal Ray[1,*] and **Priyanka Bhaje**[2]

[1] *Dr. R Ahmed Dental College and Hospital, Kolkata, West Bengal, India*

[2] *Rungta College of Dental Sciences and Research, Bhilai, Chhattisgarh 490024, India*

Abstract: Orofacial swelling is clinically a common problem found in pediatric dental patients. The causes of these swellings are mostly diverse, and the knowledge about specific clinical as well as imaging manifestations along with the most affected sites of these swelling is needed for the formulation of a differential diagnosis. Mid-facial non-progressive swelling is usually suggestive of a congenital defect (like a cephalocele, nasal glioma, epidermoid cyst or nasal dermoid). Swelling that is slowly progressive, may be indicative of a neurofibroma, hemangioma, vascular malformation, lymph angioma, pseudocyst or fibrous dysplasia. In cases of facial swellings that are rapidly progressive and associated with cranial nerve deficits, rhabdomyosarcoma, Ewing sarcoma, Langerhans cell histiocytosis, metastatic neuroblastoma and osteogenic sarcoma should also be included in the differential diagnosis.

Keywords: Congenital Defect, Differential Diagnosis, Oro-facial Swelling.

INTRODUCTION

Facial swelling is one of the common and significant clinical problems in pediatric dentistry. The etiological factors (origins) of a facial mass or swelling may vary from congenital causes to various acquired conditions like infections and conditions of soft tissue and/or bone (malignant or benign). The detailed history, physical manifestations and clinical examination are the most important factors when evaluating these facial swellings (Fig. **1**). Jaw swellings, another important problem in children, pose a major diagnostic challenge in Pediatric Dentistry. Detailed knowledge about these entities helps in the appropriate management of this condition.

Diseases of Jawbones

The diseases of jawbones are mentioned in the following Fig. (**1**):

---

* **Corresponding author Jay Gopal Ray:** Dr. R Ahmed Dental College and Hospital, Kolkata, West Bengal, India; E-mail: jaygopalray60@gmail.com

OSTEOPETROSIS	CAFFEY'S DISEASE
CHERUBISM	OSTEOGENESIS IMPERFECTA
FIBROUS DYSPLSIA	GARRE'S OSTEOMYELITIS
OSSIFYING FIBROMA	HISTIOCYTOSIS X
JUVENILE OSSIFYING FIBROMA	REILET-DAY SYNDROME
LEONTIASIS OSSEA	OSTEOMYELITIS

Fig. (1). Diseases of jawbones.

Osteopetrosis (Marble Bone Disease)

• Osteopetrosis is caused by an inherited defect in osteoclasts. Defective osteoclasts fail to resorb bone in the normal resorption remodeling cycle of the skeleton. So, all bones progressively become denser, less cellular, and less vascular. The bone foramina and marrow cavity spaces become compromised and compressed in the disease. Bone pain, fractures, anemia and thrombocytopenia, hepatosplenomegaly, and nerve dysfunction, due to compression of the nerve within foramina, ranging from hearing loss to visual disturbance to facial palsy, are possible (Fig. **2**).

• Facial deformity develops in many children. They manifest as a broad face, hypertelorism, snub nose and frontal bossing. Tooth eruption is almost always delayed. Osteomyelitis of the jaws can occur.

• Radiographically there is a highly increased density of the skull and mandible, and distinction between cortical and cancellous bone is lost [1, 2].

Treatment

• Treatment by means of bone marrow transplantation and interferon-gamma 1b and calcitriol have been advocated.
• Corticosteroid, parathormone, CSF and erythropoietin have been hypothesized.
• In cases of fracture in the pediatric age group, surgery might be required.
• Vitamin D (calcitriol) is administered in cases of osteoclastic stimulation.

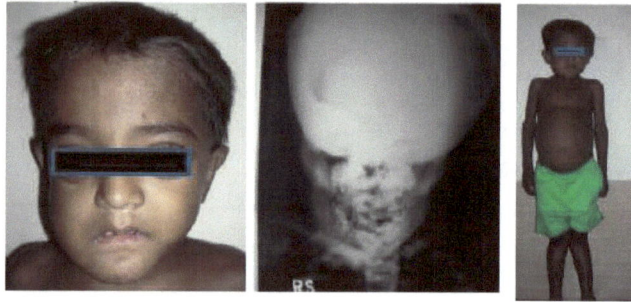

Fig. (2). Case of osteopetrosis.

Ossifying Fibroma

- Ossifying fibroma is a fibro-osseous lesion that is composed of fibrous tissue that contains a variable mixture of bony trabeculae, cementum-like spherules or both. The origin can be from odontogenic sources and PDL. The mandibular premolar molar areas are commonly affected. It usually causes a slow enlarging, asymptomatic, painless mass of the affected bone, whereas larger lesions can cause facial asymmetry and cosmetic disfigurement (Fig. **3**).
- Radiological appearance varies to some degree. The initial appearance is radiolucent, which becomes progressively radiopaque as the stroma mineralizes. Eventually, the individual radiopacities coalesce to the extent that the mature lesion may appear sclerotic. There is a presence of a well-demarcated radiologic margin.
- Histopathology shows a benign, osteogenic, well-demarcated neoplasm, within a fibroblastic stroma, composed of calcified material in the form of osteoid and/or cementoid structures with variable osteoblastic rimming along with occasional multinucleated giant cells and endothelial lined blood-filled spaces [3, 4].

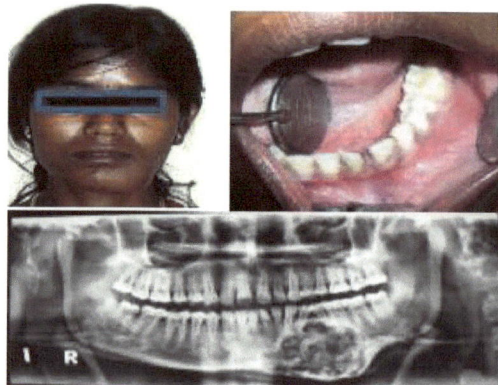

Fig. (3). Case of ossifying fibroma (Clinical photograph and corresponding OPG image).

Treatment

- Surgical enucleation/curettage is the treatment of choice for smaller lesions.
- En bloc resection for a larger lesion.

Juvenile Aggressive Ossifying Fibroma (Figs. 4a and 4b)

- It is an aggressive variant that usually affects children and young adults. It has two variants-trabecular and psamomatoid. Among these, the trabecular variant affects children in the age group of 5-15 years.
- WHO describes it as 'an actively growing lesion consisting of a cell-rich fibrous stroma, containing bands of cellular osteoid without osteoblastic rimming together with trabeculae of typical woven bone. Small foci of giant cells may also be present, and in some parts, there may be abundant osteoclasts related to woven bone. Usually, no fibrous capsule can be demonstrated.'
- The presence of nonrandom chromosomal breakpoints at Xq26 and 2q33 resulting in the translocation has been observed in psamommatoid variant [5].

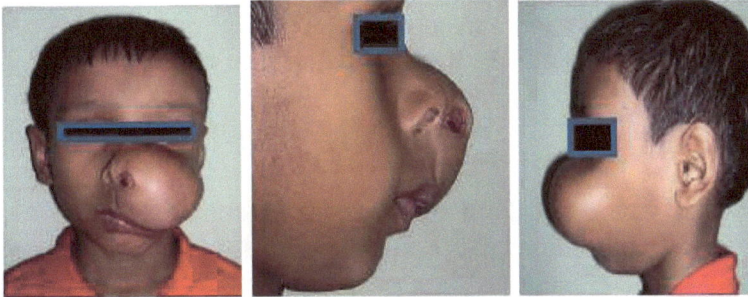

Fig. (4a). Extra-oral photograph showing deviation of left nostril.

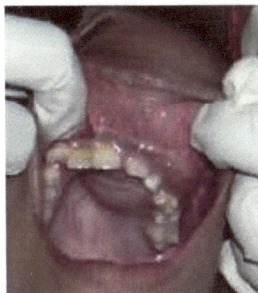

Fig. (4b). Intraoral photograph showing involvement of palate.

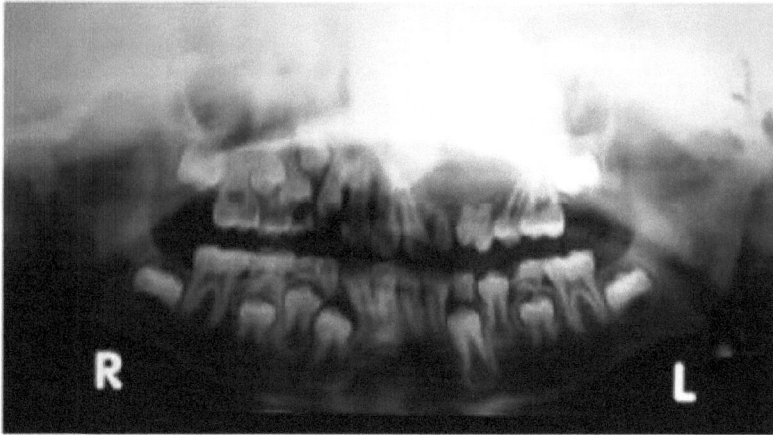

Fig. (4c). Panoramic radiograph showing displacement of maxillary anterior teeth.

Treatment

- The most preferred treatment option is surgical excision.
- Sometimes large tumors are managed with hemi sections.
- In cases of incomplete removal of lesion recurrence rate is high.

Cherubism (Fig. 5)

- Cherubism is an autosomal dominant genetic defect that affects bone remodeling in the specific anatomically confined regions of embryonic maxilla and mandible. It begins to manifest itself by the age of 2.5 years and is fully expressed by the age of 5 years. The jaws are affected bilaterally along with the expansion of the maxilla and mandible. The upward turned eyes with scleral show give a characteristic. 'Cherubic eyes towards heaven' appearance. This is due to maxillary expansion to the orbital space. The open bite caused by nasal obstruction and subsequent mouth breathing may be there.
- Histopathology shows multinucleated giant cells in a thin delicate fibro vascular connective tissue stroma. Perivascular eosinophilic cuffing of collagen fibers is also sometimes present [6].

Treatment

- Treatment is normally deferred till puberty.
- Surgical corrections and removal of ectopically impacted teeth should be done.
- Calcitonin and imatinib have been advocated in the treatment recently.

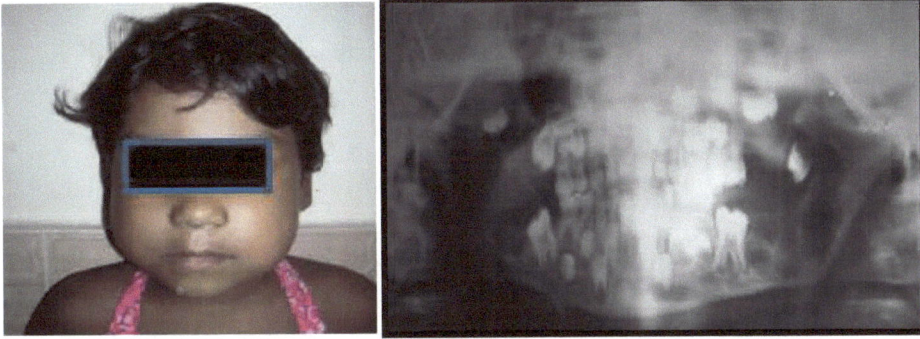

Fig. (5). Cherubism (Clinical photograph and corresponding panoramic radiograph).

Fibrous Dysplasia (Fig. 6)

- It is a developmental tumor-like condition characterized by the replacement of normal bone by an excessive proliferation of cellular fibrous connective tissue intermixed with irregular bony trabeculae, giving rise to the typical 'ground glass' radiological appearance. There is a post-zygotic mutation of the GNAS1 gene, affecting the differentiation of osteogenic precursor cells, melanocytes, and endocrine cells at various stages of embryonic life.
- Histopathology shows multiple variably shaped and sized trabeculae of immature woven bone without osteoblastic rimming, dispersed in a mature fibrous connective tissue stroma, which possesses curvilinear shapes, and are not connected to each other. These are linked to Chinese letter writing or cuneiform shapes due to their appearance [7].

Treatment

- The treatment is watchful neglect or surgical recontouring as per requirement.
- Radiation therapy is contraindicated.
- IV palmidronate can be used.

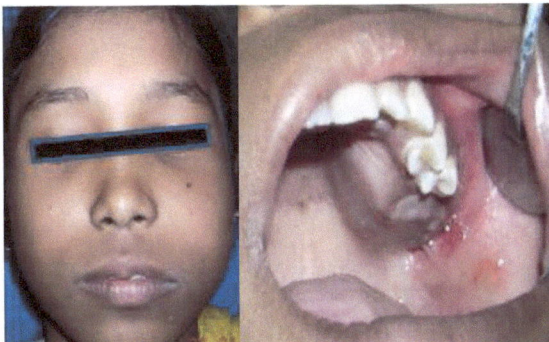

Fig. (6). Case of Fibrous dysplasia.

Osteogenesis Imperfecta (Fig. 7)

- A hereditary disorder producing abnormal quality and quantity of bone. It is characterized by impairment of collagen maturation. It is associated with genetic abnormalities which guide the formation of type 1 collagen-COLA1A gene on chromosome 17 and COLIA2 gene on chromosome 7. OI can be associated with dentinogenesis imperfecta.
- Bone fragility, blue sclera, altered teeth, hypoacusis, long bone and spine deformities and joint hyperextensibility may be present. The radiologic hallmarks of OI include osteopenia, bowing, angulation or deformity of the long bones, and multiple fractures. Mandible is more commonly affected. Radiographs typically reveal premature pulpal obliteration, although shell teeth may be seen. In affected patients, both dentitions demonstrate blue to brown translucence [8].

Treatment

- The mainstays of TT are physiotherapy, rehabilitation, and orthopedic surgery.
- IV bisphophonates can reduce bone pain and risk of fracture.

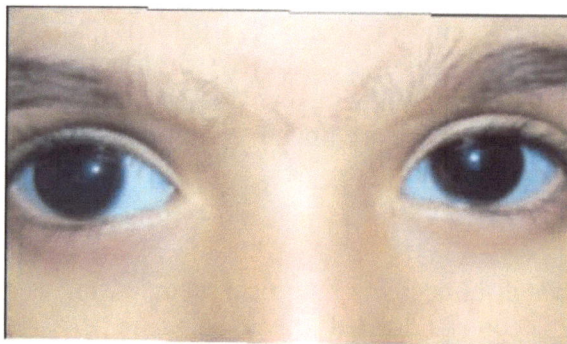

Fig. (7). Blue sclera in Osteogenesisimperfecta.

Caffey's Disease (Infantile Cortical Hyperostosis)

- It generally occurs before 6 months of age. It is due to mutations of the COLA1A gene. The mandible is affected in 75% of cases.
- The child is irritable and may have a fever, malaise, leukocytosis, anemia, increased ESR and increased alkaline phosphatase.
- The radiographs show thickening of cortex and bowing of inferior border. The swelling disappears in 3 to 10 months. Symptomatic treatment is recommended.

Treatment

- It has a good Prognosis, and therefore, only symptomatic therapy is advised.

- Nonsteroidal anti-inflammatory drugs such as Ibuprofen and Naproxen are recommended for any symptomatic treatment.

Osteomyelitis (Fig. 8)

- Osteomyelitis is usually defined as the inflammation of the bone and its marrow contents. Changes in the calcified tissue are secondary to inflammation of the soft tissue component of bone. Though osteomyelitis commonly occurs as a complication of dental sepsis, it is also seen in various other situations.
- Mandible is more commonly affected. Swelling and pain with fever, malaise, and leukocytosis persist. Draining sinus may be present.
- Predisposing factors include fractures due to trauma and RTA, gunshot wounds, radiation damage, Paget disease, and osteopetrosis. Systemic conditions like malnutrition, acute leukemia and uncontrolled diabetes may be responsible. It is a polymicrobial infection caused by *S aureus S albus, Bacteriodes, Porphyromonas etc* [9].

Treatment

- The recommended treatment options are drainage, antibiotics, and removal of the sequestrum.

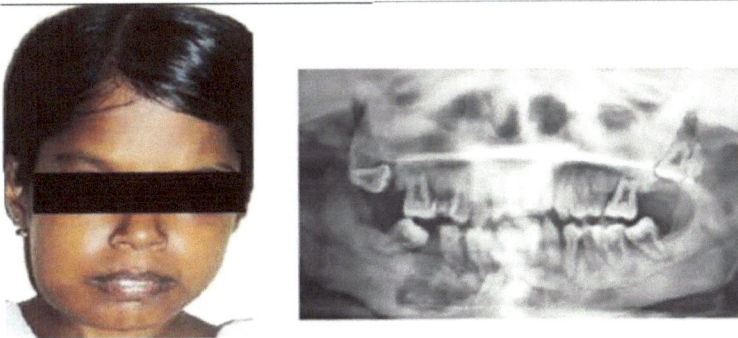

Fig. (8). Osteomyelitis of mandible (clinical and OPG image).

Garre's Osteomyelitis

- It is also known as chronic osteomyelitis with proliferative periosteitis. This is a distinct type of chronic osteomyelitis in which there is a focal gross thickening of the periosteum, with peripheral reactive bone formation resulting from mild infections or irritations. It is practically a periosteal osteosclerosis.
- It usually occurs in young person's prior to 25 years of age.
- The condition in the jaws occurs exclusively in the mandible in children and young adults, and most cases occur in the bicuspid and molar regions.
- The patient generally complains of a toothache in the jaws and a bony hard

swelling on the outer surface of the jaw. This mass is usually of several weeks' durations. Occasionally, cellulitis might move to the deeper periosteum and can cause such an infection.

- An occlusal radiograph reveals a focal overgrowth of bone on the outer surface of cortex, which may be described as a duplication of the cortical layer of bone.
- Garre's osteomyelitis is treated with the endodontic treatment of the affected tooth or removal of the carious infected tooth.

Treatment

- Conservative treatment is recommended to prevent extensive loss of developing teeth.
- Sometimes only the removal of the involved tooth and antibiotic coverage is advised in severe cases.

Langerhan's Cell Histiocytosis

- LCH is a clonal proliferation of cells of the immune system owing to its histogenesis from ubiquitous dendritic antigen-presenting and processing cells termed Langerhans cells.
- Langerhans cells are found in every organ, but they are somewhat numerous in bone marrow, lungs, mucosa, and skin. Therefore, LCH may have unifocal or multifocal presentations in any bone, most commonly the skull, facial bones, mandible, proximal femur, and ribs, but also in the lungs and either skin or mucosa, usually around the oral cavity or genitalia.
- The clinicopathologic spectrum is traditionally considered under the designation of LCH –
  - Monostotic or polyostotic eosinophilic granuloma of bone-solitary or multiple bone lesions without visceral involvement.
  - Chronic disseminated histiocytosis- a disease involving bone, skin, and viscera—Hand Schuller Christian disease.
  - Acute disseminated histiocytosis—a disease with prominent cutaneous, visceral, and bone marrow involvement occurring mainly in infants—Letterer siwe disease.
- The Hand Schuller Christian disease triad of bone lesions, exopthalmous and diabetes insipidus- is present in only a few patients. Pulmonary LCH has also been described. More than 50% of cases are seen in patients younger than age 15. Children younger than age 10 most often have a skull and femoral lesions, patients older than age 20 more often have lesions in the ribs, shoulder girdle and mandible.
- The jaws are affected in 10%-20% of all the cases. Dull pain and tenderness are often seen in bone lesions. Radiographically the lesions often appear as sharply

punched out radiolucencies without a corticated rim. Extensive alveolar destruction leading to a tooth having a characteristic floating on-air appearance is evident.

- Histopathology shows diffuse infiltration of large, pale staining mononuclear cells that resemble histiocytes. They have indistinct cytoplasmic borders and indented; vesicular coffee bean-shaped unfolded nuclei. Ultra-structurally rod-shaped Birbeck granules within the cytoplasm are a characteristic feature.

- IHC shows positivity for CD1a or CD 207 for Langerhans cells. They also show positivity for peanut-specific agglutinin [10].

Treatment

The treatment options include surgery, CT or RT, depending upon the aggressiveness of the disease process.

Odontogenic and Nonodontogenic Cysts and Tumour (Fig. 9)

Cyst is a pathologic cavity containing fluid, semifluid, or gaseous material, frequently but not always lined by epithelium, and never created due to accumulation of pus (Fig. **10**).

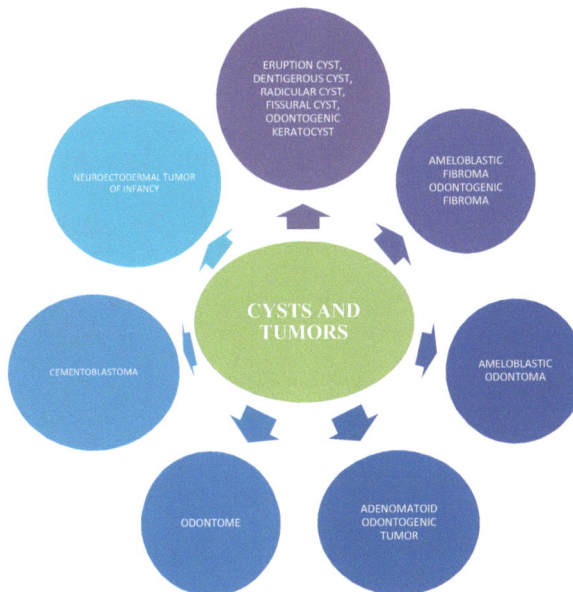

Fig. (9). Odontogenic and non-odontogenic cysts and tumour.

Eruption Cyst

- Eruption cyst is defined as an odontogenic cyst with the histologic feature of a dentigerous cyst that surrounds a tooth crown which has erupted through bone but not soft tissue and is clinically visible as a soft tissue fluctuant mass on alveolar ridges.
- The eruption cyst occurs when a tooth is impeded in its path of eruption within the soft tissues overlying the bone. The presence of particularly dense fibrous tissue in the overlying gingiva could be responsible.
- These cysts are usually found in children of different ages and occasionally in adults if there is delayed eruption. Deciduous and permanent teeth, anterior to 1st permanent molar, are normally involved. Clinically the lesion appears as a circumscribed, fluctuant, translucent swelling of the alveolar ridge over the site of the erupting tooth. When the circumscribed cystic cavity contains blood, owing to its purple or deep blue appearance, it is called as an eruption hematoma.
- Radiographically a soft tissue shadow may be present, since there is no bone involvement.
- The superficial aspect is covered by keratinized stratified squamous epithelium of the overlying gingiva. This is separated from the cyst by a strip of dense connective tissue of varying thickness, which usually shows a mild chronic inflammatory cell infiltrate. The follicular connective tissue is densely cellular, less collagenous and has a basophilic hue owing to higher content of acid mucopolysaccharide. In noninflamed areas, the epithelial lining of the cysts is characteristically reduced enamel epithelium origin, consisting of two to three layers of squamous epithelium with a few foci, where it may be a little thicker [11].

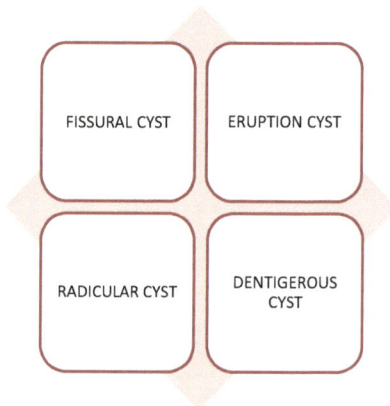

FISSURAL CYST	ERUPTION CYST
RADICULAR CYST	DENTIGEROUS CYST

Fig. (10). Cysts.

Treatment

- Majority of the cysts resolve over a period, and no treatment is required.
- Surgical exposure of the associated tooth crown may aid in the eruption procedure.

Dentigerous Cyst

- A dentigerous cyst surrounds the crown of a tooth and is a dilatation of the follicle. The cyst is attached to the neck of the tooth, prevents its eruption, and may displace it for a considerable distance. It is an odontogenic cyst, which is caused by a fluid accumulation between the enamel surface and reduced enamel epithelium. It is the second most common odontogenic cyst after a radicular cyst. These cysts usually show peak incidence in the 2nd decade of life. Most commonly occur in the posterior mandible or maxilla and are normally associated with 3rd molars. The second most frequent location is the maxillary canine.
- A dentigerous cyst may be discovered as an incidental radiographic finding or by examination of a clinical expansion. Some cases present with bony expansion and facial fullness. The cysts are not painful until secondarily infected, and their size has created a pathologic fracture. Bony resorption may be there due to the expansion of the cyst. The cyst can be compressible and translucent. Fluctuation might be present. Pain or paraesthesia might be present depending on the level of nerve involvement.
- Radio graphically, a dentigerous cyst is a well-demarcated, unilocular radio lucency associated with the crown of an unerupted tooth. The tooth may be displaced; it is not surprising to see teeth displaced to the ramus or condylar neck, the nasal floor, or high in the maxillary sinus approaching the orbit. Frequently teeth are displaced to the inferior border of the mandible and can cause a displacement of the inferior alveolar neurovascular bundle. Smooth, regular resorption of adjacent teeth has been reported.
- Grossly the dentigerous cyst surrounds the crown and is attached to the tooth at CEJ. In the uninflamed cyst, the lining resembles the reduced enamel epithelium from which it is derived and consists of two to three rows of cuboidal or flattened epithelium. Mucous cells may be present and may be prominent. The wall is fibrous, and the stroma contains abundant mucopolysaccharides such that it appears basophilic. In the wall, Odontogenic epithelial rests and dystrophic calcification may be present. Rushton bodies can be seen in the cyst lining (Fig. 11).
- Aspiration of the lesion is recommended, and if that returns a straw-colored fluid, this finding with clinical-radiographic-pathologic features provides a

strong inclination to the dentigerous cyst. The cyst is removed *via* enucleation procedure [12, 13].

Treatment

- The treatment commonly recommended is enucleation.
- In cases of large cysts, marsupialization or decompression is advised.

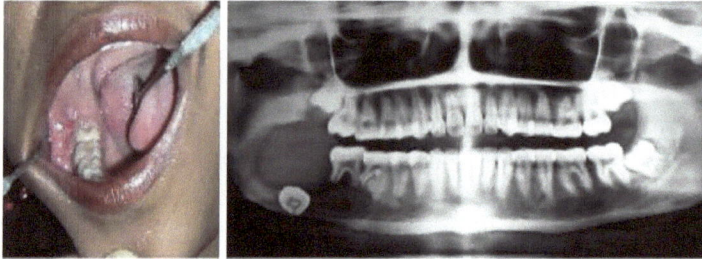

Fig. (11). Case of Dentigerous cysts.

Radicular Cyst

- The radicular Cyst is an inflammatory cyst associated with the root apex of a nonvital tooth. Because of the high incidence of pulpal pathology, it is the commonest cyst in the oral and maxillofacial regions.
- The cysts are associated with a tooth that is carious, has undergone previous restorative care, has sustained trauma, or an apparent failure of RCT therapy.
- These cysts are caused because of pulpal necrosis following caries, with an associated periapical inflammatory response. Other causes include events that may result in pulpal necrosis, such as tooth fracture and improper restorations.
- Most of the radicular cysts are asymptomatic. The tooth is seldom painful or even sensitive to percussion. Rarely cortical bone expansion. In some cases, a long-standing cyst may undergo an acute exacerbation of inflammatory response that can proceed to a cellulites or draining fistula. The radiological images of the cyst are a peri or para-apical, round, or ovoid radiolucency of variable size, which is well delineated and has a marked radiopaque rim. On aspiration reddish-brown fluid, which is sometimes glistening in nature, is yielded due to the presence of cholesterol clefts (Fig. **12**).
- Microscopic examination shows stratified squamous epithelium, which is often hyperplastic and inflamed connective tissue. Frequently, cholesterol crystals and Rushton bodies are also noted.

Treatment

- It consists of extraction of the affected teeth and careful curettage of the periapical tissue.

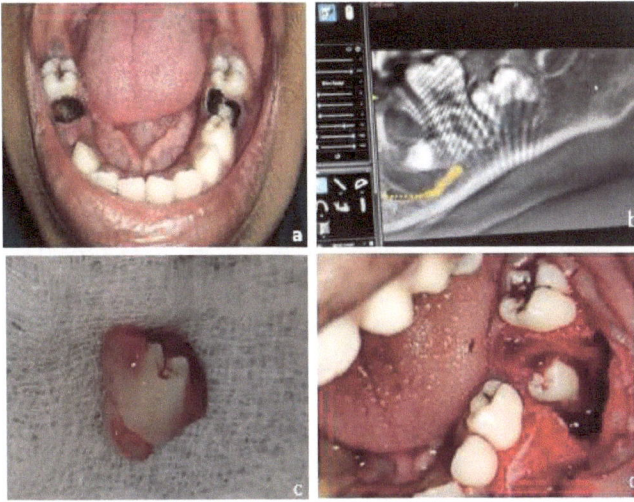

Fig. (12). Case of Radicular cyst.

Fissural Cyst

These are inclusion cysts that occur along the lines of fusion of bones or embryonic processes and are true cysts that contain fluid or semisolid material. A mid palatine cyst is a true fissural cyst [14].

Treatment

The recommended treatment is marsupialization or enucleation.

Odontogenic Keratocyst (OKC), (Fig. 13)

- It is unicystic or multicystic, benign, intraosseous tumour of odontogenic origin.
- It shows bimodal age of distribution from 10 to 40 years.
- Clinically it shows asymptomatic growth anterio-posteriorly in the medullary space with little and late bone expansion.
- Sometime paresthesia can occur due to pathological fracture.
- Radiographically it shows multilocular radiolucencies with scalloped well-defined margins.
- It shows tendency of multiplicity especially when associated with syndromes like the naevoid basal cell carcinoma syndrome or Gorlin Gotz syndrome.
- It shows high occurrence rate due to incomplete removal of cyst lining, the presence of satellite cysts in the connective tissue of the cystic wall, which remain even after enucleation.
- Odontogenic keratocyst is derived from the dental lamina and its remnants, traumatic implantation or down of basal layer of the surface epithelium, reduced enamel epithelium or Hertwig epithelium root sheath.

- This lesion shows aggressive behaviour with its ability to extend in adjacent bone and soft tissue.
- Histopathological features of OKC are parakeratinized epithelium with corrugated epithelium and daughter cysts/satellite cysts.

Treatment

- It includes conservative or aggressive management depending upon the extent of the lesion.
- Conservative management includes marsupialization.
- The aggressive management includes enucleation, enucleation with carnoys solution, margical or surgical resection and bone implantation.

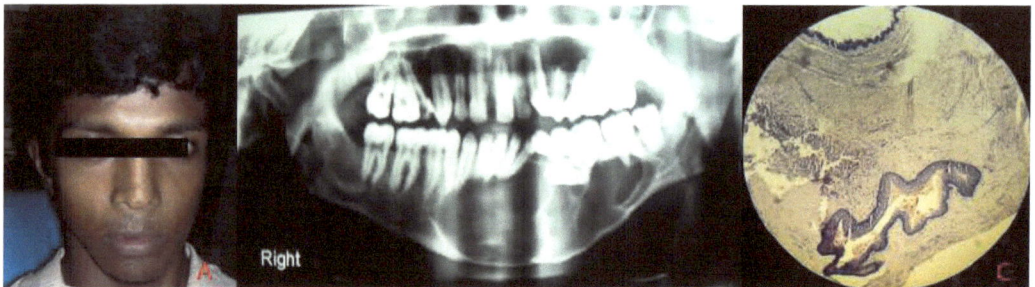

Fig. (13). Case of OKC, **A**- Extraoral photograph without any obvious facial deformity, **B**- corresponding OPG image showing associated root resorption of the regional teeth and displacement, **C**- Histopathology image showing parakeratinized and corrugated epithelium and daughter cysts / satellite cysts.

Odontogenic Tumors (Fig. 14)

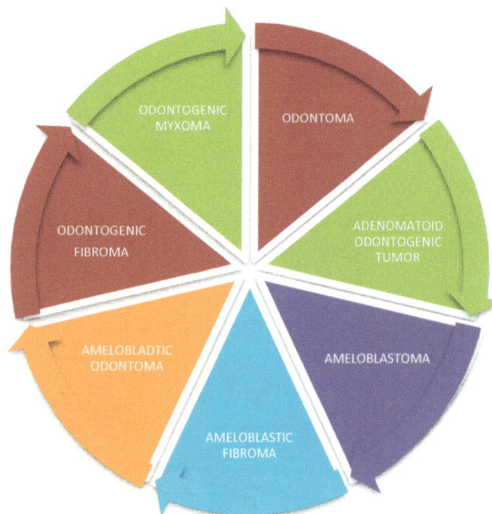

Fig. (14). Odontogenic tumors.

Ameloblastoma

- The ameloblastoma is a benign but locally invasive neoplasm comprising characteristic odontogenic epithelial proliferations supported by a mature stroma of fibrous tissue. It is agreed that most SMA occurs as growths arising from remnants of odontogenic epithelium, more specifically rest of the dental lamina.
- It is a slowly enlarging painless mass with a high rate of recurrence if not removed adequately. It is located intraosseously within the jaws, and there are little or no clinical signs in the early stages. Later, there is gradually increasing facial deformity, loosening of teeth, and spontaneous fracture may occur in cases where only a rim of bone is remaining in the mandible. The affected part of the jaw is bony hard and bulky. Pain might occur because of secondary trauma or infection or due to compression of a nerve.
- Radiographically, the typical picture is of a multilocular radiolucent lesion. Although unilocular appearance can occur. The bone is replaced by a number of small, or large, well-defined radiolucent areas, giving the whole lesion a honeycomb or soap bubble appearance. In the unilocular type, there is a well-defined area of radiolucency associated with unerupted tooth (Fig. **15**).
- It is a polymorphic neoplasm consisting of proliferating odontogenic epithelium, usually occurring in two main patterns. In the follicular type of growth, the tumor consists of enamel organ-like islands or follicles of epithelial cells, while in the plexiform type, the epithelium forms continuous anastomosing bands or chords. In both types of epithelial tumor, components are embedded in a mature fibrous connective tissue stroma.
- The histologic variants are follicular, plexiform, acanthomatous, desmoplastic, granular cell, basal cell, keratoameloblastoma and hemangiomatous ameloblastoma. Also, there is unicystic ameloblastoma, with the variant being luminal, intra luminal, mural, and intramural. In the plexiform pattern, the tumor epithelium is arranged as a network that is inbound by a layer of cuboidal to columnar cells and includes cells resembling stellate reticulum [15]. Cyst formation can take place owing to stromal degeneration. The cut surface of ameloblastoma may show a variable amount of grayish-white soft tissues and cystic spaces of different sizes interspersed with bone.

Treatment

- The solid multi-cystic ameloblastomas require radical surgical intervention while unicystic ameloblastomas need surgical enucleation.

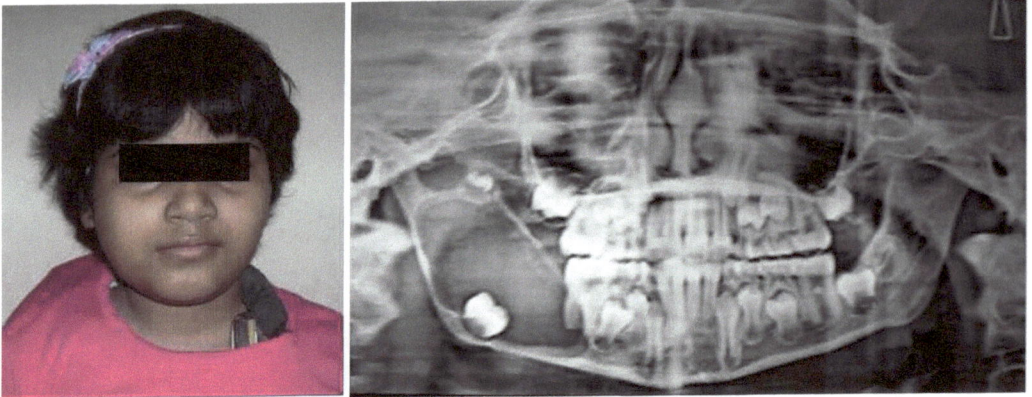

Fig. (15). Case of Plexiform Ameloblastoma (extraoral photograph and corresponding OPG image).

Adenomatoid Odontogenic Tumor (Fig. 16)

- The AOT is a benign, hamartomatous non-neoplastic lesion with a slow but progressive growth, which may present as intraosseous and peripheral forms.
- Philipsen *et al.* strongly argued that AOT arises from dental lamina or its remnants. It commonly affects the anterior portion of the jaws, particularly maxilla.
- Radiologically as well-defined unilocular radiolucency involves an unerupted tooth, and permanent impacted maxillary canine. It mimics like that of a dentigerous or follicular cyst or often a globulomaxillary cyst, because of its location. Occasionally, flecks of minute radiopacities may be present. It is usually diagnosed in the 2nd decade of life. Females are affected more than males. Cortical expansion and tooth displacement might be present. The lesion may be partly cystic and, in some cases, the solid tumerous masses may be present on the cystic wall. Characteristic tubular or ductlike structures lined by a single row of cuboidal or low columnar epithelial cells are prominent histological features. Rosette-like structures, calcific bodies of dentinoid or calcified osteodentin producing a Liessagang ring pattern or eosinophilic amorphous materials are other common findings.

Treatment

- The treatment modality of choice includes conservative surgical enucleation or curettage.

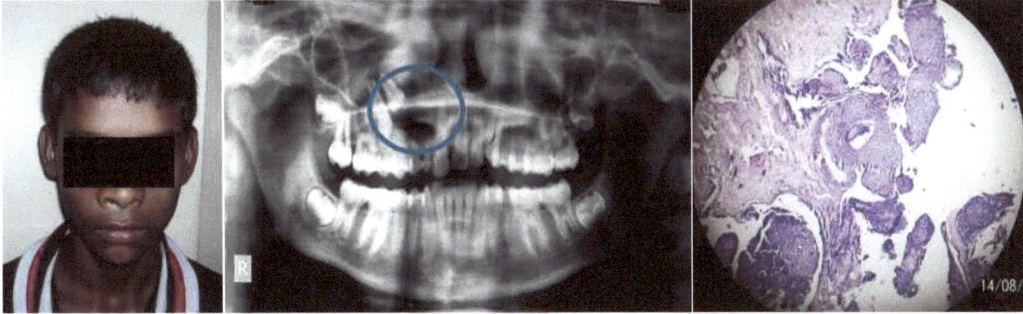

Fig. (16). Adenomatoid odontogenic tumour (clinical photograph, corresponding OPG and histological image.

Odontoma (Fig. 17)

- Odontomas are the most common odontogenic tumors and represent a hamartomatous malformation rather than a neoplasm. It is a mixed odontogenic tumor as it has both epithelial and ectomesenchymal components.
- The etiologies may include local trauma, infection, familial history, and genetic mutation. Abnormal proliferation of cells of enamel organs may be noted with differentiation of both epithelial and mesenchymal components.
- The individual hard tissues may be well developed, resulting in the well-organized tooth-like structures or masses of disorganized odontogenic tissues.
- Accordingly, WHO has classified odontomas into two types-
- Compound odontoma ---- In this, all the dental tissues are present in an orderly fashion with similarity to the normal tooth.
- Complex odontoma---Little or no similarity to the normal tooth exists. The diffuse mass of disorganized dental tissue is often referred to as complex composite odontoma.
- Complex odontomas are located commonly on the posterior mandible, while a majority of the compound odontomas are seen in the anterior maxilla.
- Histologically it may show irregularly formed dental hard structures like enamel matrix or mineralized masses of dentin with islands of pulpal tissues and nests of the odontogenic epithelium [16].

Treatment

- Conservative enucleation is the recommended treatment.

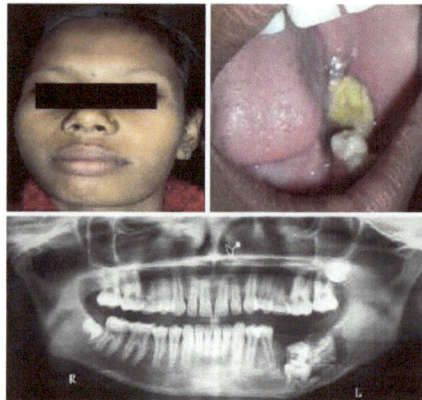

Fig. (17). Case of odontoma (clinical photograph, corresponding OPG and histological image).

Neuroectodermal Tumor of Infancy (Fig. 18)

It is a benign tumor, which occurs during the first year of life, in females, and 80% of lesions occur in the maxilla [17].

Treatment

It is treated by conservative surgical enucleation.

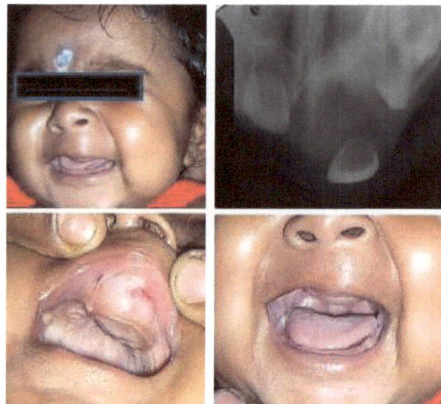

Fig. (18). Case of melanotic neuroectodermal tumor of infancy.

Ameloblastic Fibroma

- This is a true mixed odontogenic tumor in which both the epithelial and ectomesenchymal components are neoplastic.
- It is commonly seen in the mandible in the premolar molar area. Age predilection is in the first two decades of life.
- It appears as a painless slow-growing expansile lesion of the jaws with the occasional association of impacted tooth. Radiologically it appears as multifocal

radiolucency with the expansion of the cortex and tooth displacement in some instances.
- The tumor mass is surrounded by a thin capsule macroscopically. The tumor is histologically composed of strands, or chords or islands of odontogenic epithelium in the connective tissue stroma, which has rounded or angular or stellate-shaped ectomesenchymal cells with delicate collagen fibrils, resembling dental papilla.
- It can recur or undergo malignant transformation.

Treatment

- Due to the high rate of malignant transformation, it should be treated with wide excision and regular checkup.

Odontoameloblastoma (Fig. 19)

- The odontoameloblastoma is an extremely rare tumor consisting of simultaneous occurrence of the ameloblastoma and composite odontome, formerly known by different names such as soft and calcified odontoma and ameloblastic odontoma.
- It usually occurs in the first decade of life, involving the posterior mandible and males are more affected than females.
- They are slow, progressive growing lesions like SMA. They can also be expansile, centrally destructive lesions with progressive alveolar bone swelling, dull pain, and delayed teeth eruption.
- Radiographically the OA appears as well defined unilocular or multilocular radiolucency containing varying degrees of radiopaque substances and associated with an unerupted tooth. Microscopy reveals proliferating odontogenic epithelium, arranged in islands and rosettes, embedded in a mature fibrous connective tissue stroma, like SMA.
- There is also a presence of the odontogenic ectomesenchyme, inducing inductive changes, leading to the formation of dysplastic dentin and enamel in a haphazard manner, whilst rudimentary teeth also may be present [18].

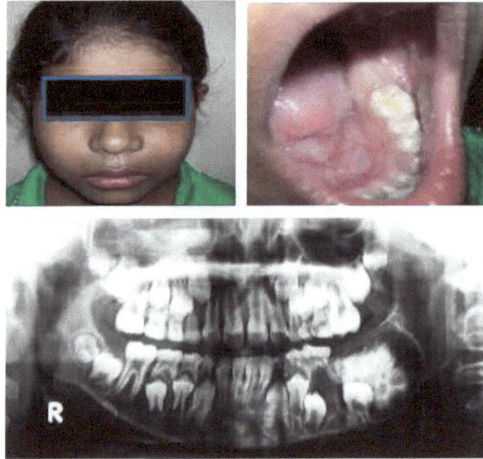

Fig. (19). Case of odontoameloblastoma.

Treatment

- A radical treatment is normally performed in this case.

Odontogenic Fibroma

- It is a rare tumor comprising about 23% of all odontogenic tumors of the jaws. Topographically two variants can be distinguished-intraosseous or central and extraosseous or peripheral variants. Some authors believe the COF to be derived from the ectomesenchymal tissue of the PDL, dental papilla, or dental follicle. It affects the mandible in the premolar molar regions, and the maxillary anterior regions.
- The mean age of diagnosis is 39 years. Females are more affected than males.
- The tumor produces a slow, progressive, painless swelling that can result in cortical expansion and mobility of regional teeth.
- Radiographically, a unilocular radiolucent area, occasionally exhibiting varying degrees of calcifications, with well-defined sclerotic borders may be noted.
- Lesions may be associated with the crown of unerupted molar, premolar, or incisor teeth. The gross specimen has a gray to brownish color. Cutting through the tissue mass, the pathologist may notice calcified mass.
- It is a benign neoplasm composed of cellular connective tissue. It often occurs in fibroblastic strands that are interwoven with less cellular areas in which numerous small blood vessels are present.
- Foci of the calcified collagenous matrix, resembling dysplastic cementum, osteoid or dysplastic dentin-like material can occur. Islands of inactive-looking odontogenic epithelium are an integral component of COF.
- However, in simple type, odontogenic epithelial islands are absent.

Treatment

• Enucleation followed by vigorous curettage is a recommended treatment approach for Odontogenic fibroma.

Odontogenic Myxoma (Fig. 20)

• Myxomas of the jaws are believed to arise from odontogenic ectomesenchyme. Researchers believe that OM can have multiple sources of origin, including fibroblastic, fibroblastic-histiocytic, myofibroblastic and myxoblastic sources.
• It usually affects mandible in the premolar molar region, in the 2nd-4th decade of life, and the females are affected more than males. Smaller lesions may be asymptomatic, but larger lesions are associated with a painless expansion of affected bone, which may cause facial asymmetry.
• Radiologically, a multilocular radiolucent lesion with scalloped margins, having thin, wispy bone trabeculae arranged at right angles to each other, giving a characteristic 'soap bubble' or 'tennis racket' appearance might be evident.
• The cut surface of the lesion has a grayish-white sticky gelatinous mucoid substance. Microscopically, OM is characterized by loose, abundant mucoid stroma, having delicate collagen fibrils, akin to primitive mesenchyme, rich in glycosaminoglycans that contain rounded, angular or spindle-shaped cells.
• Cellular and nuclear polymorphisms are rare. IHC exhibits that the myxoma cells show positivity for vimentin and occasionally for muscle specific actin [19].

Treatment

• It involves variety of approach depending upon extent of involvement from local excision, curettage, or enucleation to radical excision.

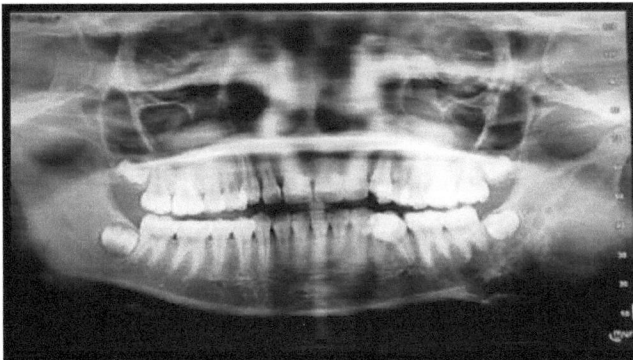

Fig. (20). Odontogenic myxoma: ill-defined radiolucency seen in left posterior ramus region.

Cementoblastoma

- Cementoblastoma is an odontogenic neoplasm of cementoblasts, and many authorities believe that this neoplasm represents the only true neoplasm of cementum.
- It mostly affects the mandible, with most of the cases arising in the premolar molar region. Almost 50% of cases involve the 1st molars.
- It occurs in children and young adults, usually below 2nd decades of life. Pain and swelling are present in approximately two-thirds of reported cases.
- Locally aggressive behavior, including bony expansion, cortical erosion, displacement of adjacent teeth and infiltration to the pulp chamber and root canals might be there. Radiographically the tumor appears as a radiopaque mass fused to one or more tooth roots and is surrounded by a thin radiolucent rim, and the root outline of the involved tooth is obscured.
- Most of the tumor consists of sheets and thick trabeculae of mineralized material with irregularly placed lacunae and prominent basophilic reversal lines dispersed in cellular fibrovascular tissue. Multinucleated giant cells often are present.

Treatment

- Surgical excision along with the extraction of involved teeth is a treatment of choice.
- There is no recurrence after surgical removal.

NON-ODONTOGENIC TUMORS [20]

Congenital Granular Cell Tumor (Congenital Epulis of the Newborn)

- The congenital granular cell tumor is a specific lesion representing a hamartomatous proliferation of granular cells rather than a true neoplasm. It is thought to be derived from Schwann cells or neuroendocrine cells.
- It is more common in females than in males. Within the oral cavity, the dorsal surface of the tongue is the commonest site, followed by buccal mucosa and anterior part of the maxillary gingiva.
- It is usually present at birth as a mass emanating from mucosa, which is painless and possesses a narrow stalk. Some can attain very large sizes and interfere with feeding. Histologically, the characteristic features are granular cells, being composed of granular eosinophilic cytoplasm due to the presence of enlarged lysosomes.
- The tumor is covered by a thin stratified squamous epithelium, and pseudoepitheliomatous hyperplasia is absent. Increased vascularity is present. Ultra structurally, it shows smooth muscle features [21].

Treatment

- Excision is the treatment of choice.

Ewing Sarcoma (Fig. 21)

- Ewing sarcoma is a distinctive primary malignant tumor of bone that is composed of small, undifferentiated round cells of uncertain histogenesis.
- It is a notoriously aggressive and destructive malignancy of bone. There is a unique reciprocal translocation between chromosomes 11 and 22.
- The peak prevalence of Ewing sarcoma is in the second decade of life. Males are affected slightly more than females. White people are exclusively affected.
- The long bones, pelvis and ribs are affected most frequently. Mandible, particularly the posterior region, is more commonly affected. Dull to severe pain, often associated with swelling, is the most common symptom.
- Fever, leukocytosis may be there. The tumor commonly penetrates the cortex, resulting in a tissue mass overlying the affected area of bone.
- Paraesthesia and mobility of teeth might be there. Ewing sarcoma often has been reported to produce a multilayered periosteal reaction that has been described as an onion skin appearance. A CT scan or PET scan is useful for assessing the metastasis to the lung, which is the commonest metastatic site. Histopathologically, it is composed of densely packed, small, monotonous, sheets of uniform cells with little intercellular stroma. The nuclei are round to oval with defined nuclear borders and a finely granular chromatin pattern.
- The cytoplasm is indistinct and may be vacuolated. There might be considerable hemorrhage and necrosis.CD99 is a potent IHC marker regarding the small round cells of Ewing sarcoma. RT PCR and FISH may be used as sensitive methods to detect genetic translocation [22].

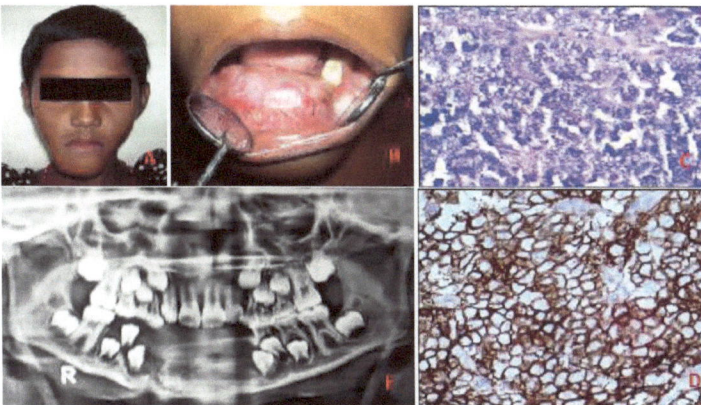

Fig. (21). A-Extraoral photograph, **B-**Intraoral photograph, **C-**H/E section showing round cells, **D-**Immunohistochemistry showing CD99 positive, **E-** Corresponding OPG image.

Treatment

• Combined surgery, radiotherapy and multidrug CT are the treatment of choice.

Burkitt's Lymphoma

• Burkitt's lymphoma is a malignancy of B lymphocyte origin, caused by Epstein Barr virus that represents an undifferentiated lymphoma.
• It was first described by a missionary doctor, Dennis Burkitt, in young east African children. As it was seen frequently in Sub-Saharan Africa, the term *African Burkitt lymphoma* has been applied to the disease.
• In the case of the African-endemic subtype, individuals develop the well-known jaw tumors associated with the development of permanent molar teeth, whilst abdominal masses have been reported in cases of *American Burkitt* lymphoma. There is a known chromosomal translocation (8:14). In some cases, mutation of the tumor suppressor gene is also responsible.
• About 50-70% of endemic Burkitt's lymphoma is present in the jaws. The malignancy usually affects children about 7 years of age who live in Central Africa, and a male predilection is reported. The posterior quadrants of the jaws, especially the maxilla, are commonly affected.
• The tendency for jaw involvement seems to be age-related; 90% of 3-year-old patients have jaw lesions, in contrast to the only 25% of patients older than age 15.
• Facial swelling and proptosis along with mild degrees of pain, tenderness and paresthesia are noted.
• Aggressive destruction of alveolar bone and marked tooth mobility might be present. Gingival and alveolar process enlargement may be seen.
• The radiographic features show radiolucent destruction of bone with ragged, ill-defined margins. Patchy loss of lamina dura can be seen. Microscopy shows a classic 'starry sky' appearance, a pattern caused by interspersed histiocytic cells with abundant cytoplasm (stars) set against a background of malignant, darkly staining lymphoma cells (night sky).

Treatment

• It consists of an intense chemotherapeutic regime, especially cyclophosphamide. The prognosis is quite poor.

Osteosarcoma (Fig. 22)

• Osteosarcomas represent malignant neoplasms arising from mesenchymal stem cells or their early progeny, causing the production of tumor bone from a malignant cellular stroma. It is the commonest malignancy to originate within the bone. Genetic findings show that osteosarcoma development is related to loss of p53, Rb and the development of independence from regulation by PDGF.

- Extra gnathic OS exhibit a bimodal age distribution. Most arise in patients between 10 to 20 years of ages, and a lesser number in older adults above 50 years of age. Most OS arise in the distal femoral and proximal tibial metaphysis. OS in the jaws is uncommon.
- They mostly tend to occur in the 3rd-4th decade of life. The maxilla and mandible are involved with equal frequency and mandibular tumors arise far more frequently in the posterior body and horizontal ramus.
- Maxillary lesions are seen more commonly in the inferior portion- the alveolar ridge, sinus, floor, and palate. Swelling and pain are the most common symptoms. Loosening of teeth, paresthesia and nasal obstruction can be noted.
- OS may produce the often described- sun ray appearance. A widening of the PDL space, called Garrington's sign, is noted. Codman's triangle can be there. Most radiographs and CT scans show a mottled radiopaque or mixed radiolucent radiopaque appearance in the medullary space.
- Extracortical bone formation is commonly responsible for the sun ray appearance. Cortical bone destruction is characteristic. PET scan or CT SCAN to detect metastatic foci in the body is necessary.
- Microscopically there will be a direct formation of osteoid from a sarcomatous stroma. The quantity of neoplastic osteoid varies greatly-from too little to a great amount. The stromal cells may be osteoblastic, chondroblastic or fibroblastic. In the jaws, the chondroblastic pattern usually prevails. A myxoid stroma is frequently seen. Some OS are heavily ossified, and in these cases, there may be entrapment of tumor cells within the sclerotic osteoid, which show varying degrees of nuclear and cellular pleomorphism, nuclear hyperchromatism, cellular atypia, increased and/or abnormal mitotic figures. Occasional areas of necrosis and hemorrhage may be noted. Multinucleated giant cells may be noted. A small round cell variant is also there. A telangiectatic variant with numerous widely dilated vascular channels is there.
- Alkaline phosphatase and galectin 1 are essential markers of OS [23].

Treatment

- The jaws are ideally treated with initial chemotherapy followed by surgery, which is followed by two to three additional doses of CT.

Rhabdomyosarcoma (Fig. 23)

- Rhabdomyosarcoma is a malignant neoplasm that is characterized by skeletal muscle differentiation. This primarily occurs during 1st decade of life but also may occur in teenagers and young adults.
- The variants of rhabdomyosarcoma are embryonal, alveolar, undifferentiated,

and anaplastic.

- Embryonal RS is most common in the first 10 years of life and accounts for almost 60% of the cases. Most head and neck lesions are alveolar and embryonic types.
- The tumor is most often a painless, infiltrative mass that can grow rapidly. In the head-neck region, the face and orbit are the most frequent locations, followed by the nasal cavity. The palate is the most frequent intraoral site, and the maxillary sinus can also be involved.
- Embryonal forms are cellular with immature rhabdomyoblasts that fail to show cross striations.
- The cells are oval, with occasional spindle-shaped forms scattered. The alveolar type is represented by organoid grouping or clustering pertaining to ovoid rhabdomyoblasts, whereas the pleomorphic variety manifests a very wide array of cell types, including racket, strap, and giant cells. Tandem nuclei are occasionally encountered.
- Two important translocations have been identified in alveolar RS (PAX3-FKHR and PAX7-FKHR). Embryonal RS is characterized by a consistent loss of heterozygosity in chromosome 11p15.

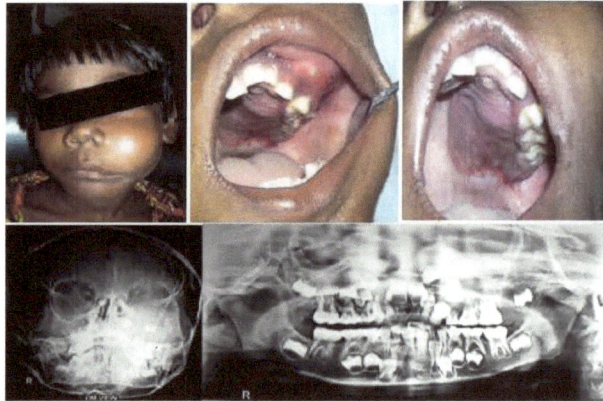

Fig. (22). Case of Osteosarcoma.

Treatment

- It includes local surgical excision followed by multiagent CT.
- Postoperative radiotherapy.

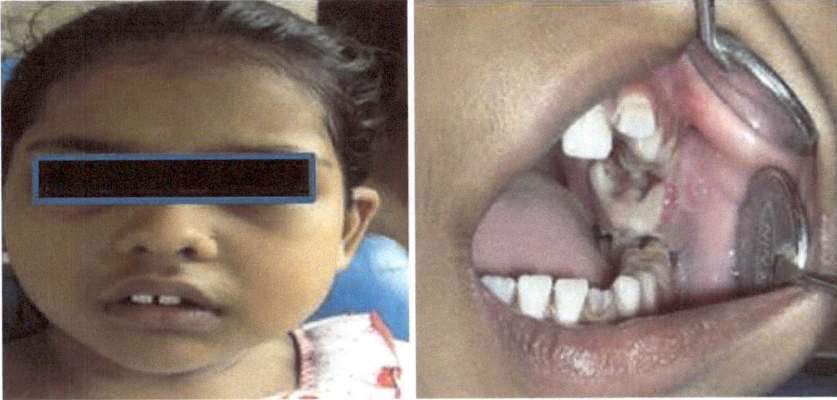

Fig. (23). case of Rhabdomyosarcoma.

Mesenchymal Chondrosarcoma (Fig. 24)

- It is an uncommon and distinctive tumor of bone and soft tissue showing a biphasic histologic pattern.
- MC affects the individuals during the 2nd -3rd decade of life, and the jaws are the most frequently involved sites.
- Swelling and pain are the most common symptoms. Radiographically the tumor demonstrates a radiolucency with infiltrative margins.
- Microscopically MC reveals sheets of small, undifferentiated, spindle or round cells surrounding discrete nodules of cartilage.
- In some cases, a prominent branching vascular pattern akin to hemangiopericytoma may be present.

Treatment

- Surgical excision with wide margins is the most appropriate therapy.

Lymphangiomas (Fig. 25)

- These are hamartomatous tumors of lymphatic vessels that can cause macroglossia of tongue, macrocheilia of lip and hemifacial hypertrophy of the face.
- It can also affect infants and about 90% develop by 2 years of age.
- can leads to macroglossia
- It can be of three types-capillary, cavernous and cystic types. It most commonly affects the anterior two-thirds of the tongue, resulting in the formation of a pebbly, vesicle-like appearance.
- Dilated lymphatic vessels beneath the epithelium filled with lymphatic proteinaceous fluid and in the deep connective tissues may be seen. Microscopically the submucosal CT is traversed by dilated vascular channels

lined by a single stratum of compressed endothelial cells lacking a muscular coat. IHC using D2-40, LYVE-1, and Prox-1 markers is helpful to discriminate lymphatic from vascular endothelium [24, 25].

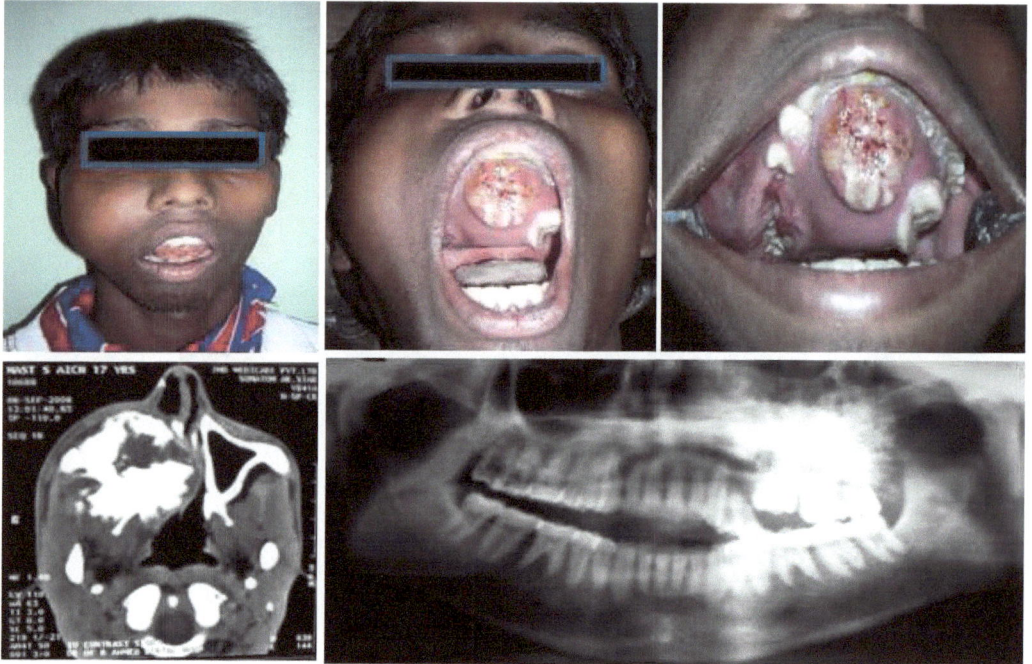

Fig. (24). Case of Mesenchymal chondrosarcoma (Clinical photograph and corresponding CT scan and OPG image).

Treatment

- Excision if possible; also, sclerotherapy or observation.
- Intralesional bleomycin therapy may be an effective alternative to surgery

Conditions Affecting the Salivary Glands [26]

Due to the common habit of cheek chewing and lip biting, both lesions of minor&minor salivary glands affect patients of the pediatric group.

Mumps

- Mumps is an infection caused by the paramyxovirus family, which causes a diffuse disease of exocrine glands. Although the salivary glands are the best-known sites for involvement, the pancreas, choroid plexus and mature ovaries and testes are also involved.
- The mumps virus can be transmitted by urine, saliva, or respiratory droplet.
- It most frequently occurs in the 5-11 years age group. The incubation period

usually is 16-18 days.
- Approximately 30% of mumps infections are subclinical.
- In symptomatic cases, prodromal features of low-grade fever, headache, anorexia, and myalgia arrive first. Most frequently these nonspecific findings are followed within 1 day by significant salivary gland changes.
- The parotid glands are involved most frequently bilaterally, but the submandibular and sublingual glands can also be affected.
- Painful, firm, elastic, rubbery swelling associated with discomfort can occur involving the lower half of the external ear and extends down the posterior inferior border of adjacent mandible.
- The enlargement typically peaks within 2-3 days and pain is most intense during periods of maximal enlargement.
- Chewing movements of the jaw and eating the saliva stimulating foods increase pain.
- There is associated redness and enlargement of Stenson's and Wharton's duct. Less commonly, meningoencephalitis, cerebellar ataxia, hearing loss, pancreatitis, arthritis, carditis and decreased renal function can take place, male sterility can occur.
- Demonstration of mumps-specific IgM or a fourfold increase in mumps-specific IgG titer when measured during the acute phase and about 2 weeks later.

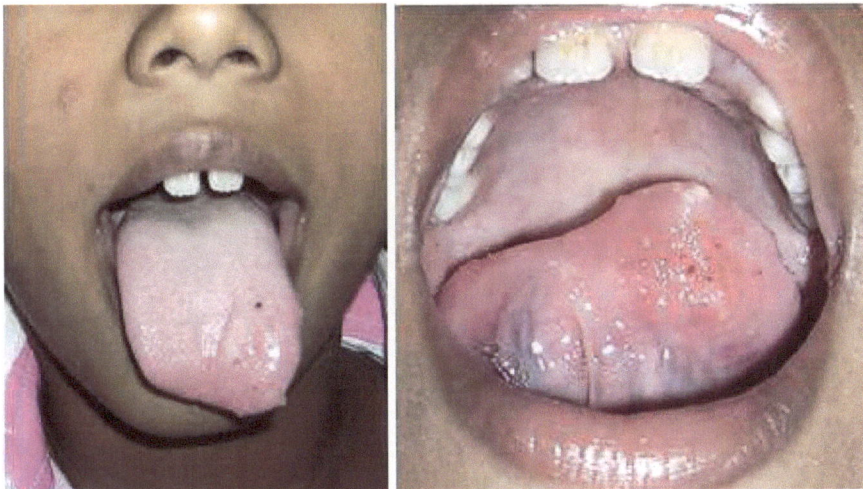

Fig. (25). Case of lymphangioma of tongue.

Treatment

- Treatment of mumps is palliative.
- Frequently non aspirin analgesics and antipyretics are administered.
- Avoidance of sour foods and drinks and lots of hydration must be there.

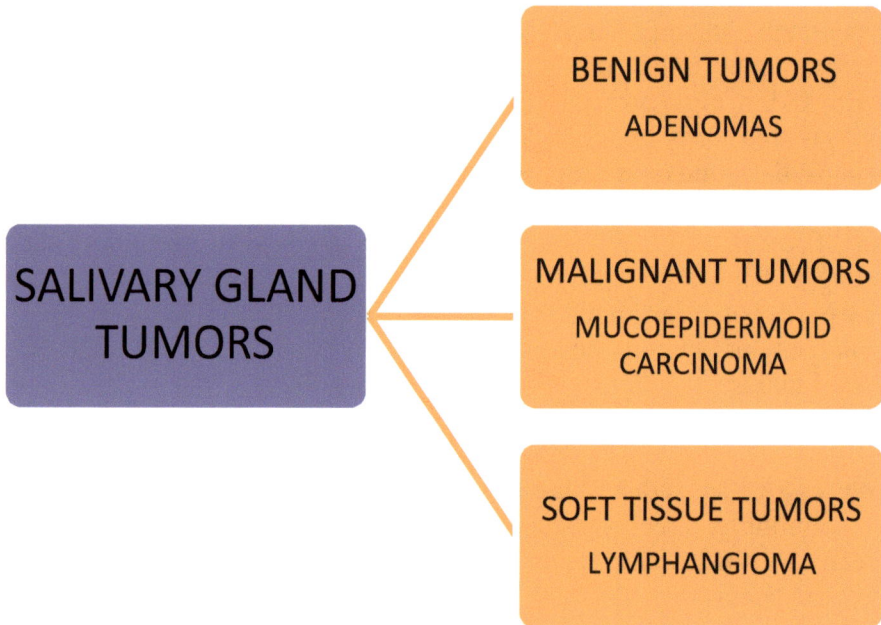

Fig. (26). Tumors of salivary glands.

Tumors of Salivary Glands (Fig. 26)

These are a distinct group of tumors affecting children.

As compared to the tumor of the later years, lesions found in children are exclusively mesenchymal in origin and benign in nature.

The parotid gland is more frequently involved than other glands.

Juvenile hemangioma, adenoma, juvenile xanthoma, lymphangioma, mucoepidermoid tumors and juvenile xanthoma are some of the tumors affecting the salivary glands in children (Figs. **27a** and **27b**).

Treatment

Surgical excision is advised for most salivary gland tumours.

Chemotherapy or radiotherapy is sometimes recommended either alone or in combination as an aide procedure.

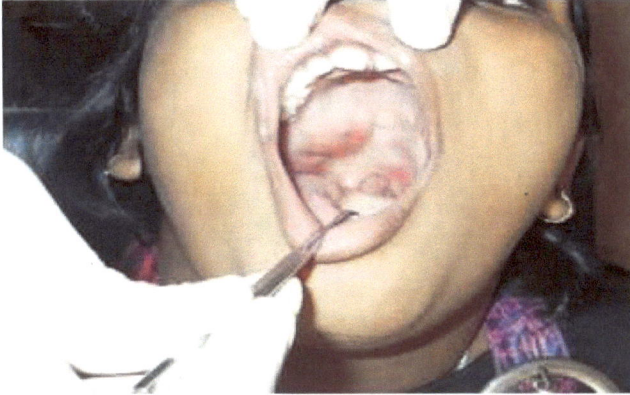

Fig. (27A). Palatal growth of mucoepidermoid carcinoma.

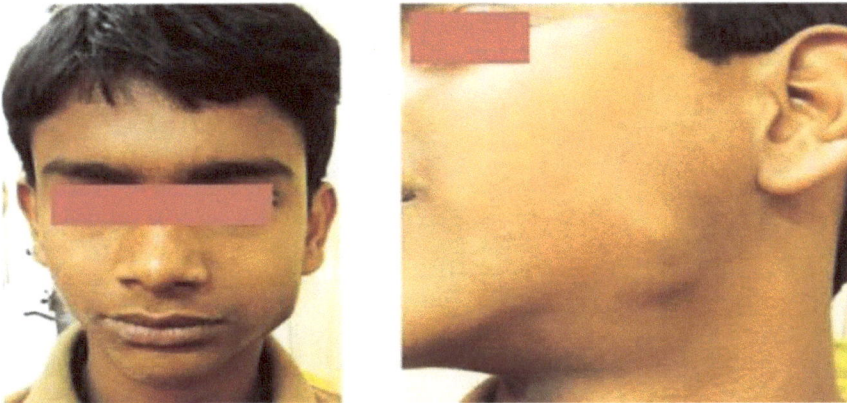

Fig. (27B). Lymphangioma of left parotid gland.

CONCLUSION

Oro-facial swelling in pediatric patients can be associated with a wide variety of causes. Detailed knowledge of the location, clinical characteristics of a lesion and clinical examination helps to formulate a differential diagnosis. The most common cause of facial swelling is infection. Imaging is indicated if there is a concern about an underlying abscess which might require surgical drainage. Mid-facial and non-progressive swellings require consideration for a congenital or developmental cause. Rapidly progressive lesions with associated cranial nerve deficits are mostly suggestive of malignancy.

CONSENT FOR PUBLICATION

Not applicable.

CONFLICT OF INTEREST

The authors declare no conflict of interest, financial or otherwise.

ACKNOWLEDGEMENT

Declared none.

REFERENCES

[1]   Stark Z, Savarirayan R. Osteopetrosis. Orphanet J Rare Dis 2009; 4(1): 5-17.
        [http://dx.doi.org/10.1186/1750-1172-4-5] [PMID: 19232111]

[2]   Reddy MH R. Osteopetrosis (Marble Bone Disease): A Rare Disease in Children. Int J Clin Pediatr
        Dent 2011; 4(3): 232-4.
        [http://dx.doi.org/10.5005/jp-journals-10005-1115] [PMID: 27678232]

[3]   Liu Y, Wang H, You M, *et al.* Ossifying fibromas of the jaw bone: 20 cases. Dentomaxillofac Radiol
        2010; 39(1): 57-63.
        [http://dx.doi.org/10.1259/dmfr/96330046] [PMID: 20089746]

[4]   Owosho AA, Hughes MA, Prasad JL, Potluri A, Branstetter B. Psammomatoid and trabecular juvenile
        ossifying fibroma: two distinct radiologic entities. Oral Surg Oral Med Oral Pathol Oral Radiol 2014;
        118(6): 732-8.
        [http://dx.doi.org/10.1016/j.oooo.2014.09.010] [PMID: 25457891]

[5]   Keles B, Duran M, Uyar Y, Azimov A, Demirkan A, Esen HH. Juvenile ossifying fibroma of the
        mandible: a case report. J Oral Maxillofac Res 2010; 1(2): e5.
        [http://dx.doi.org/10.5037/jomr.2010.1205] [PMID: 24421970]

[6]   Hero M, Suomalainen A, Hagström J, *et al.* Anti-tumor necrosis factor treatment in cherubism —
        Clinical, radiological and histological findings in two children. Bone 2013; 52(1): 347-53.
        [http://dx.doi.org/10.1016/j.bone.2012.10.003] [PMID: 23069372]

[7]   Boyce AM, Chong WH, Yao J, *et al.* Denosumab treatment for fibrous dysplasia. J Bone Miner Res
        2012; 27(7): 1462-70.
        [http://dx.doi.org/10.1002/jbmr.1603] [PMID: 22431375]

[8]   Esposito P, Plotkin H. Surgical treatment of osteogenesis imperfecta: current concepts. Curr Opin
        Pediatr 2008; 20(1): 52-7.
        [http://dx.doi.org/10.1097/MOP.0b013e3282f35f03] [PMID: 18197039]

[9]   Mylona E, Samarkos M, Kakalou E, Fanourgiakis P, Skoutelis A. Pyogenic vertebral osteomyelitis: a
        systematic review of clinical characteristics. Semin Arthritis Rheum 2009; 39(1): 10-7.
        [http://dx.doi.org/10.1016/j.semarthrit.2008.03.002] [PMID: 18550153]

[10]   Langerhans histiopalm- Buchmann L, Emami A, Wei JL Primary head and neck Langerhans cell
        histiocytosis in children. Otolaryngol Head Neck Surg 2006; 135(2): 312-317OD.

[11]   DhawanP,KoccharGK,ChachraS,AdvaniS.Eruptioncysts:Aseriesoftwocases.DentResJ 2012; 9(5): 647.

[12]   Zhang LL, Yang R, Zhang L, Li W. MacDonald- JankowskiD,PohCF.Dentigerouscyst:aretrospective
        clinicopathological analysis of 2082 dentigerous cysts in British Columbia, Canada. Int J Oral
        Maxillofac Surg 2010; 39(9): 878-82.
        [http://dx.doi.org/10.1016/j.ijom.2010.04.048] [PMID: 20605411]

[13]   Debone MCZ, Brozoski MA, Traina AA, Acay RR, Homem MGN. Surgical management of
        dentigerouscyst and keratocystic odontogenic tumor in children: a conservative approach and 7-year
        follow-up. J Appl Oral Sci 2012; 20(2): 268-71.
        [PMID: 22666849]

[14]   Allmendinger A, Gabe M, Destian S. Median palatine cyst. J Radiol Case Rep 2009; 3(7): 7-10.
        [PMID: 22470670]

[15]   Chapelle KAOM, Stoelinga PJW, de Wilde PCM, Brouns JJA, Voorsmit RACA. Rational approach to
        diagnosis and treatment of ameloblastomas and odontogenic keratocysts. Br J Oral Maxillofac Surg
        2004; 42(5): 381-90.
        [http://dx.doi.org/10.1016/j.bjoms.2004.04.005] [PMID: 15336762]

[16]   Sheehy EC, Odell EW, Al-Jaddir G. Odontomas in the primary dentition: literature review and case
        report. J Dent Child (Chic) 2004; 71(1): 73-6.
        [PMID: 15272662]

[17]   Demir A, Gunluoglu MZ, Dagoglu N, *et al.* Surgical treatment and prognosis of primitive
        neuroectodermal tumors of the thorax. J Thorac Oncol 2009; 4(2): 185-92.
        [http://dx.doi.org/10.1097/JTO.0b013e318194fafe] [PMID: 19179894]

[18]   Lúcio PSC, Cavalcante RB, Maia RN, Santos ES, Godoy GP. Aggressive ameloblastic fibro-odontoma
        assessment with CBCT and treatment. Eur Arch Paediatr Dent 2013; 14(3): 179-84.
        [http://dx.doi.org/10.1007/s40368-013-0032-9] [PMID: 23633233]

[19]   Kawase-Koga Y, Saijo H, Hoshi K, Takato T, Mori Y. Surgical management of odontogenic myxoma:
        a case report and review of the literature. BMC Res Notes 2014; 7(1): 214-22.
        [http://dx.doi.org/10.1186/1756-0500-7-214] [PMID: 24708884]

[20]   Becker M, Stefanelli S, Rougemont AL, Poletti PA, Merlini L. Non-odontogenic tumors of the facial
        bones in children and adolescents: role of multiparametric imaging. Neuroradiology 2017 59(4): 327-
        42.
        [http://dx.doi.org/10.1007/s00234-017-1798-y]

[21]   Eghbalian F, Monsef A. Congenital epulis in the newborn, review of the literature and a case report. J
        Pediatr Hematol Oncol 2009; 31(3): 198-9.
        [http://dx.doi.org/10.1097/MPH.0b013e31818ab2f7] [PMID: 19262247]

[22]   Vaccani JP, Forte V, de Jong AL, Taylor G. Ewing's sarcoma of the head and neck in children. Int J
        Pediatr Otorhinolaryngol 1999; 48(3): 209-16.

[23]   Chaudhary M, Chaudhary S. Osteosarcoma of jaws. J Oral Maxillofac Pathol 2012; 16(2): 233-8.
        [http://dx.doi.org/10.4103/0973-029X.99075] [PMID: 22923896]

[24]   Krainick-Strobel U, Krämer B, Walz-Mattmüller R, *et al.* Massive cavernous lymphangioma of the
        breast and thoracic wall: case report and literature review. Lymphology 2006; 39(3): 147-51.
        [PMID: 17036636]

[25]   Yetiser S, Karaman K. Treatment of lymphangioma of the face with intralesional bleomycin: case
        discussion and literature review. J Maxillofac Oral Surg 2011; 10(2): 152-4.
        [http://dx.doi.org/10.1007/s12663-011-0210-4] [PMID: 22654368]

[26]   Thariat J, Vedrine PO, Orbach D, *et al.* Salivary gland tumors in children. Bull Cancer 2011; 98(7):
        847-55.
        [http://dx.doi.org/10.1684/bdc.2011.1399] [PMID: 21690035]

CHAPTER 2

Oral Examination and Diagnostic Aids in Pediatric Dentistry

Ashita Kalaskar[1,*] and **S. Jayachandran**[2]

[1] *Professor and Head, Department of Oral Medicine and Radiology, Govt. Dental College and Hospital, Nagpur, India*

[2] *Professor and Head, Department of of Oral Medicine and Radiology, Tamil Nādu Govt. Dental College and Hospital, Chennai, Tamil Nadu 600 003, India*

Abstract: The oral examination of the pediatric patients involves detailed evaluation and assessment along with comprehensive history taking. The pediatric history involves prenatal history, birth history, past medical history, past dental history, and family history. The examination part includes a general examination, extra oral examination and intra oral examination. The pediatric examination specifically includes dental caries, eruption pattern, shedding pattern, type of dentition, occlusion, supernumerary teeth, missing teeth *etc*. Various new diagnostic modalities have been introduced in the pediatric oral examination for both the hard tissues and soft tissues. Early diagnosis is mandated for precise treatment and proper prognosis for any disease which can be achieved by thorough examination through conventional and modern diagnostic techniques.

Keywords: Diagnosis, Dental caries, Examination, History, Pediatric.

INTRODUCTION

For successful treatment plan of a child patient, it is important to get a detailed medical, family, and dental history followed by thorough clinical and oral examination, appropriate investigations, correct diagnosis and accordingly an appropriate treatment plan and follow up. The prenatal and birth history plays a key role in the pediatric population with ages from birth through three years. They aid information about the presence of any infections at the time of birth, natal teeth at or around the time of birth *etc*. The family history, especially maternal history, can aid information on many congenital or birth defects. Maternal history, including habits, drugs and infection during pregnancy period must be recorded.

* **Corresponding author Ashita Kalaskar:** Professor and Head, Department of Oral Medicine and Radiology, Govt. Dental College and Hospital, Nagpur, India; E-mail: kalaskarshita@gmail.com

In contrast to taking the case history in an adult patient, the case history in children and especially in young children must be taken through another person, often one of the parents. This has two important implications.

The information obtained from the accompanying person may not necessarily be a valid reflection of the situation of the child. Most often it is, but the dentist should keep in mind that the adult is talking on behalf of the child when evaluating pain, for example in the case of traumatic injuries, the pediatric dentist should be especially aware of atypical lesions that do not seem to correspond with the information obtained in the history to identify cases related to child abuse.

The complete evaluation of the pediatric patients involves:

1. Recording history
2. Clinical and oral examination

This enables to arrive at a provisional diagnosis and after appropriate investigations final diagnosis could be obtained and treatment planning could be done.

CASE HISTORY

- Personal information
  1. Name- if child is called by his or her name, it may help maintain a good rapport with the child. Sometimes calling by nick name may alleviate apprehension. It is also useful for communication and record purpose.
  2. Patient registration number should be mandatorily recorded for:
     a. Record maintenance
     b. Medico-legal aspects
     c. Billing purposes
  3. Date - for reference and record maintenance
  4. Age
     a. As a growth assessment parameter
     b. To recognize the disparities between the dental – chronological age
     c. Aid in treatment planning
     d. Appropriate use of behavioral management technique- it differs according to the age of the patient. In case of pediatric patients, the dentist must deal with the child as well as with the parent; hence in pediatric dentistry, the approach is 1:2; while in case of adults, the approach is 1:1.
     e. Helps in forensic odontology
     f. Child dose- it differs by age. It is used to calculate the drug dosage

5. Gender
   a. As an aid in treatment planning *e.g.*, Growth spurts in girls are ahead of boys
   b. Sex related diseases like hemophilia, G6PD deficiency (causes hemolytic anemia), pubertal gingivitis seen in adolescent females.
   c. In trauma: – Boys sustain more injuries than girls – Ratio approx. – 2:1
   d. Child abuse—sexual abuse or exploitation is more common in case of females.
6. Address
   a. For communication purpose
   b. Record maintenance
   c. Medicolegal cases
   d. To rule out endemic diseases *e.g.*, goiter, skeletal or dental fluorosis
7. Occupation of parents – determines the socioeconomic status of parents

• Chief complaint – it is the concern about what made the patient to visit the dentist. It should always be in patient's own words. To have good rapport with child, it is better to ask the child about his/her chief complaint before the involvement of parent. But it is also necessary to get information from parents.

• History of present illness – it is a detailed description of chief complaint. Information should be collected by asking questions that includes:
   ○ Duration and mode of action
   ○ Cause of onset
   ○ Progress
   ○ Severity nature
   ○ Aggravating or relieving factors
   ○ Any medications or treatment taken for same

All these give a hint towards a disease/condition.

History of pain should be elicited in detail that include location of pain, origin or mode of onset, intensity, nature, progression, duration, radiation of pain, effect on functional activity and association with any systemic effects.

Detailed history of swelling should include mode of onset, progress, symptoms, associated features, secondary changes, impairment of function and any medication taken.

• Family history – it should include information about
   ○ genetic diseases in family if any (like hemophilia, sickle cell disease)
   ○ Co-morbidities /systemic diseases present with family members
   ○ housing conditions
   ○ parents' education and occupation

- number of children in family (nutritional deficiencies, malnourishment *etc.*)
- social background of child and parents
- consanguineous marriages (birth defects, diabetes mellitus, congenital heart diseases)

Medical history – This includes history of systemic diseases the patient has been diagnosed earlier. Also, many systemic diseases have their oral manifestations so all systems should be incorporated while taking medical history like

- Cardiovascular system (congenital heart diseases, rhematic fever *etc.*)
- Endocrine system (GH deficiency, diabetes)
- Respiratory system (Asthma)
- Central nervous system (epilepsy, cognitive delay)
- Hematological system (bleeding or clotting disorders, anemia)
- Urogenital system

This includes details about the drugs that patient is currently on, any drug being used for systemic diseases, duration of drugs being used and allergic reactions to any medicine should be recorded.

- Past dental history –It helps to evaluate
    - Child's experience of dental treatment
    - Factors that have been responsible for existing dental problem
    - Dietary habits like breastfeeding, bottle feeding at bedtime (nursing bottle caries)
    - Conditions like rampant caries, attrition.
    - Parent's attitude towards their child's dental health [1]
- Personal history
    - Habits

ORAL HYGIENE AND BRUSHING TECHNIQUE

Pressure habits—thumb sucking, lip sucking, and finger sucking may lead to anterior proclination of maxillary anterior teeth.

Tongue thrusting—it may lead to anterior and posterior open bite and proclination of anterior teeth.

Mouth breathing—it may lead to anterior marginal gingivitis and caries.

Other habits—nail biting, pencil and lip biting, lead to proclination of upper anterior and retroclination of lower anterior teeth.

- Patient's appetite- type of diet
- Bowel and micturition habit—Is it regular or irregular?
- Sleep pattern: Helps to identify apnea cases.
- Masochistic habit—some children use the fingernail to strip away the gingival tissue from the labial surface of a lower cuspid. If not discontinued, the marginal and attached gingival tissue will be stripped away exposing the alveolar bone [2, 3].

GENERAL CLINICAL EXAMINATION

Assessment of general appearance should start before the child is seated in the dental chair. It forms a first impression of the child's stature, body proportions, general posture, head posture, gait, and physical capability. This assessment may indicate growth disturbances, central nervous system disorders, neuromuscular disorders, or orthopedic problems worthy of further examination.

1. Height and weight- it depicts developmental and nutritional status of child. (Figs. **1** and **2**) [4].
2. Posture- look for any abnormality. *e.g.*, bowing of legs in rickets, cerebral palsy, scoliosis, *etc*.
3. Gait – Gait analysis assesses musculoskeletal abnormalities. Look for any abnormality. 'Head to toe' approach should be preferred to observe anatomical and functional features in all three planes. Conditions in which abnormal gait could be present are –pes planus, leg length discrepancy, tibial torsion, toe walking and bowlegs.
4. Vital signs
    a. Pulse (Table **1**).
       Assess
          - Rate: The number of pulses occurring per minute
          - Rhythm: The pattern or regularity of pulses
          - Volume: The perceived degree of pulsation
          - Character: An impression of the pulse wave form or shape

The rate and rhythm of the pulse are usually determined at the radial artery; use the larger pulses (brachial, carotid, or femoral) to assess the pulse volume and character.

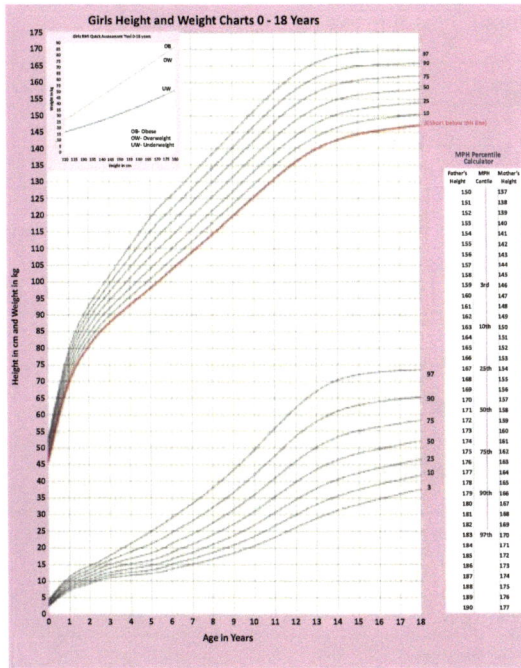

Fig. (1). Girls' height and weight chart 0-18 years.

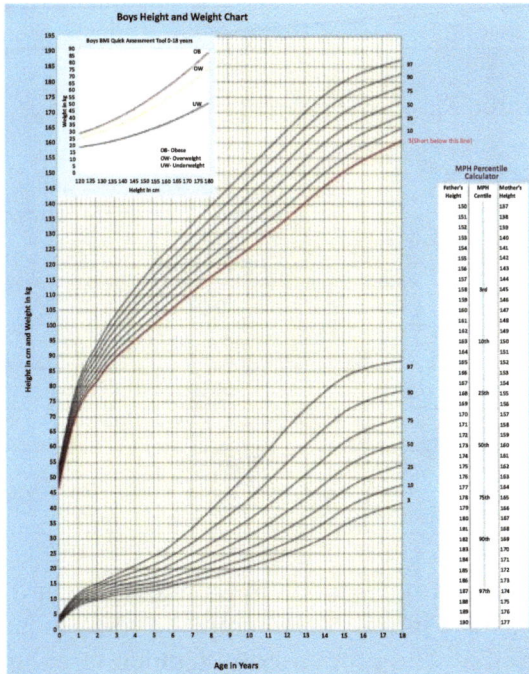

Fig. (2). Boys' height and weight chart.

Table 1. Pulse rate (beats/min) according to age.

Age	Pulse rate (beats/min)
1 to 2	80 to 130
3 to 4	80 to 120
5 to 6	75 to 115
7 to 9	70 to 110
10 or more	60 to 100

b. Respiratory rate should be recorded accurately as these differ in children at different ages until these reach adult value (Table **2**).

Table 2. Respiratory rate according to age.

Children at Different Ages	Respiratory Rate
Infant	30–60 rate/minute
Toddler	24–40
Preschooler	22–34
School–Aged Child	18–30
Adolescent	12–16

c. Blood pressure- [Table **3**].

Table 3. Blood pressure according to age.

Age	Systolic (mm of Hg)	Diastolic (mm of Hg)
Neonate	60–90	20–60
Infant	87–105	53–66
Toddler	95–105	53–66
Preschooler	95–110	56–70
School–Aged Child	97–112	57–71
Adolescent	112–128	66–80

5. Temperature- — it is normally taken in the mouth or in the axilla by keeping mercury thermometer for a minute. The temperature of mouth is about 1 degree higher than that of axilla. The normal body temperature varies from 36 degree Celsius to 37.5 degree Celsius. The lowest temperature being between 2-4 am and highest in the afternoon. The normal oral temperature is 37°C. Example:

Remittent fever- Typhoid, Intermittent fever- malaria [1].

• Extraoral examination – The dentist should assess:
  ○ Shape of head- it can be classified as:
    1. Mesocephalic – average shape of head
    2. Dolichocephalic- long and narrow head, often due to premature closure of the sagittal suture
    3. Brachycephalic- broad and short head
  ○ Facial form-it can be classified as:
    1. Mesoprosopic – average facial form
    2. Euryprosopic – broad and short facial form
    3. Leptoprosopic – long and narrow facial form
  ○ Facial profile – it can be straight, convex, or concave.
  ○ Facial symmetry - the size, location, tenderness, ulceration all should be inspected first followed by palpation of swelling for size, consistency, tenderness. Thorough history and proper examination play a significant role in making correct diagnosis. Causes for facial asymmetry:
    ▪ Congenital/ acquired facial nerve palsy
    ▪ Cleft lip/palate
    ▪ TMJ ankylosis
    ▪ Craniosynostosis
    ▪ Condylar hypoplasia or hyperplasia
    ▪ Facial tumors
  ○ Examination of the skin-
    a. Color- It is checked for anemia and jaundice. (Generalized pallor—it is seen in severe anemia, Lemon yellow tint—a pale lemon-yellow tint in hemolytic jaundice and dark yellow or orange tint in obstructive jaundice is seen
Yellowness of skin—yellowness of skin is seen in carotenemia.
    a. Texture—it is thickened, greasy and loose in acromegaly. In dehydration, skin is dry and inelastic so that it can be pinched into ridge
    b. Pigmentation, bullae, scarring, dryness, and scaling may indicate the presence of systemic disease.
    c. The hands should be examined with emphasis on, webbing of fingers, polydactyly, syndactyly, arachnodactyly (Fig. **3**) (indicative of a syndrome) [5], and evidence of any pressure habits like callus formation on thumb in patient having thumb sucking habit.
    d. The quality and the shape of the nails should be assessed. In ectodermal disorders the nails may be missing or be of inferior quality. In chronic respiratory diseases or congenital heart diseases, the fingernails may be markedly convex, and the fingers clubbed.

- Examination of lips - lips should be examined for any abnormal color, swelling, malformation, competent or noncompetent. Lip abnormalities- Cleft lip, developmental lip pits (Van der woude syndrome), pigmentations like in Addison's disease.
- Examination of Temporomandibular joint (TMJ)
  a. Functional examination of TMJ should be conducted by palpation and auscultation of TMJ and muscles of mastication.
  b. Any clicking, crepitus, deviation, pain should be noticed. Causes for TMJ abnormalities -Trauma, Ankylosis of TMJ (Fig. **4**), Juvenile arthritis, condylar hypoplasia/ hyperplasia [6].
  c. Mouth opening should be checked, normal values for children: – 35-45 mm; Lateral movements- 8 – 12 mm
- Lymph node examination- lymphadenopathy is common in children. All groups of lymph nodes should be inspected and palpated thoroughly.
  - Palpate one side at a time, using the fingers of each hand in turn.
  - Compare with the nodes on the contralateral side.
  - Assess:
    ○ Site
    ○ Size
  - Determine whether the node is fixed to:
    ○ Surrounding and deep structures
    ○ Skin
    ○ Check consistency
    ○ Check for tenderness
  - Examine the cervical and axillary nodes with the patient sitting.
  - From behind, examine the submental, submandibular, preauricular, tonsillar, supraclavicular, and deep cervical nodes in the anterior triangle of the neck.
  - Palpate for the scalene nodes by placing your index finger between the sternocleidomastoid muscle and clavicle.
  - Ask the patient to tilt their head to the same side and press firmly down towards the first rib.
  - From the front of the patient, palpate the posterior triangles, up the back of the neck and the posterior auricular and occipital nodes.

Causes of lymph nodes enlargement could be:

Inflammatory—acute lymphadenitis, chronic lymphadenitis, septic, tuberculosis, Hematological—Hodgkin's disease, non-Hodgkin lymphoma [1, 2].

INTRAORAL EXAMINATION

It should begin with "Tell-show-do approach" *i.e.*, first tell child what you are going to do, then show the instruments, so that he/she gets familiar to them and then perform examination. Intraoral examination should be conducted under adequate light. A small depressor can also be used for observation and inspection.

The examination of a newborn or infant is usually "lap to lap" with informed consent from the parent/guardian.

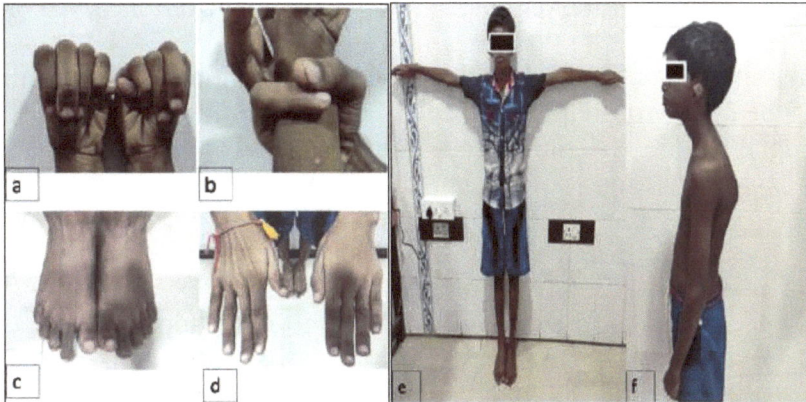

Fig. (3). A thirteen-year-old child of Marfans syndrome. There was presence of **a**. The Steinberg sign, **b**. The Walker-Murdoch sign (There was a grip of the wrist with the opposite hand), **c** and **d**. Arachnodactyly of hand and feet fingers and **e** and **f**. Armspan: height was more than 1.05. Disproportionately long arms and legs with hindfoot deformity present.

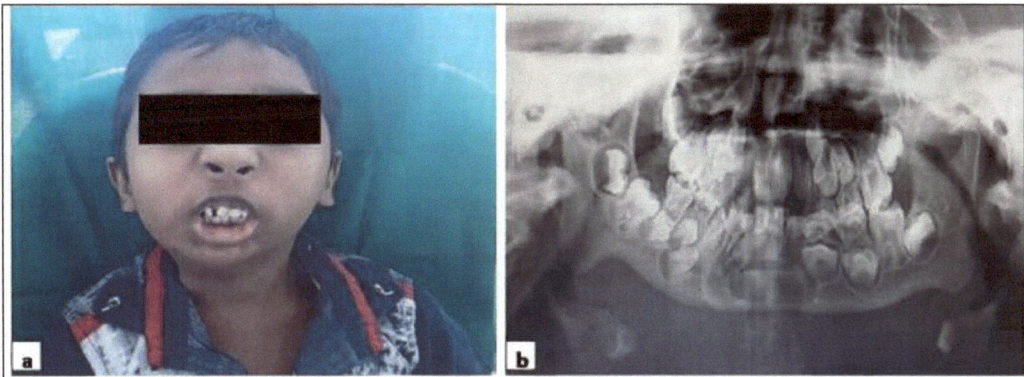

Fig. (4). a) A six-year-old child who had a severely restricted mouth opening, deviation of mandible and bird chin appearance. b. The orthopantomogram revealed bilateral TMJ ankylosis.

Soft Tissue Examination

a. It includes complete inspection and palpation of oral mucosa. An abnormal appearance of oral mucosa like change in colour and appearance should be recorded as this may indicate underlying systemic disease or nutritional deficiency (Tables **4** and **5**).

b. Palate- it needs be looked for congenital cleft, perforation, ulceration, swelling, fistula, Bohn's nodules.

Cleft examination—in case of congenital cleft, note the extent of the cleft (involving only the uvula, only the soft palate or part or whole of the hard palate). Whether the nasal septum is hanging free or attached to one side of the cleft. It may be associated with Pierre's robin syndrome and Vander woude's syndrome.

Tongue- colour, texture, papillae, mobility should be checked, *e.g.*-congenital fissures,

-massive tongue due to lymphangioma, hemangioma and neurofibroma,

-If the child with impaired speech fails to protrude the tongue, it is due to tongue-tie; look for short frenum linguae called as ankyloglossia.

-Tongue thrusting—note tongue thrust on swallowing.

c. Gingiva—

  ▫ Child's marginal gingiva is thicker and rounded than adults.
  ▫ Attached gingiva shows less stippling and keratinization, is red in color with presence of interdental clefts and retrocuspid papillae compared to adult gingiva.
  ▫ The interdental gingiva is pyramidal shape
  ▫ The common pathologies observed are juvenile periodontitis and inflammatory gingival enlargement. Less common condition is granulomatous involvement of gingival (Fig. **5**) [7].

d. Frenum

-High labial frenae may cause Midline diastema. Incision of the papilla is advisable.

-Tongue Tie can lead to speech defects and poor hygiene maintenance in the adjacent teeth (Fig. **6**).

-Blanch test is performed for confirmation.

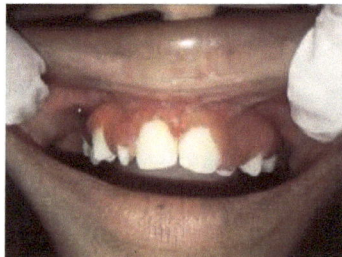

Fig. (5). Represents generalized gingival enlargement of the maxillary gingiva including the interdental gingiva and attached gingiva of an eleven-year-old child. The gingiva is soft, hemorrhagic, and friable which was representative of strawberry gingivitis.

Table 4. Normal and pathological findings of soft tissues of oral cavity.

Parts of Moutd (Oral Cavity)	Common Findings Normal and Pathological
Gingiva	• Eruption cyst or hematoma • Normal pigmentation • Patdologic pigmentation • Gingival cyst of newborn • Retrocuspid papillae • Parulis ("gum boil") • Gingival overgrowtd • Pyogenic Granuloma • Localized Juvenile Spongiotic Gingival Hyperplasia • Peripheral Giant Cell Granuloma • Peripheral Ossifying Fibroma • Giant Cell Fibroma
Tongue	• Ankyloglossia ("tongue-tie") • Fissured tongue • Macroglossia • Ankyloglossia • Congenital lingual melanotic macules • Geographic tongue • Benign Migratory Glossitis • Strawberry Tongue • Mucocele • Lingual Tonsil
Lips/labial	• Herpes labialis
Mucosa	• Ranula
-	• Angular cheilitis (Iron deficiency)
-	• Mucocele
-	• Riga fede disease
-	• Congenital pits
Buccal Mucosa	• Bohn's nodules • Fordyce spots • Epstein pearls • Irritation fibromas • Traumatic ulcers • Aphtdous ulcers

(Table 4) cont.....

Parts of Moutd (Oral Cavity)	Common Findings Normal and Pathological
Teeth	• Dental caries • Gemination • Fusion • Twinning • Supernumerary teetd • Macrodontia • Microdontia • Enamel hypoplasia • Resorption • Pigmentation
-	• Natal teetd • Neonatal teetd • Otder developmental anomalies [1]

Table 5. Common infections in children.

Type of Infection	Common Finding in Children which Shows Oral Manifestations
Bacterial	• Impetigo • Scarlet fever • Actinomycosis (rarely)
Viral	• Herpetic gingivostomatitis • Chicken pox (Herpesvirus) • Mumps • Measles • Rubella • EBV/CMV (rarely)
Fungal	• Candidiasis

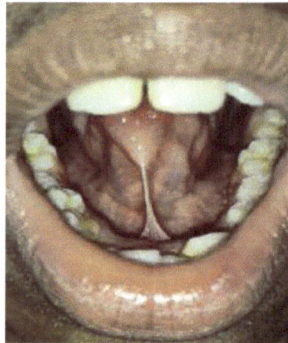

Fig. (6). Ankyloglossia of a twelve-year-old male. There was partial ankyloglossia of the lingual frenum which mildly restricted the movements of the tongue but not much alteration of speech was evident [8].

e. Tonsils – examine the tonsils for swelling and inflammation.

• The palatine tonsils are simply referred to as 'the tonsil'- in between the anterior

& posterior pillars of oropharynx
- The Nasopharyngeal tonsils or the adenoids- in the nasopharynx.
- The tubal tonsils- near opening of eustachian tubes.
- The Lingual tonsils- in the base of the tongue [3].

Hard Tissue Examination

Overall condition of dentition should be evaluated. Variations in number, morphology and colour of teeth should be noted. Teeth should be evaluated for-

- Caries
- Fractured teeth (trauma)
- Hypoplastic teeth (nutritional deficiency (vitamins A, C, and D); exanthemata's diseases (*e.g.*, measles, chickenpox, scarlet fever); congenital syphilis; hypocalcaemia; birth injury, prematurity, Rh hemolytic disease; local infection or trauma; ingestion of chemicals (chiefly fluoride); and idiopathic causes.)
- Retained teeth
- Delayed eruption may be associated with certain systemic conditions, including rickets, cretinism, and cleidocranial dysplasia (q.v.). Local factors like cystic lesions (Fig. **7**) or circumstances may also delay eruption, as in the case of fibromatosis gingivae, in which the dense connective tissue will not permit eruption [9].
- Teeth number – Anodontia, hypodontia or oligodontia [10] *e.g.*, Ectodermal dysplasia (Fig. **8**).
- Tooth structure affected in conditions like amelogenesis imperfecta, dentinogenesis imperfecta (Fig. **9**), dentin dysplasia, dental fluorosis [9, 11].
- Premature eruption: Deciduous teeth that have erupted into the oral cavity are occasionally seen in infants at birth and are called natal teeth in contrast to neonatal teeth (**Fig. 10**), which have been defined as those teeth erupting prematurely in the first 30 days of life [12].
- Supernumerary teeth – A supernumerary tooth is an additional entity to the normal series and is seen in all the quadrants of the jaw. In a survey of 2,000 schoolchildren, Brook found that supernumerary teeth were present in 0.8% of primary dentition and in 2.1% of permanent dentition. Different morphological forms-
    - ° Conical
    - ° Tuberculate
    - ° Supplemental
    - ° Odontome
- Submerged teeth—are deciduous teeth, most commonly mandibular second molars, which have undergone a variable degree of root resorption and then have become ankylosed to the bone.

- Orthodontic evaluation
    i. Alignment- molar and canine relationship, crowding/spacing, skeletal discrepancies, midline deviation, incisal relationship should be evaluated.
    ii. Tooth position- it involves ectopic eruption, transposition, impaction, failure of primary teeth eruption
    iii. Occlusion in deciduous dentition—it is evaluated by following ways
        1. Flush terminal plane—the distal surface of maxillary and mandibular second molar are in straight plane.
        2. Mesial step—distal surface of mandibular second molar is more mesial to maxillary second molar.
        3. Distal step—distal surface of mandibular second molar is more distal to maxillary second molar [3, 13].
            - Provisional diagnosis—

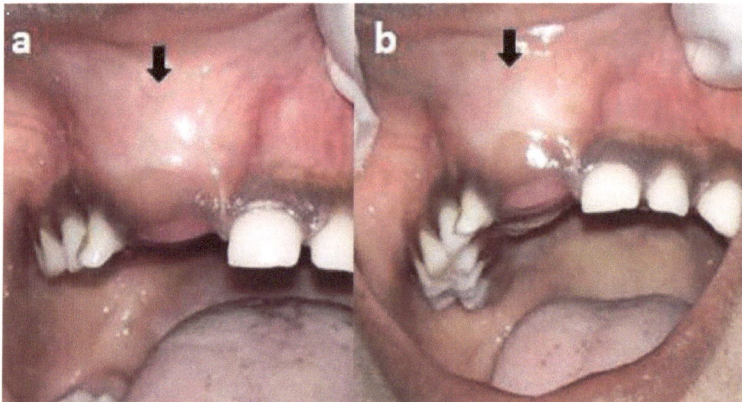

Fig. (7). A seven-year-old male child with a chief complaint of swelling in the upper right front region of the jaw and delayed eruption of upper front tooth. The surgical excision and histopathology revealed dentigerous cyst.

After clubbing all records and clinical examination, clinician should be able to form a provisional diagnosis along with the differential diagnosis. Accordingly, appropriate investigations should be carried to confirm diagnosis.

Investigations

Laboratory investigations help to come to the final diagnosis, *e.g.*, in case of caries (proximal) the provisional diagnosis will be mesial or distal caries. Radiograph will confirm the diagnosis and help us to differentiate it into incipient, moderate, advanced, and severe type. The common investigation methods are radiological, hematological investigations, urine analysis, biochemical investigations, histopathological investigations, microbiological investigations, and special investigations like sialography, MRI, *etc.*

Special Diagnostic Aids [2]

Diagnosis is a process by which the practitioner differentiates between normal and abnormal and determines the etiology of abnormal conditions.

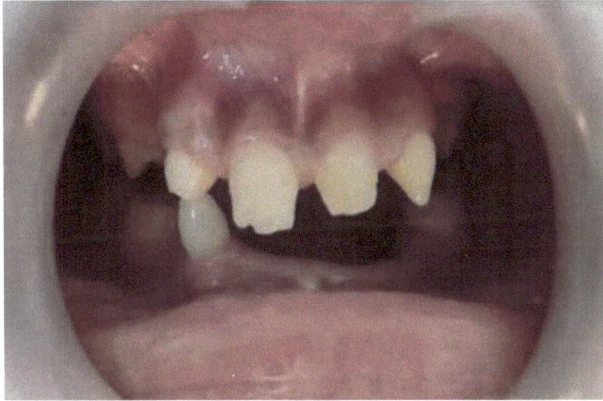

Fig. (8). The oral manifestation of ectodermal dysplasia of a six-year-old patient which reveals multiple missing teeth. There is partial loss of enamel with altered morphological structures. The patient also had sparse hair and brittle nail which was suggestive of ectodermal dysplasia.

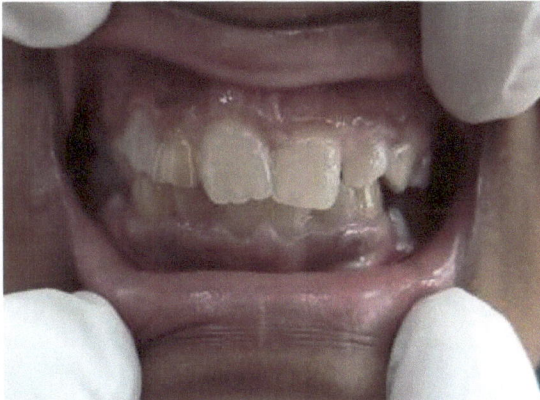

Fig. (9). A ten-year-old child with discoloration of all present teeth. There is complete loss of enamel which exposed the dentin. The teeth were yellowish brown, smooth and glossy. The patient also complained of sensitivity.

The various diagnostic aids can be categorized as:

- Routine diagnostic aids - The clinical intraoral examination is performed systematically in a clean, dry, well-illuminated mouth using the mouth mirror, explorer, and periodontal probe.
- Specialized diagnostic aids - These are used for the diagnosis of specific dental problems like detection of dental caries, pulpal diseases, and orthodontic

problems.
- Advanced diagnostic aids- like CBCT, MRI
    - Methods of clinical diagnosis of dental caries
- Clinical method (visual-tactile method): Use of a mirror and blunt probe is the most common method of diagnosing tooth decay. A sharp probe can break the intact tooth surface in one of the enamel lesions causing a cavity.
- Radiographic methods: conventional radiographs like bitewing and intraoral periapical radiograph are most frequently used for the detection of caries. During the primary dentition, the occlusal surface is most susceptible to caries attack, but with the eruption of first permanent molars the incidence of proximal lesions increases. In such situation, bitewing radiographs are absolutely required to detect proximal lesions. Advanced radiographic techniques like digital radiography can also be helpful.
- Tooth separation: Orthodontic modules or bands can be used to achieve slow separation and by separating the teeth one can visualize the proximal surfaces.
- Fibre-optic transillumination diagnoses proximal lesions in anterior teeth and posterior teeth by utilizing fibre-optic light source with the beam reduced to 0.5 mm in diameter. When this method is combined with digital camera, it is called as digital imaging fibreoptic transillumination (DIFOTI).
- Caries detector dyes, such as silver nitrate, methyl red and alizarin stain have been used to detect carious sites by change of colour.
- Ultrasonics utilizes a sonar device in which a beam of ultrasound waves is directed against the tooth surface and, if reflected, is picked up by an appropriate receiver. This method can be readily adopted to easily accessible areas but not for interproximal surface.
- Advanced techniques include electroconductivity measurements (ECM), direct digital radiography (DDR), and endoscopic filtered fluorescence method (EFF) [14]. Based on the fluorescence of the organic components of teeth the Quantitative Light Induced Fluorescence and Infrared Fluorescence techniques have been develop.
- Carbon Dioxide Laser

When carbon dioxide laser is applied to an incipient lesion of caries, the organic contents evaporate leaving a black carbonized residue behind whereas the inorganic substance of sound enamel containing minimum amount of water is less affected by the laser beam [14].

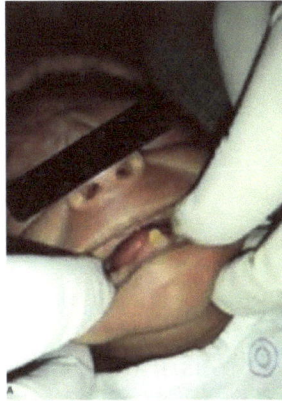

Fig. (10). The presence of neonatal teeth in the mandibular anterior region of a 24-day-old male preterm baby.

Final Diagnosis

The final diagnosis is made by chronologic organization and critical evaluation of the information obtained from the patient history, physical examination, and the result of radiological and laboratory examination. The parents should be informed about the findings of examination, diagnosis, results of tests and treatment planning. This should be followed by taking an informed consent

Informed Consent

The informed consent form should include the following:

1. Legal name and date of birth of pediatric patient.
2. Legal name and relationship to the pediatric patient/legal basis on which the person is granting permission on behalf of the patient.
3. Patient's diagnosis.
4. Nature and purpose of the proposed treatment in simple terms.
5. Potential benefits and risks associated with that treatment.
6. Professionally-recognized or evidence-based alternative treatment – including no treatment
7. Place for parent to indicate that all questions have been asked and answered.
8. Places for signatures of the parent, dentist, and an office staff member as a witness [15].

Treatment Plan

When staging treatment, it can be helpful to order treatments in the following ways:

1. Emergency phase: management of dental pain and/or trauma should take precedence, and a quick assessment of the child's coping ability is necessary to deem whether a timely referral is required for sedation or general anesthetic. *e.g.*,
   - Emergency Treatments like maxillofacial trauma,
   - swelling,
   - systemic infection,
   - severe pain
2. Systemic phase: Premedication, antibiotic prophylaxis managing anticoagulants adrenal/thyroid insufficiency cases.
3. Prevention/preparatory phase: this involves a tailored oral health promotion plan, which may include the following
   - Caries risk assessment
   - Oral hygiene counselling
   - Diet counselling
   - Pit &Fissure sealants
   - Fluoride application
   - Behavioral management
   - Caries control
   - Oral Prophylaxis
   - Preventive orthodontics
   - Extraction of unrestorable teeth
   - Pre-prosthetic treatment
4. Restorative/definitive phase: Start with smaller less-invasive procedures to build confidence *e.g.*, preventive resin restoration on first permanent molars, small occlusal restorations, or Hall Technique crowns, before the introduction of local anesthetic for pulp therapy or extractions. Again, staging treatment to prioritize strategic teeth can help structure this phase, particularly for the child experiencing multiple progressing carious lesions. *e.g.*
   - Restorative and Pulpal treatment
   - Prosthetic rehabilitation
   - Orthodontic interventions – serial extractions, space management, tooth movements
   - Orthognathic surgery
   - Periodontal therapy
5. Maintenance phase: as previously mentioned, consideration of the child's caries risk allows appropriate maintenance care pathways to be followed with respect to dental recall interval [as per National Institute for health and clinical excellence (NICE) guidelines], bitewing radiograph frequency [as per Faculty of General Dental Practitioners (FGPD) guidelines] and frequency of topical fluoride application.

- 3-6 month recalls
- review checkup of oral health indices
- repeat caries activity tests
- reinforcement of home care measures
- motivation and re-counselling of the parent
- follow up of treatment procedures

Natal Teeth / Neonatal Teeth

Natal teeth are defined as the teeth present at birth. Natal teeth are also called as congenital teeth [15]. The presence of natal teeth/neonatal teeth leads to Riga fede disease which is traumatic ulceration of labial mucosa due to the incisal edges. Managing a child born with natal tooth can be challenging as it poses problems in feeding, increased risk of aspiration, and causes ulceration of the tongue [16]. It is discussed in detail in another chapter.

General Drug Usages (American Academy of Pediatric Dentistry Guidelines)

- Acetaminophen is associated with hepatotoxicity in children and hence it is limited to 325 mg per dosage unit.
- Naproxen can be used at 200 mg naproxen base/220 mg naproxen sodium. As it has decreased adverse effects.
- Clavulanic acid can be used at its lowest dose with amoxicillin to decrease gastrointestinal adverse effects.
- Azithromycin is used on children with penicillin/ cephalosporin antibiotics. This drug must be used in caution with patients with previous cardiac history.
- Cephalexin is also commonly used but in caution due to penicillin allergy.
- Clindamycin is also commonly used on children with penicillin/cephalosporin antibiotic as it is effective against gram-positive aerobic bacteria and gram-positive or gram-negative anaerobic bacteria
- Doxycycline may cause permanent tooth discoloration, hypoplasia (enamel), and hyperpigmentation. Pregnant women and children below eight years of old should not use this drug
- Metronidazole is a used along with other antibiotics when broad coverage of anaerobic bacteria is needed.
- Fluconazole is prescribed occasionally. It requires acidic pH for absorption and hence the absorption is decreased by few other medications.
- Acyclovir is used in caution during viral infection [17].

CONCLUSION

History taking is the principle way of appropriately analyzing and finalizing the correct treatment plan. The clinician must use proper techniques for child patients as and when required. Documentation of the observed findings is necessary for providing competent and quality oral health care. It serves as an information source for the care provider and patient. This is so because it helps to establish records, for further medico legal purposes and provides definite base line criteria against which the future conditions can be compared. Thus, the patient record provides the history and details of patient assessment and communications between dentist, patient, and caregiver, as well as specific treatment recommendations, alternatives, risks, and care provided.

CONSENT FOR PUBLICATION

Not applicable.

CONFLICT OF INTEREST

The authors declare no conflict of interest, financial or otherwise.

ACKNOWLEDGEMENT

Declared none.

REFERENCES

[1]   American Academy of Pediatric Dentistry Periodicity of examination, preventive dental services, anticipatory guidance/ counseling, and oral treatment for infants, children, and adolescents. The Reference Manual of Pediatric Dentistry. 2020; 232-42.

[2]   American Academy of Pediatric Dentistry Record-keeping. Pediatr Dent 2017; 39(6): 389-96.
        [PMID: 29179380]

[3]   Harris EJ. The Pediatric History and Physical Examination. Switzerland. 2020; 1-42.
        [http://dx.doi.org/10.1007/978-3-030-29788-6_1]

[4]   Parekh BJ, Khadilkar V. Pediatrician-Friendly IAP Growth Charts for Children Aged 0–18 Years. Indian Pediatr 2020; 57(11): 997-8.
        [http://dx.doi.org/10.1007/s13312-020-2021-5] [PMID: 33231172]

[5]   França EC, Abreu LG, Paiva SM, Drummond AF, Cortes ME. Oral management of Marfan syndrome: an overview and case report. Gen Dent 2016; 64(6): 54-9.
        [PMID: 27814256]

[6]   Mittal N, Goyal M, Sardana D, Dua JS. Granulomatosis with Polyangiitis (Wegener's Granulomatosis): Evolving Concepts in Treatment.Semin Respir Crit Care Med 2018 2019; 47(7): 1120-33.
        [http://dx.doi.org/10.1016/j.jcms.2019.03.029] [PMID: 31027859]

[7]   Lynch JP III, Derhovanessian A, Tazelaar H, Belperio JA. Granulomatosis with polyangiitis(Wegener'sgranulomatosis):evolvingconceptsintreatment.InSeminarsinrespiratory and critical care medicine Thieme Medical Publishers. 2018; 39: 434-58.

[8]   Lisonek M, Liu S, Dzakpasu S, Moore AM, Joseph KS. Changes in the incidence and surgical treatment of ankyloglossia in Canada. Paediatr Child Health 2017 2017; 22(7): 382-6.
        [http://dx.doi.org/10.1093/pch/pxx112]

[9]   Martinelli-Kläy CP, Martinelli CR, Martinelli C, Macedo HR, Lombardi T. Unusual imaging features

of dentigerous cyst: a case report. Dent J 2019; 7(3): 76.
[http://dx.doi.org/10.3390/dj7030076] [PMID: 31374841]

[10]   Wimalarathna AAAK, Weerasekara WBMCRD, Herath EMUCK. Comprehensive Management of Ectodermal Dysplasia with Interceptive Orthodontics in a Young Boy Who Was Bullied at School. Case Rep Dent 2020; 2020: 1-7.
[http://dx.doi.org/10.1155/2020/6691235] [PMID: 33489382]

[11]   Wright JT, Carrion IA, Morris C. The molecular basis of hereditary enamel defects in humans. J Dent Res 2015; 94(1): 52-61.
[http://dx.doi.org/10.1177/0022034514556708] [PMID: 25389004]

[12]   Sadaksharam J, Jeba Priya JS. Natal tooth: a histomorphologic variant, a rarity. Ann Natl Acad Med Sci 2019; 55(4): 210-2.
[http://dx.doi.org/10.1055/s-0039-3401468]

[13]   Martins-Júnior PA, Vieira-Andrade RG, Corrêa-Faria P, Oliveira-Ferreira F, Marques LS, Ramos-Jorge ML. Impact of early childhood caries on the oral health-related quality of life of preschool children and their parents. Caries Res 2013; 47(3): 211-8.
[http://dx.doi.org/10.1159/000345534] [PMID: 23257929]

[14]   Yılmaz H, Keleş S. Recent methods for diagnosis of dental caries in dentistry. Meandros Medical and Dental Journal 2018; 19(1): 1-8.
[http://dx.doi.org/10.4274/meandros.21931]

[15]   American Academy of Pediatric Dentistry. Guideline on informed consent 2015; 37(5): 95-7.
[PMID: 26531081]

[16]   Lewis C. Treatment Planning in Pediatric Dentistry-a Structured Approach. Dent Health (London) 2020; 59: 28-9.

[17]   American Academy of Pediatric Dentistry Useful Medications for Oral Conditions 2018; 40: 108.

CHAPTER 3

Dental Radiology in Pediatric Dentistry

Jayachandran Sadaksharam[1,*] and **Ashita Kalaskar**[2]

[1] *Professor & Head, Department of Oral Medicine & Radiology, Tamil Nadu Government Dental College & Hospital, Chennai, Tamil Nadu, India*

[2] *Department of Oral Medicine & Radiology, Government Dental College & Hospital, Nagpur, India*

Abstract: Dental radiology occupies a pivotal role in pediatric dentistry and acts as an aid in the diagnosis of oral health and disease states. It is used in conjunction with clinical examination for the final diagnosis. It includes the intraoral radiograph, extraoral radiograph, and specialized radiographs like Cone Beam Computed Tomography (CBCT), computed tomography (CT) *etc.* The Intra Oral Periapical Radiograph (IOPA) and orthopantomogram (OPG) are commonly used in the dental setting owing to the low exposure and broad coverage of the areas. Radiation protection includes many entities, which must be provided for both the patient and the accompanying person. The radiographic requirements differ for neonates, children, and adolescents. This chapter emphasizes the importance of dental radiology in pediatric dentistry and the various aspects of radiology from the perspective of the pediatric population

Keywords: Cone beam computed tomography, Diagnosis, Digital radiography, Orthopantomogram, Pediatric.

INTRODUCTION

Radiographs are valuable diagnostic aid for proper and detailed examination of the oral cavity of infants, children, adolescents, and individuals with special health care needs (Fig. **1**). It also helps the clinician to arrive at a precise diagnosis and proper treatment planning. American Academy of Pediatric Dentistry developed guidelines (Table **1**) [1, 2].

---

* Corresponding author Jayachandran Sadaksharam: Professor & Head, Department of Oral Medicine & Radiology Tamil Nadu Government Dental College & Hospital Chennai, India; E-mail: drsjayachandranmds@ yahoo.com

Dental Caries	History of pain	Pulpal and periapical pathology	History of trauma to teeth and traumatic injuries
Postoperative evaluation	Problems of eruption	Familial history of dental problems	Developmental anomalies
Unexplained discolouration of teeth	Orthodontic treatment planning	Evidence of swelling	Unexplained tooth mobility
Unexplained bleeding	Fistula formation	Unusual spacing or migration of teeth	Lack of response to conventional dental treatment
Unusual tooth morphology, calcification or colour	Evaluation of growth abnormalities	Altered occlusal relationship	Aid in diagnosis of systemic disease

Fig. (1). Common conditions for indicating dental radiographs.

Table 1. Criteria for recommending dental radiographs.

Patient Age and Dental Developmental Stage			
Type of Encounter	A child with Primary Dentition before the eruption of the first permanent tooth)	A child with Transitional Dentition (after the r eruption of the first permanent tooth)	An adolescent with Permanent Dentition (before the option of third molars)
New patient being evaluated for dental diseases and dental development	Selected periapical/occlusal views and/or posterior bitewings if proximal surfaces cannot be visualized or probed. Patients without evidence of disease and with open proximal contacts may not require a radiographic exam at this time.	Posterior bitewings with panoramic exam or posterior bitewings and selected periapical images.	Posterior bitewings with panoramic exam or posterior bitewings and selected periapical images. A full mouth intraoral radiographic exam is preferred when the patient has clinical evidence of generalized dental disease or a history of extensive dental treatment.

(Table 1) cont.....

Patient Age and Dental Developmental Stage		
Recall patients with clinical caries or at increased risk for caries	Posterior bitewing exam at 6–12-month intervals if proximal surfaces cannot be examined visually or with a probe.	
Recall patient with no clinical caries and not at increased risk for caries	Posterior bitewing exam at 12-24 months intervals if proximal surfaces cannot be examined visually or with a probe.	Posterior bitewing exam at 18-36 months intervals.
Recall patient with periodontal disease	Clinical judgment as to the need for and type of radiographic images for the evaluation of periodontal disease. Imaging may consist of but is not limited to, selected bitewing and/or periapical images of areas where periodontal disease (other than nonspecific gingivitis) can be identified clinically.	
Patient for monitoring of growth and development.	Clinical judgment as to the need for and type of radiographic images for evaluation and/or monitoring of dentofacial growth and development	Clinical judgment as to the need for and type of radiographic images for evaluation and/or monitoring of dentofacial growth and development. Panoramic or periapical exam to assess developing third molars.
Patients with other circumstances including, but not limited to, proposed or existing implants, pathology, restorative/endodontic needs, treated periodontal disease and caries remineralization	Clinical judgment as to the need for and type of radiographic images for evaluation and/or monitoring in these circumstances.	

Radiation Biology

X-rays are the ionizing radiation that can cause biological damage, the severity of which is proportional to the dose. Biological effects or damage occur at molecular levels and are exhibited as direct effects or indirect effects. In the direct effect, the biological macromolecule is directly affected, whereas, in the indirect effect, the water molecules in the biological system are ionized, forming free radicals (hydrogen and hydroxyl free radicals), which further undergo biological damage [3].

At cellular levels, effect on the nucleus is seen more in the cytoplasm as it is more radiosensitive. DNA and chromosomes are the sensitive sites in the nucleus. When DNA condenses to form chromosomes at the time of mitosis, chromosomal aberrations are observed the most. Thus, the dividing or proliferating cells are the ones to be targeted by the radiation. Children, therefore, are more concerned because most of the biological system is under the growth phase exhibiting a greater number of proliferating cells. These cells are thus more radiosensitive due to their high mitotic rate and ability to undergo much future mitosis [3]. Apart from this, the other reasons for the high risk of radiation exposure as compared to adults to the child's organs could be due to the following reasons:

- Children have a longer life span.
- Children might require a greater number of radiographs because of the high prevalence of caries.
- Effects of radiation are cumulative and lasting for a longer time [4].

In general, the dose received from dental radiology is quite minimal than the dose required to cause chromosomal aberrations or the genetic doubling dose for the mutation (0.46Sv-1.25Sv) [3]. Table **2** shows the radiation dose by different radiological examinations [5].

Table 2. Effective radiation dose by different radiological examinations [5].

X-ray examination	Effective Dose (mSv)
Intraoral Periapical Radiograph	0.001- 0.008
Panoramic	0.004-0.03
Lateral cephalometrics	0.002-0.003
CT	0.1 – 3.3
CBCT	0.045 – 0.65

Radiation Protection

Dentists should be concerned about the radiation effects while exposing patients to radiographs and always follow the three basic rules of safe radiation exposure, which are justification, limitation and optimization (Fig. **2**) [4]. Justification means ensuring that radiographs are the only ways to obtain the necessary information, limitation means following the ALARA principle, and optimization means that the image quality should be as high as possible. The ALARA principle is "as low as reasonably achievable," which means that without compromising the diagnostic quality of the radiographic image, the lowest possible radiation exposure should be done [4, 6].

Thus, X-rays should not be taken routinely. Dental and Medical status should be examined first before ordering radiographs. Also, the number and types of radiographs depend on the age of the child, the presence and amount of visual decay, the child's and family's history of dental treatment, and spaces between teeth. Additionally, copies of prior radiographs, if available, should be obtained [7].

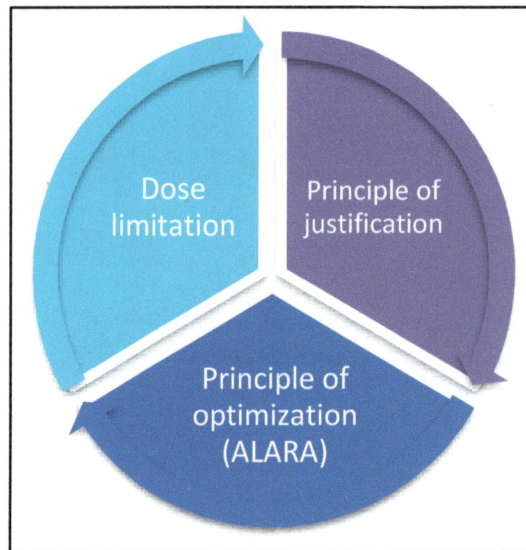

Fig. (2). Rules of safe radiation exposure.

Many techniques have been achieved to reduce the dose received by patients and personnel in radiology centres [3, 7, 8] (Fig. **3**). These are:

- Use of faster films (E and F speed films) and double pack films (preferably).
- The use of a long-distance between the patient and the source of radiation can be achieved by using a position indicating device (PID).
- The use of protective devices for the sensitive body's organs (lead aprons and thyroid collars).
- Collimation of X-ray beam.
- Use the manufacturer's recommended time and temperature for processing.
- Anti-scatter grid should be used judiciously for children when high image quality is of prime concern.
- For the desired X-ray, tube current and time product (mAs), should use the shortest exposure time.
- Additional filters, if provided by design, should be used [8].
- Quality control of equipment: It should be ensured that dose assessment is performed regularly primarily to keep patient exposure within the recommended levels and secondarily to identify any equipment malfunction or inadequate technique [7].

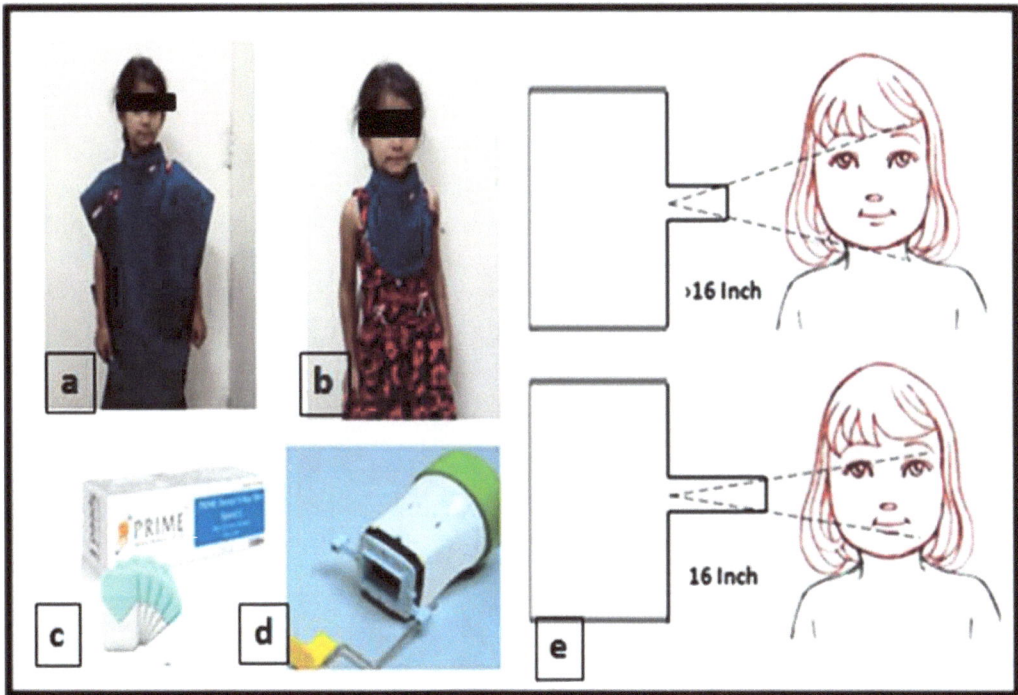

Fig. (3). Various means of radiation protections **(a)** Lead apron **(b)** Thyroid collar **(c)** Faster films (E/F)**(d)** Collimator **(e)** Preferred 16 inches position indicating device (PID).

In addition to the above, it is advisable to select the correct technique, radiograph, and film holding device along with efficient patient behaviour management protocol to minimize errors and retakes. The common errors encountered as shown in Table **3**.

Table 3. Common radiographic errors.

Radiographic Errors	Reasons
Cone cutting or area of interest not exposed	The improper film, object or x-ray beam alignment is caused by the displacement of any of the above either due to an uncooperative child or gag reflex.
Overlapping of the contact area	Incorrect horizontal angulations
Foreshortening or elongation of images.	Improper vertical angulations
Blurred images	Movement of the patient because of repetition of radiographic examination or an uncooperative child.
Improper contrast of the image	Overexposure or underexposure

Exposure Parameters and Infection Control

- Children have thinner skull and tissue than adults, which warrants decreased exposure parameters in children.
- Exposure parameters like operating mA, kVp or exposure time should be appropriately adjusted to compensate for the variations in size and thickness of the pediatric patient. Nowadays, X-ray units have a pre-set child exposure setting available which helps in reducing radiation doses by up to 50%.
- Policies and procedures used to prevent or reduce the potential for disease transmission should be strictly adhered to as there is an increased risk of acquiring TB, herpes infection, hepatitis, URI, AIDS, and the novel void-19pandemic. This can be achieved by breaking the chain of transmission of infection from the oral cavity to the frequently touched surfaces and *vice versa* by following proper asepsis protocol, for example, using disposable surface covers for the frequently touched surfaces, film barriers, disposable protective gears used by the operators, sterilization of holding devices and regular disinfection of the radiology unit [3, 6].

X-Ray Dose Measurement

- Most of the X-ray units come with a control panel having a display of the amount of radiation dose the patient has been exposed to while taking the radiograph.
- Whereas for the operator, portable dosimeters like the thermo-luminescent dosimeter (TLD)containing Lithium fluoride or calcium fluoride-containing manganese are indicated to be used as a personal monitoring device to monitor the quantity of radiation exposure. Their small size, accuracy and easy handling characteristics make them the preferred devices [3].

Management of Child Behavior While Taking Radiograph [2, 9, 10]

A. In Infants

- It is quite challenging to perform radiographs on an infant below 3 years of age, thus, the dental office should be prepared with techniques to reduce any psychological trauma.
- The size zero intraoral periapical films are always recommended for the exposure.
- For a child of three years, it is advisable to let the child sit in the parent's lap while exposing the radiograph.
- The clinician must tell, enact, and use various techniques to explain to the child that a tooth camera will be used to take a picture of their tooth.
- The child is allowed to touch and examine the radiographic film and camera.

▪ Children may have difficulty holding the film in their mouth for an extended period; therefore, a positioning device such as a Snap-A-Ray can be used to aid the parent in positioning and securing the film (Fig. **4**).

▪ For the uncooperative child, desensitizing techniques like "Lollipop Radiograph" can be performed. The child is given a sugarless lollipop to lick. After a few licks, the lollipop is taken from the child, and a radiograph is attached to the lollipop with an orthodontic rubber band on the lingual side of the film. The lollipop with the attached film is returned to the child, who is told to lick the lollipop again. After a few licks, the child is told to hold the lollipop in his mouth and exposure is made. The child has now associated the radiograph procedure with a pleasurable experience (the licking of the lollipop) and has been desensitized to the extent that the more difficult posterior radiographs can be attempted. Posterior radiographs can be made more pleasant by associating them with a pleasurable taste such as bubble gum [9].

▪ If the child is very uncooperative, then additional restraint by a second adult may be used to successfully obtain the radiograph. The second adult stabilizes the child's head with one hand while the other hand positions the Snap-A-Ray instrument in the patient's mouth.

▪ If a second adult is not available, it may be necessary to restrain the child in a "papoose board." This frees the parent to stabilize the child's head and properly position the radiograph in the child's mouth.

▪ If the child is still uncooperative, it may be necessary to manage the child pharmacologically with inhalation, oral, or parental sedatives.

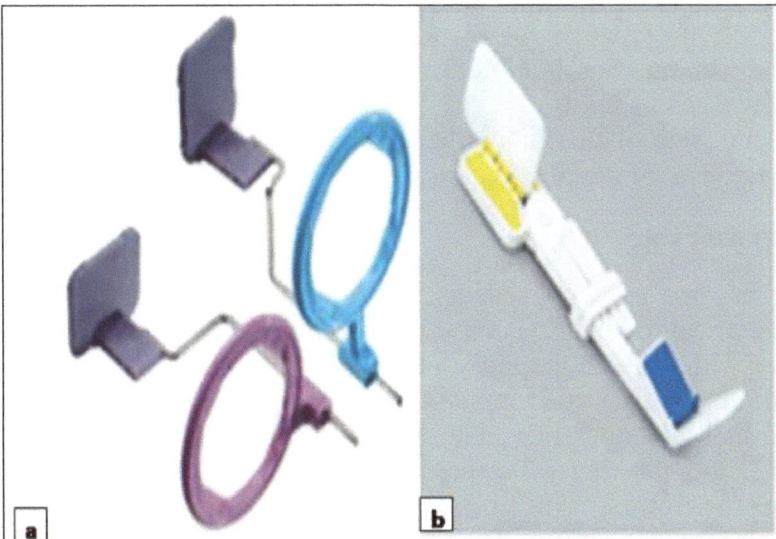

Fig. (4). Film holding devices **(a)** Rinn XCP for paralleling technique **(b)** Snap A Ray for bisecting angle technique.

B. Older Children

May also be uncooperative for a variety of reasons. These can range from the jaw being too small to accommodate the radiograph, fear of swallowing the radiograph, fear of the procedure itself, or a severe gag reflex.

C. Child with Small Jaw

- In a child with a small mouth, the smallest size film (size 0) is used.
- The other alternatives for children with a small mouth
  - Roll the film (do not place sharp bends) to allow the film to accommodate the shape of the jaw and not impinge on the soft tissues. Excessive rolling should be avoided as it increases the distortion of the radiographic image at its edges.
  - Size one film with Snap-A-Ray instrument as a bitewing tab will reduce impingement on the soft tissue. (Snap-A-Ray device with #0 size film is usually not recommended because it reduces the amount of detectable tooth structure on the radiograph).

D. Children with Fear of Swallowing

Can be managed by using a Snap-A-Ray instrument in which biting on the large positioning device and watching in a mirror can assure them that they will not swallow the radiograph.

E. Mentally Disabled Children

- To control film position in children with limited ability, an intraoral film with bitewing tabs can be used.
- An 18-inch length of floss could be attached through a hole made in the tab to facilitate retrieval of the film.

F. Children with Gag Reflex

- Gagging has been interpreted as an effort by the child to defend himself consciously against the invasion of the oral cavity. So, the patient should be acquainted with the radiographic procedure before taking radiographs.
- One of the most effective methods of reducing gagging is a distraction. The child is asked to concentrate intensely on other activities like raising one leg, and his/her toes making a fist holding his/their breath. Also, examination of children in the morning with an empty stomach helps in reducing gagging.
- Pharmacological techniques for managing gag response include the use of sedatives and topical anaesthetic. The patient's palate and tongue can be coated with a topical anaesthetic using a cotton tip applicator, to reduce the sensation of

the radiograph. Few agents that have been recommended for decreasing the gag reflex include phenothiazine derivatives, antihistamines, barbiturates, and nitrous oxide.
- Film size and manner of placement may also reduce gag reflex during radiography. Children having smaller jaws with shallow lingual vestibule require the use of smaller films.
- The film could be placed in such a manner so that it does not meet the palate or tongue. This is accomplished by either extraoral placement of a #4-sized film (occlusal film) or placing the film between the cheek and the tooth. The film is then exposed from the other side of the jaw.

G. Handicapped Children

In these children, usually, parents hold the intraoral radiographs for positioning in the child's mouth. A holding device may be used to fix the film in position while the patient occludes. Such patients may not co-operate while opening their mouths for radiographic procedures. In these cases, extraoral radiographs like panoramic, lateral jaw or 45° projections are used.

Types of Radiographs Used in Dental Radiology for Pediatric Population

- Intraoral radiograph
  - Intra oral periapical radiograph (IOPA)
  - Bitewing radiograph
  - Occlusal radiograph
- Extra oral radiograph
  - Orthopantomogram (OPG)
  - Extra oral views
    - Lateral view
    - Lateral oblique view
    - Antero-posterior view
    - Postero-anterior view
    - Paranasal sinus view
    - Submento vertex view
    - Reverse Townes view
- Cone Beam Computed Tomography (CBCT)
- Computed Tomography
- Magnetic Resonance Imaging
- Ultrasonography
- Others like Nuclear medicine, Positron emission tomography *etc.*

Intra – Oral Radiography in Pediatric Dental Practice [2, 3]

The commonly used intraoral radiographs are Intra Oral Periapical (IOPA) Radiograph, Bitewing radiograph and Occlusal radiograph (Table **4** and Fig. **5**).

Table 4. Film sizes used for intra-oral radiography [3].

Size	Uses
Size 0 (22X35mm)	Used for bitewing and IOPA of small children.
Size 1 (24X40mm)	Anterior teeth in adults
Size 2 (31X41mm)	The standard film is used for posterior IOPA and bitewings in mixed and permanent dentition.
Occlusal films (57x76 mm)	Used for maxillary or mandibular occlusal radiographs.

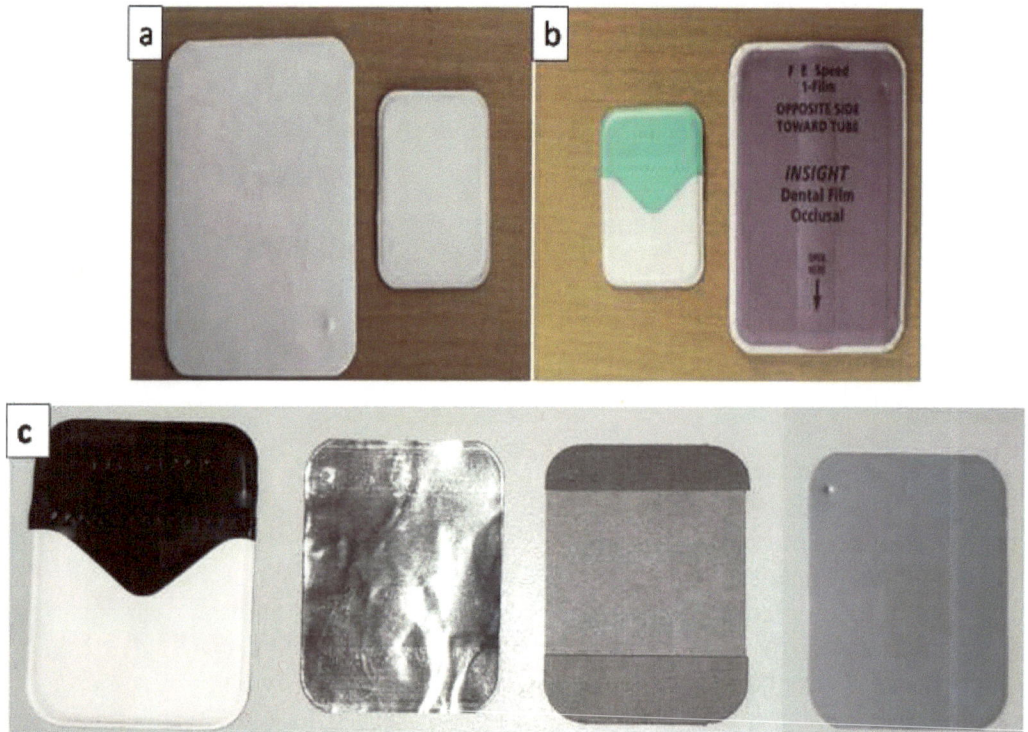

Fig. (5). Radiographic films: **(a)** and **(b)** Intraoral periapical radiograph and occlusal radiograph and **(c)** Components of the film packet.

Intra Oral Periapical (IOPA) Radiograph

These radiographs are indicated when the tooth /teeth (2-3) of interest, along with the periapical areas, are to be visualized. Periapical radiographs can be obtained by two methods: Bisecting angle technique (Fig. **6**) –Based on Cieszynski's rule of isometry) and Paralleling technique (Figs. **7 a and b**).

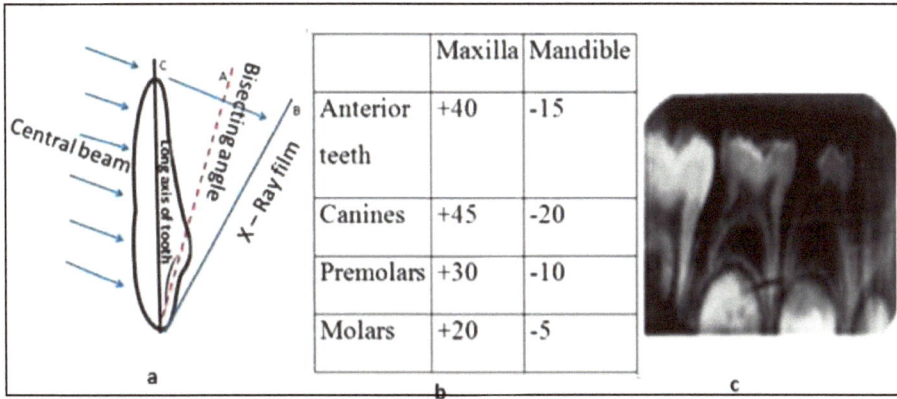

	Maxilla	Mandible
Anterior teeth	+40	-15
Canines	+45	-20
Premolars	+30	-10
Molars	+20	-5

Fig. (6). Details of Bisecting angle technique **(a)** Diagrammatic representation **(b)** Angulations **(c)** Radiograph by bisecting angle technique.

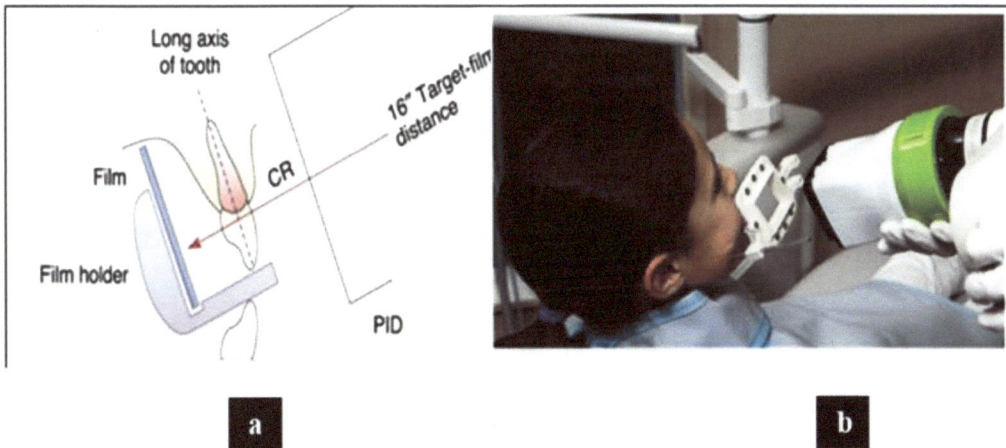

Fig. (7). Details of paralleling technique **(a)** Diagrammatic representation and **(b)** Patient's position for paralleling technique.

Indications for Periapical Radiograph

• Detection of pathologic changes like apical infection/inflammation or internal resorption associated with primary teeth.
• After trauma to the dentoalveolar structure.
• Developmental abnormalities,
• evaluation of the presence and position of unerupted teeth

- evaluation of the periodontal status,
- evaluation of root morphology before extractions,
- Detailed evaluation of apical cysts and other lesions within the alveolar bone,
- In endodontic/pulp treatment (Preoperative, Working length estimation, Post condensation, Review).

Occlusal Radiograph

- This is indicated to reveal the skeletal or pathologic anatomy of either the floor of the mouth or the palate. It is taken with a large film (3X2.3 inches) and the patient is asked to gently bite on it (Fig. **8**).

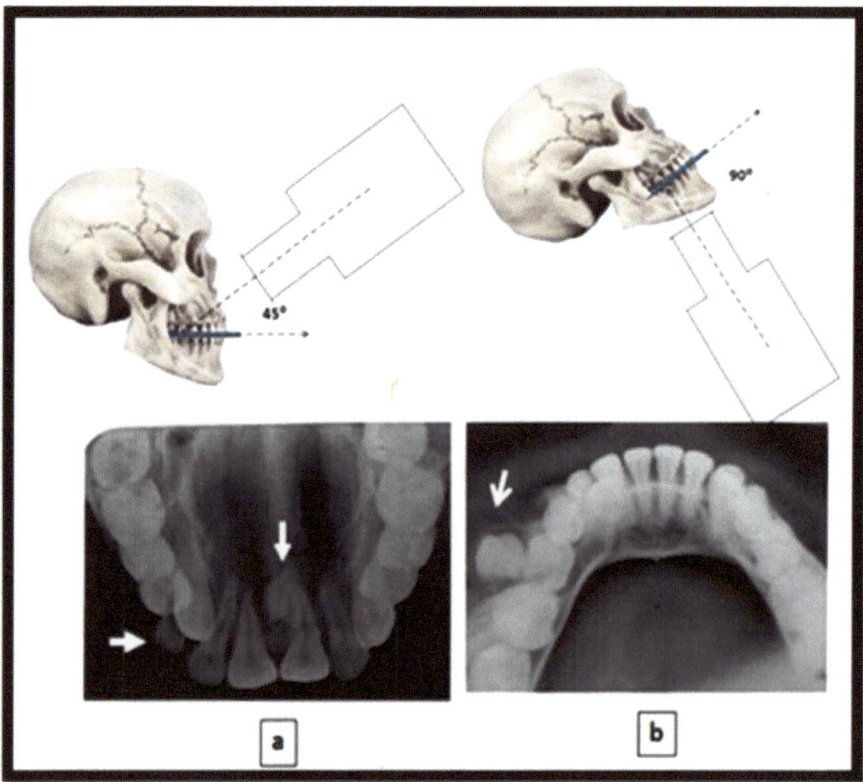

Fig. (8). Occlusal radiography: **(a)** Maxillary anterior and **(b)** Mandibular cross-sectional occlusal radiographs.

Types

Maxillary occlusal view

a. Cross-sectional (65⁰)
b. Topographic (45⁰)

c. Lateral

Mandibular occlusal view

a. Cross-sectional (90^0)
b. Topographic (55^0)
c. Lateral

Indications for Occlusal Radiography in Pediatric Patients

1. Determine the presence, shape, and position of supernumerary teeth.

2. Determine impaction of canines.

3. Assess the extent of trauma to teeth and anterior segments of the arches.

4. In case of trismus and trauma, where the patient cannot open the mouth completely.

5. Determine the medial and lateral extent of cysts and tumours.

6. To localize foreign bodies in jaws and stones in ducts of salivary glands.

7. To obtain information about the location, nature, extent, and displacement of fractures of the maxilla and mandible.

Bite-Wing Radiograph (Fig. 9)

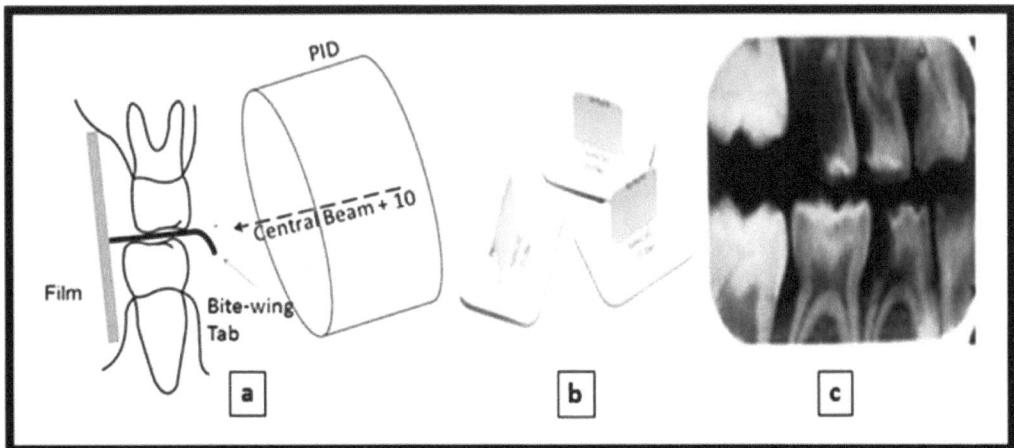

Fig. (9). Bitewing radiography **(a)** Diagrammatic representation of bitewing radiography technique **(b)** Size 2 films along with the bitewing tabs **(c)** Bitewing radiograph showing caries involving multiple teeth.

Bite-wing radiographs include the crowns of upper and lower teeth up to the middle third of the roots, including the interdental alveolar bone. They are the best radiographs for screening caries periodically. The intervals to the next bitewing examination in children are as shown in Table **5**.

Table 5. Intervals to the next bitewing examination in children.

Baseline Bitewing Examination	Interval to Next Nitewing Examination	
At Age	Low Caries Risk	High Caries Risk
5 years	3 years	1 year
8 or 9 years	3-4 years	1 year
12 to 16 years	2 years	1 year
16 years	3 years	1 year

The indication for bite-wing radiographs is:

- Detect proximal caries
- Determine pulp chamber configuration
- Detect secondary caries under old restorations

Digital Intraoral Radiography

- Digital radiography offers many advantages over the use of conventional x-ray films in pediatric dentistry.
- Several categories of innovative intraoral digital imaging technologies have been introduced into dentistry (Fig. **10**).
  - Based on the sensor – CCD (Charge Couple Device)
    - CMOS (Complementary Metal Oxide Sensor)
    - PSP (Phosphor Storage Plate)
  - Based on presence or absence of wire – Wired (CCD and CMOS)
    - Wireless (PSP)
  - Direct radiography and indirect radiography (computed radiography)
- Wireless digital sensor is the most popular and advantageous over wired sensor, especially in children. The thickness of wire in wired sensors is 4-6 mm, which results in empty interocclusal space preventing effective imaging of the crestal bone. Compared to these, the wireless sensors are very convenient to place in pediatric patients.
- Direct digital radiographs are acquired using CCD or CMOS-based chips, which after exposure, can display the image directly on the screen (example RVG - Radio visiography), whereas indirect radiography (computed radiography) uses a photostimulable phosphor plate sensor which, after exposure, needs to be scanned by a laser before the image can be displayed (example Scan X system)

on the screen. Photostimulable phosphor plate sensors are thin and flexible (compared to CCD or CMOS sensors). This makes it very convenient to place in a pediatric patient's oral cavity.

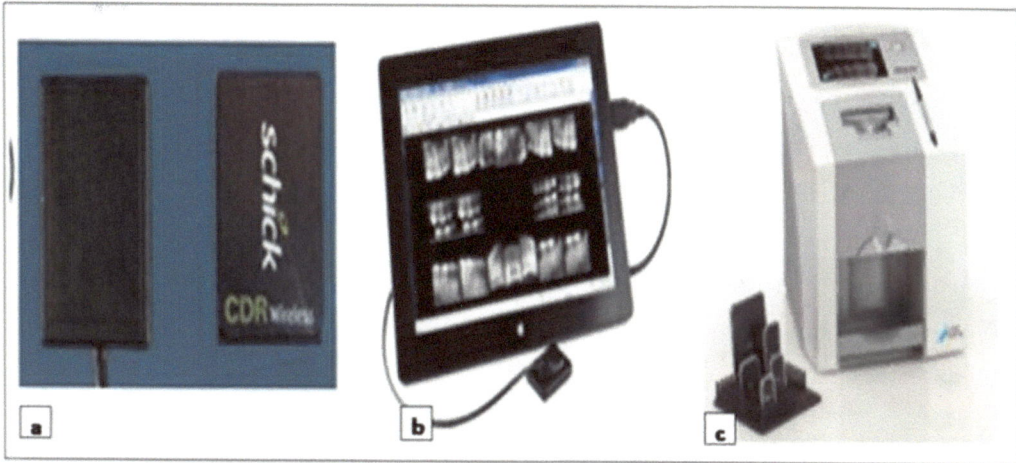

Fig. (10). Digital intraoral radiography system **(a)** Wired and wireless sensors **(b)** Direct imaging system (RVG) **(c)** Indirect imaging system (Scan X).

Advantages

- Less radiation exposure
- High-quality radiographs
- More efficient
- Patient and parent education
- Convenient in telemedicine and tele-radiography
- Saving time/money

Limitations

- Sensor and wire thickness can compromise patient comfort.

Extra – Oral Radiography in Pediatric Dental Practice [10]

- If intraoral radiographs cannot be obtained or the area of interest is large enough to be incompletely visualized in small intraoral radiographs, then extraoral radiographs are advisable.
- In extraoral radiography, both the image detector and the X-ray machine are placed outside the patient's mouth. The X-ray source and the image detector must be aligned to generate the desired image quality.

Panoramic Imaging

- The dental panoramic tomography or orthopantomography (OPG) gives a complete visualization of both the jaws (Fig. **11**).

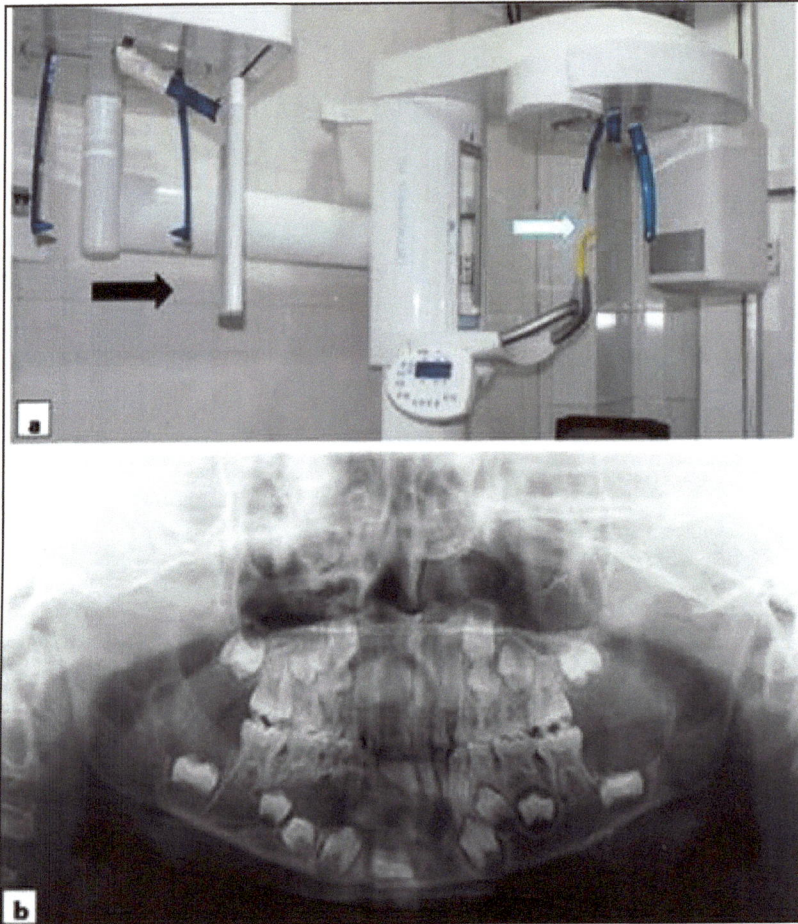

Fig. (11). Panoramic radiography **(a)** digital orthopantomogram with cephalogram. The white arrow indicates the orthopantomogram section and the black arrow indicates the cephalogram, **(b)** digital OPG reveals multiple radiolucencies in the mandible of a 7-year-old child in bilateral posterior body and ramus of the mandible, which was later diagnosed as Gorlin-Goltz syndrome. The radiograph reveals a mixed dentition stage with erupting molars and premolars.

Technique Details

- The technique implies that the X-ray source and the image detector move synchronously in opposite directions. This synchronous movement of the tube head and the film produces a focal trough, in which structures lying within are clearly demonstrated on a panoramic radiograph.

- The X-ray beam used in panoramic radiography is a vertical narrow slit beam, which can be adjusted (collimated) in height to accommodate adult or pediatric settings. This helps in reducing unnecessary radiation exposure to other parts of the head and neck.
- While patient positioning, if the machine cannot be lowered enough, then the patient can be placed on a step stool.
- Instructions or patient education about the procedure is necessary as the revolving machine could be distressing for some patients. A mock demo could be beneficial in this regard.
- Once the appropriate positioning has been done, the patient should be locked in that position, with the lips closed and the tongue against the hard palate. Additional immobilization could be achieved with the help of the head stabilizer.

Panoramic or Extraoral Bitewings

- Some panoramic machines allow extraoral bitewing radiographs (Fig. **12**).
- This is a suitable alternative for patients who cannot cope with intraoral bitewings.

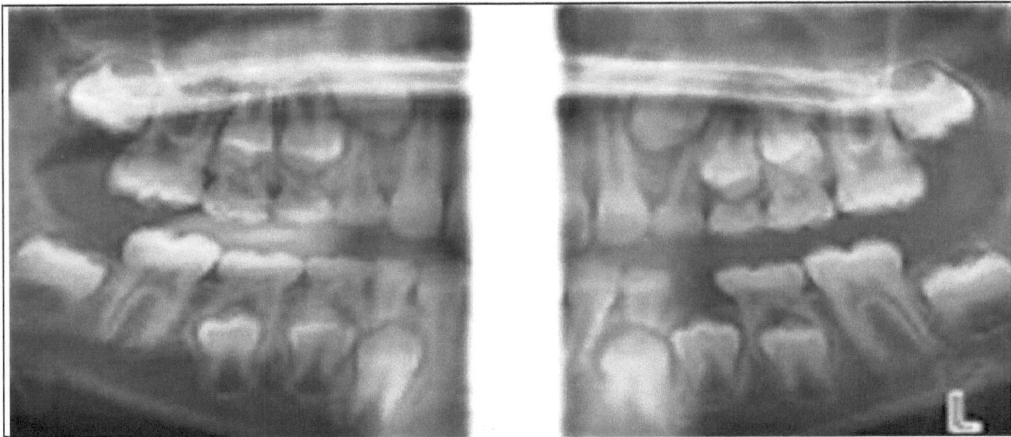

Fig. (12). Pan-bitewing.

Cephalometric Imaging

- This imaging provides a reproducible lateral skull view.
- This radiograph is important to obtain structures in the skull, especially the Sella turcica, which can be used as a reference to verify the growth or impact of disease or in orthognathic surgery.

Oblique Lateral Radiograph

- This technique can be considered an alternative for a panoramic radiograph or a periapical or bitewing radiograph in cases where patients are not able to cope with the procedures (Fig. **13**).
- This technique can also be used under general anaesthesia. The cassette can be taped around the patient's head instead of someone holding it in place.
- The main limitation is distortion, especially if X-rays are not perpendicular to the cassette.

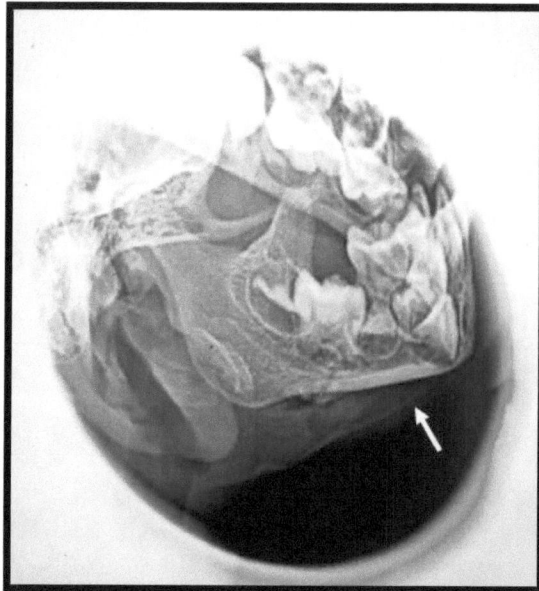

Fig. (13). Lateral oblique radiograph showing suspected fracture of body of mandible involving molar area.

Other radiographs which could also be advisable for certain conditions are as follows:

Posteroanterior View

- In this view, the central x-ray beam is directed from behind and through the skull (Fig. **14**).
- It is used to evaluate the skull, along with the maxilla and mandible for any pathology, trauma, or developmental anomalies.
- It gives a good mediolateral view.

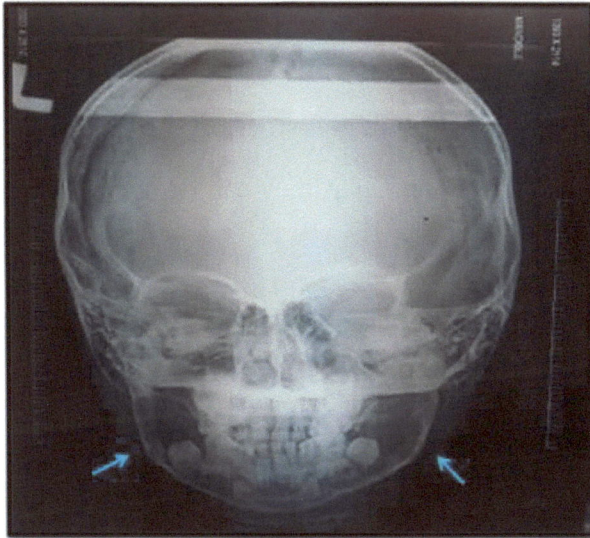

Fig. (14). PA view showing the bilateral expansion of ramus due to multilocular lesion.

Paranasal Sinus View

- PNS view is a variation of the PA view and is indicated for visualization of a paranasal sinus, orbits, and zygomaticofrontal sutures.
- In this projection, the head is tilted 45° upwards with the central x-ray beam directed through the occiput to exit at the maxillary sinus region.

Reverse – Towne Projection

- Mainly indicated to evaluate the suspected cases of condylar neck fractures.
- This radiograph is taken in an open-mouth position.
- This projection is like the PNS view, but here, the head should be tilted downward.

Submentovertex View

- A submentovertex view is taken by directing the central x-ray beam through the floor of the mouth to exit at the vertex of the skull.
- This radiograph helps in the visualization of the condylar fractures, sphenoid sinus, and curvature of the mandible.

Computed Tomography [11]

- The term "computed tomography" or CT uses a motorized x-ray source that rotates around the circular opening of a doughnut-shaped structure called a gantry.
- In this computerized x-ray imaging procedure, a fan-shaped X-ray beam is

aimed at a patient and quickly rotated around the body, producing signals that are processed by the machine's computer to generate cross-sectional images or "slices" of the body.

- These slices are called tomographic images and contain more detailed information than conventional x-rays. Once several successive slices are collected by the machine's computer, they can be digitally "stacked" together to form a three-dimensional image of the patient that allows for easier identification and location of basic structures as well as tumours or abnormalities. Additional images could be visualized in coronal, axial, and sagittal sections.
- Unlike bone, soft tissue has limited ability to stop X rays thus, may appear faint. Therefore, Contrast CT is usually indicated in pathology involving soft tissue.
- Contrast agents contain substances that are better at stopping x-rays and, thus, are more visible on an x-ray image. Intravenous (IV) contrast agents have been developed which are safe to use in patients.

Indications of CT in Pediatric Dentistry

- Craniofacial injury
- Neoplasms or developmental anomalies involving the craniofacial region

Advantage

- High contrast resolution

Limitation

- The ionizing radiation doses delivered by CT are 100 to 500 times higher than conventional radiography. Therefore, children in the growing phase are highly susceptible to changes due to ionizing radiation.
- Costly equipment
- Fear of closed chamber or claustrophobia is more common in children. This could prevent effective imaging.

Cone Beam Computed Tomography (CBCT) [3, 11]

- CBCT is an advanced imaging method specially designed for dentistry, which provides a three-dimensional representation of the maxillofacial skeleton with minimal distortion and improved image sharpness.
- Principle – It uses a cone-shaped beam and a reciprocating solid-state flat panel detector, which rotates once around the patient, 180-360 degrees, covering the defined anatomical volume in one swipe. This significantly reduces the radiation dose (Fig. **14**). Furthermore, CBCT facilitates exposure of a small volume (few teeth) to a large volume covering the entire maxillofacial area, thus allowing

limited exposure to radiation as per the requirements. Thus, it could be an efficient alternative for CT in the pediatric population. Table **6** shows the differentiating points between CBCT and CT.

Table 6. Difference between CBCT and CT.

CBCT	CT
Single rotation is required to acquire the image	Multiple rotations are required
Isotropic voxels	Anisotropic voxels
The radiation dose is lower (cone-shaped beam)	The radiation dose is higher (fan-shaped beam)
Low cost	High cost
Good spatial resolution	Better contrast resolution
Cannot display soft tissue	Soft tissue evaluation is possible
Scatter radiation is high	Scatter radiation is low

Indications of CBCT in Pediatric Dentistry

- Malocclusions and craniofacial anomalies, including cleft lip and palate.
- To determine the position of the unerupted teeth, especially for the canines in the upper arch
- To determine the extent of root resorption.
- Assessment of treatment planning and its outcome
  - Cyst and tumour involving the oral cavity
  - Dental trauma
  - Implant planning
  - Diagnosis of supernumerary teeth
  - Endodontic applications
  - TMJ disorders
  - Patients undergoing orthodontic treatment
  - Forensic odontology

Advantages

1. It is less expensive and involves a smaller system.

2. The X-ray beam is limited.

3. Accurate images are obtained.

4. The scan time is rapid.

5. As compared to conventional CT, CBCT has a reduced dosage

6. Image quality of CBCT scans is superior to helical CT

7. Basic image manipulations and measurements are possible.

8. Artifact suppression algorithms are available which results in a low level of the metal artefact. (Figs. **15 a-e** & **16 a-c**).

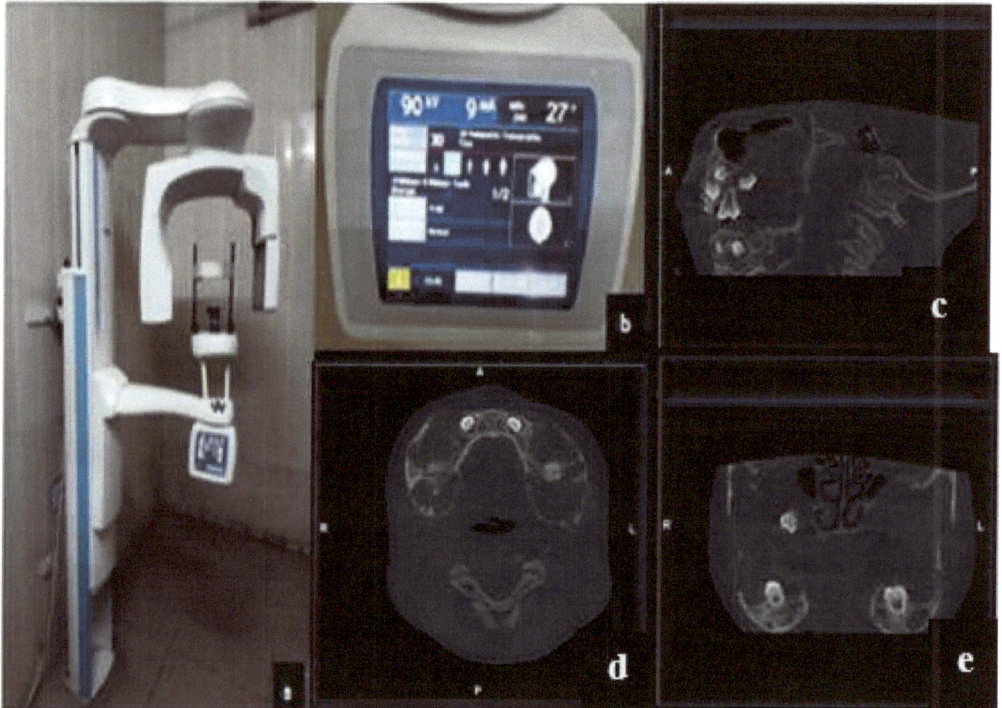

Fig. (15a). CBCT machine **(b)** Control panel showing a selection of pediatric mode **(c)** CBCT images showing cherubism with a multilocular lesion involving bilateral posterior region of the mandible in different views **(c)** axial, **(d)** sagittal **(e)** coronal.

Limitations

1. If effective artefact suppression algorithms are not available radiographic artefacts reduce the diagnostic yield of the images.

2. Unable to detect carious lesions in metal restored crowns and teeth with radiopaque restorations.

3. More radiation exposure compared to conventional radiography. Therefore, the principle of Justification, Limitation and Optimization should be strictly followed.

4. Inability to accurately represent soft tissue lesions.

5. Limited correlation with Hounsfield units (of CT which accurately determines density).

6. Patient movement during the scan might adversely affect the sharpness of the final image.

7. The resolution of CBCT is inferior compared to conventional dental radiography.

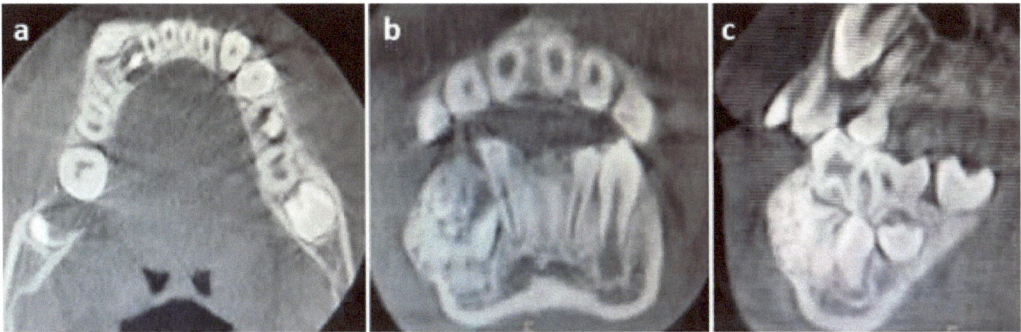

Fig 16 (a, b, c). The figures reveal the axial (a), coronal (b) and sagittal (c) section images in CBCT of the mandibular anterior region in a nine-year-old female which shows a mixed density lesion. Multiple small globular masses of hypodense area coalesced together in the mandibular anterior region within a well-defined hyperdense area suggestive of complex odontome.

Magnetic Resonance Imaging (MRI) [11]

An MRI scan is a radiology technique that uses non-ionizing radiation from the radio frequency band of the electromagnetic spectrum (10.9-10.11 nm of wavelength) for imaging soft tissues (Fig. 17).

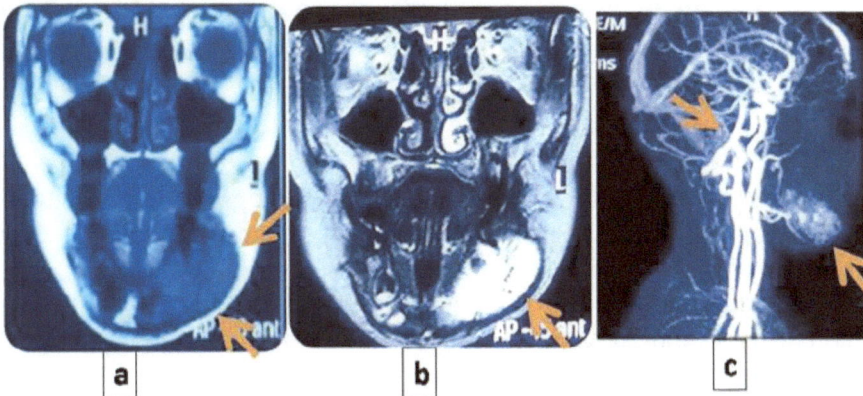

Fig. (17). MRI images of intraosseous hemangioma of the left body of mandible showing (a) isointense T1 weighted coronal image, (b) hyperintense on T2 weighted coronal image and (c) STIR (Short-T1 Inversion Recovery) images of MR angiography showing branches of the external carotid artery as feeder's vessels.

- It is a non-invasive imaging modality that uses electrical signals generated from the response of hydrogen nuclei to a strong magnetic field and radio wave/radiofrequency pulses to produce a three-dimensional image displayed on a computer to allow specialists to explore various soft tissue pathologies without the use of X-ray.
- The resultant images can be visualized as T1 images showing the fat planes and T2 images showing the fat and water planes.
- To enhance the visualization contrast agent, gadolinium can be injected which provides a clear view of the vascular areas.

Indications in Pediatric Patients

- It is indicated for assessing intracranial lesions, especially those involving the posterior cranial fossa, the pituitary, and the spinal cord.
- Trauma to the brain can be seen as bleeding or swelling.
- Staging the tumour *i.e.*, evaluating the size, site and extent of all soft tissue tumours and tumour-like lesions involving all areas, including the salivary gland, pharynx, larynx, and orbit.
- Tongue tumour for lingual tumour for the definition of boundaries and degree of vascularity.
- Extent of soft tissue tumours and tumour-like lesions involving the salivary gland, the pharynx, and the larynx.

Advantage

- It does not require ionizing radiation.

Limitation

- More costly and time-consuming, and produces a lower spatial resolution than CT.
- Evaluation of bony lesions is not possible.

Xeroradiography [3, 9]

- Xeroradiography is a highly accurate electrostatic imaging technique that uses a modified xerographic copying process to record images produced by diagnostic X-rays.
- The xerographic process was invented and first used in 1937.
- The main advantage of xeroradiography includes the simultaneous evaluation of multiple tissues.

CONCLUSION

The basis of a precise conclusion and treatment plan is based on thorough medical and dental records, a comprehensive clinical examination, and diagnostic radiographs. Radiographs and other imaging modalities are used to monitor oral diseases, dentofacial development and the progress or prognosis of therapy. Radiographs are the most reliable and valuable diagnostic tools. They help in proper treatment planning. The timing of the initial radiographic examination should not be based upon the patient's age but upon each child's individual needs. Each patient is unique, and the need for dental radiographs can be determined only after reviewing the patient's medical and dental histories, completing a clinical examination, and assessing the patient's vulnerability to environmental factors that affect oral health. The investigative imaging of children presents numerous tasks. Imaging children is unique to imaging adults. These faces must be addressed step by step, beginning with the choice of the most suitable imaging mode, performing the technique suitable for age and clinical indication, and properly interpreting the image in a pediatric context. All the advances made in maxillofacial radiology have been directed to make radiographic investigations more accurate and safer for both the child and the Pediatric Dentist, completing a clinical examination and assessing the patient's vulnerability to environmental factors that affect oral health.

CONSENT FOR PUBLICATION

Not applicable.

CONFLICT OF INTEREST

The authors declare no conflict of interest, financial or otherwise.

ACKNOWLEDGEMENT

Declared none.

REFERENCES

[1]   American Academy of Pediatric Dentistry. Prescribing dental radiographs for infants, children, adolescents, and individuals with special health care needs The Reference Manual of Pediatric Dentistry. Chicago, Ill.: American Academy of Pediatric Dentistry 2020; pp. 248-51.

[2]   Espelid I. Mejàr.E I, Weerheijm K. Eapd Guidelines for Use of Radiographs in Children. Eur J Paediatr Dent 2003; 1: 40-8.
[PMID: 12870988]

[3]   Mallya SM. Radiation Biology and Safety and Protection. White and Pharoah's- Oral Radiology, 2nd South Asia edition.. Elsevier India 2016; pp. 26-39.

[4]   Kühnisch J, Anttonen V, Duggal MS, *et al.* Best clinical practice guidelines for prescribing dental

radiographs in children and adolescents: an EAPD policy document. Eur Arch Paediatr Dent 2019; 25: 1-2.
[PMID: 31768893]

[5]   Karimi M. Dental Radiography and Radiation Damage to Children Article Review. EC Dental Science 2019; 18(8): 1836-43.

[6]   Council on Scientific affairs, American Dental association.. Dental Radiographic Examinations: Recommendations for Patient Selection and Limiting Radiation Exposure. US Department of Health and Humans Services Public Health Service Food and Drug Administration 2012. http://www.fda.gov/media/84814/download

[7]   Horner K, Rushton VE, Tsiklakis K, Hisrchmann PN, Steltvander P. European guidelines on radiation protection in dental radiology; the safe use of radiographs in dental practice. European Commission, Directorate-General for Energy and Transport. European Spine Journal 2004. 2014; pp. 20-9.

[8]   Safety Code No AERB. AERB/RF-MED/SC-3 (Rev 2) Radiation safety in manufacture, supply, and use of medical diagnostic x-ray equipment. Mumbai: Approved by Atomic Energy Regulatory Board 2016; pp. 20-4. https://www.aerb.gov.in/images/PDF/RF-MED-SC-3.pdf

[9]   Schwartz S. Radiographic techniques for the pediatric patient. J Contemp Dent Pract 2000; 1(4): 60-73.
[PMID: 12167951]

[10]   Aps J. Extraoral Radiography in Pediatric Dental Practice. Imaging in Pediatric Dental Practice . Springer, Cham. 2019; pp. 31-49.

[11]   Madan K, Baliga S, Thosar N, Rathi N. Recent advances in dental radiography for pediatric patients: A review. Journal of Medicine, Radiology, Pathology & Surgery 2015; 1(2): 21-5.
[http://dx.doi.org/10.15713/ins.jmrps.11]

CHAPTER 4

Cephalometrics in Pediatric Dentistry

N.B. Nagaveni[1,*]

[1] *Professor of Pediatric Dentistry, College of Dental Sciences, Davanagere, Karnataka, India*

Abstract: Cephalometrics, introduced by BROADBENT in the year 1931, plays a crucial role in Pedodontics and Dentofacial Orthopaedics. It has made it easier and economical to predict the post-orthodontic results of the patient using this as a tool. This chapter outlines the basics of cephalometrics, including the indications, limitations, *etc.*, with special emphasis on its role in Pediatric Dentistry. It lays down the recent guidelines given by the American Academy of Pediatric Dentistry for using cephalometrics in children. It provides details regarding various tools, equipment required, and methodology of tracing as well as analysing the cephalometric radiographs. It also enlists the skeletal and dental landmarks and planes needed for the analysis. Details regarding Down's, Steiner's, Tweed's, and Wit's analyses have been explained in this chapter.

With the new era of digitalization, this chapter also highlights the recent advances made in Cephalometrics, providing information about the different computer-based programs and smartphone applications available for efficient landmark identification and analysis. The fundamental essence of the chapter is to help both undergraduate and even post-graduate pediatric students to have the basic knowledge and information about Cephalometrics, including its advancements made.

Keywords: Cephalometrics , Cephalometric analysis, Cephalograms, Dentofacial pedodontics, Orthodontic.

INTRODUCTION

The American Academy of Pediatric Dentistry (AAPD) emphasizes the significance of dealing with a child's developing dentition and occlusion, as well as the effect on their general wellbeing. Early detection and treatment of emerging malocclusions are critical since it has both short-term and long-term advantages when achieving occlusal harmony, function, and dentofacial aesthetics objectives. Cephalometrics is radiographic health assistance that is used to investigate malocclusion as well as underlying skeletal anomalies and disproportions.

* **Corresponding author N.B. Nagaveni:** Professor of Pediatric Dentistry, College of Dental Sciences, Davanagere, Karnataka, India; E-mail: nagavenianurag@gmail.com

Satyawan Damle, Ritesh Kalaskar & Dhanashree Sakhare (Eds.)

Orthodontists and Pediatric Dentists must also consider how significant functional features of the face, such as the cranial base, jaws, and teeth, interact [1].

Components of Cephalometric Radiography

Cephalostat, x-ray apparatus, image receptor system, and film cassette holder are major components of cephalometric radiography (Figs. **1** - **3**).

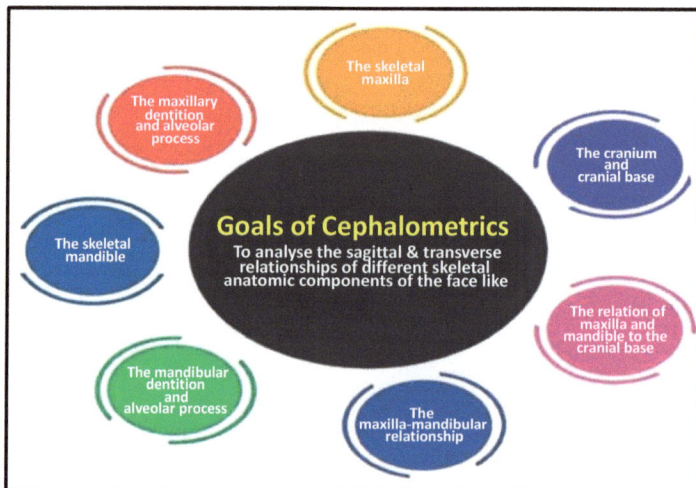

Fig. (1). Goals of cephalometrics in pediatric dentistry.

The Technique of Cephalometric Radiography (Figs. 2 and 3)

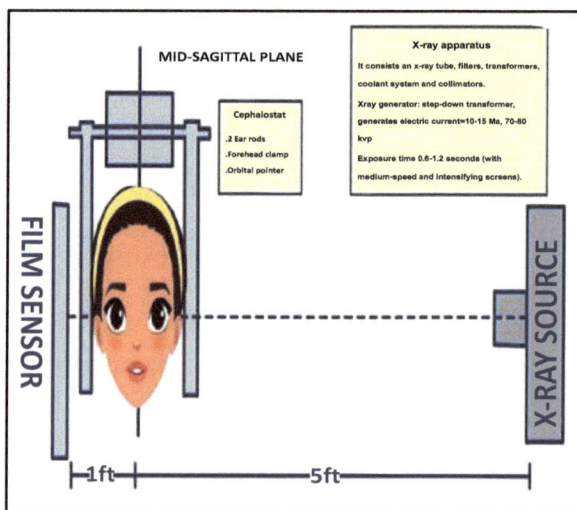

Fig. (2). Components of Cephalometric radiography.

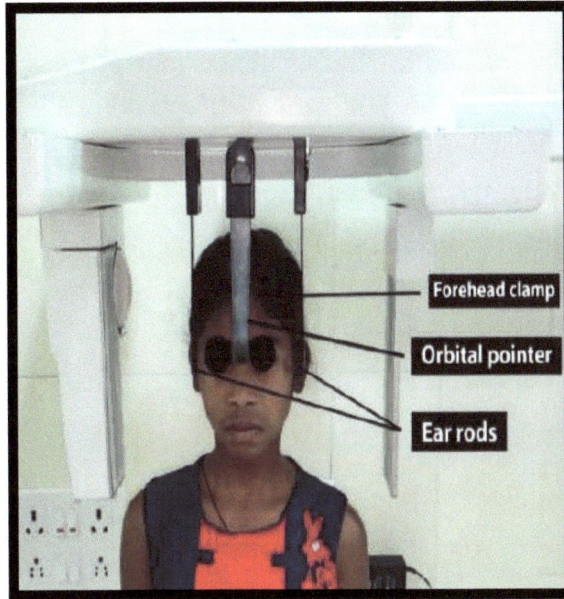

Fig. (3). Technique of cephalometric radiography.

Types of Cephalogram

There are two types of cephalogram, Lateral and Postero-Anterior (Frontal) cephalogram.

Lateral

This provides a lateral view of the skull. Taken from the x-ray source with the head in a standardized, repeatable position.

Uses

- For the skeletal and dental growth analysis of the patient.
- Evaluation of final treatment outcome.
- Diagnosis and treatment planning.

Frontal

This provides the anteroposterior view of the skull.

Uses

- Provide information related to various dimensions of the craniofacial complex like the width of the skull and other proportions of oral structures.
- Allows gauging abnormalities in the growth and symmetry of the skull.

Cephalometric Landmarks/Reference Points

Cephalometric landmarks (Tables **1** - **3**) are described as a set of points, which are typically identified as locations on a physical structure, but sometimes as constructed points such as the intersection of two planes or as extreme points.

Table 1. Lateral Cephalometric Reference points (Fig. 5).

Point	Description	Symbol
Anterior Nasal Spine	The anterior tip of the sharp bony process of the maxilla at the lower margin of the anterior nasal opening.	ANS
Articulare	Point of intersection of the dorsal contour of mandibular process and temporal bone.	Ar
Subspinale	The most posterior midline point in the concavity between the ANS and the Prosthion, the most inferior point on the alveolar bone overlying the maxillary incisors.	Point A
Basion	The lowest point is on the anterior rim of the foramen magnum.	Ba
Supramentale	The most posterior midline point in the concavity of the mandible between the most superior point on the alveolar bone overlying the mandibular incisors (infradentale) and Pog.	Point B
Bolton point	The highest point of retrocondylar fossa.	Bo
Condylion	Most superior point on the articular head of condyle.	Co
Glabella	Anterior most point on the frontal bone.	G
Gonion	The point on the curvature of the angle of the mandible located by bisecting the angle formed by lines tangent to the posterior ramus and the inferior border of the mandible.	Go
Gnathion	Point located by taking the midpoint between the anterior (pogonion) and inferior (menton) points of the bony chin.	Gn
Infradentale	Point of the alveolar contact with the lower central incisors.	Id
Nasion	The most anterior point on the frontonasal suture in the mid sagittal plane.	N
Orbitale	The lowest point is on the inferior rim of the orbit.	Or
Pogonion	The most anterior point on the bony chin.	Pog
Porion	The most superiorly positioned point of the external auditory meatus located by using the ear rods of the cephalostat.	Po
Posterior nasal spine	The posterior spine of the palatine bone constituting the hard palate.	PNS

(Table 1) cont.....

Point	Description	Symbol
Prosthion	The point of the upper alveolar process that projects most anteriorly, a point on the alveolar arch midway between the median upper incisor teeth.	**Pr**
Pt point	Intersection of inferior border of foramen rotundum with posterior wall of Ptm.	**Pt**
Pterygomaxillare	The contour of the pterygomaxillary fissure formed anteriorly by the retromolar tuberosity of the maxilla and posteriorly by the anterior curve of the pterygoid process of the sphenoid bone.	**PTM**
Registration point (Broadbent)	Midpoint of perpendicular from center of sella turcica to Bolton plane.	**R**
Spheno-occipital synchondrosis	Upper-most point of suture	**SO**
Sella turcica	Midpoint of hypophyseal fossa	**S**

Table 2. Posterior- anterior (FRONTAL) Cephalometric Reference Points (Fig. 6).

Point	Description	Symbol
Antegonial points	Points at inferior margin of antegonial protuberances.	**LAG/RAG**
Anterior nasal spine	Anterior tip of the sharp bony process of the maxilla in the midline of the lower margin of the anterior nasal opening.	**ANS**
Condylar	Superior most point of the condylar head.	**Cd**
Coronoid	Superior most point of the coronoid process.	**cor**
Incision inferior frontale	Midpoint between the two mandibular central incisors at the level of the incisal edge.	**iif**
Incision superior frontale	Midpoint between the two maxillary central incisors at the level of the incisal edge.	**isf**
Jugal process	Bilateral points on jugal processes at the junction of maxillary tuberosity and zygomatic buttress.	**LJ/RJ**
Lateral piriform aperture	Most lateral aspect of the piriform aperture.	**lpa**
Mandibular midpoint	Point obtained by projecting the mental spine on the inferior mandibular border.	**m**
Maxillary molar	The lateral most point on the buccal surface of the first permanent maxillary molar or second deciduous maxillary molar.	**um**
Mandibular molar	The lateral most point on the buccal surface of the first permanent mandibular molar or second deciduous mandibular molar.	**lm**
Medio-orbitale	The median most point of the medial orbital margin.	**mo**
Mastoid	Lowest point of the mastoid process.	**ma**

(Table 2) cont.....

Point	Description	Symbol
Mental foramen	Centre of the mental foramen.	mf
Point zygomatic arch	The lateral most of the centre of the zygomatic arch.	Za
Top nasal septum	The highest point of the nasal septum.	tns
Zygomaticofrontal medial suture point in	Point at the medial margin of zygomaticofrontal suture.	mzmf
Zygomaticofrontal lateral suture point out	Point at the lateral margin of zygomaticofrontal suture.	lzmf

Table 3. Soft tissue landmarks (Fig. 7).

Landmark	Description	Symbol
Cervical point	The innermost point between the submental area and the neck located at the intersection of lines drawn tangentially to the neck and submental areas.	C
Columella point	The most anterior point on the columella of the nose.	Cm
Glabella	The most prominent point in the midsagittal plane of the forehead.	G
Inferior labial sulcus	The point of greatest concavity in the midline of the lower lip between labrale inferius and menton.	Ils
Labrale inferius	A point indicating the mucocutaneous border of the lower lip.	Li
Labrale superius	A point indicating the mucocutaneous border of the upper lip.	Ls
Menton soft tissue	The constructed point of intersection of a vertical coordinate from menton and inferior soft-tissue contour of the chin.	Ms
Nasion soft tissue	The point of deepest concavity of the soft-tissue contour of the root of the nose.	Ns
Pogonion (soft tissue)	The most anterior point on the soft-tissue chin.	Pg'
Pronasale	The most prominent point of the nose.	Pn
Subnasale	The point at which the nasal septum merges with the upper cutaneious lip in the mid-sagittal plane.	Sn
Superior labial sulcus	The point of greatest concavity in the midline of the upper lip between labrale superius and subnasale.	Sls
Stomion superius	The lowest point on the vermilion of the upper lip.	Stms
Stomion inferius	The uppermost point on the vermilion of the upper lip.	Stmi

On the other hand, it is a cephalometric point that is used as a reference for constructing planes. These are points in relation to the bone and teeth that enable quantitative evaluation of the skeletal discrepancy. There are no fixed points in the skull of a living person and usually depend on age, sex, maturation rate, ethnic background, and other factors. These can be either anatomic or constructed (derived). Constructed landmarks are those points of intersection of tangents to the surface of the bone. The detailed classification of cephalometric landmarks is illustrated in Fig. (**4**).

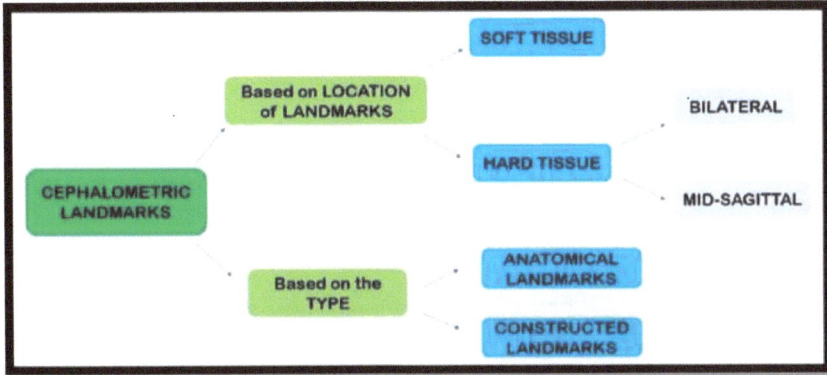

Fig. (4). Classification of Cephalometrics landmarks.

Requirements of Cephalometric Landmarks

1. Should be uniform in outline.

2. Easily visible on a radiograph.

3. Should be reproducible.

4. It should enable one to achieve accurate quantitative measurements of lines and angles.

5. There should be a strong association between the growth vectors of particular areas.

Cephalometric Reference Planes

Cephalometric Reference planes are obtained by joining two lines (linear assessment) or by joining three lines (angular assessment) with various cephalometric landmarks (at least 2 or 3 landmarks). Two types of reference planes are used: horizontal and vertical planes (Table **4**). These planes together help in the quantitative assessment of the cephalometric radiographs. Every cephalometric analysis has a reference plane to which the positions of the jaws are compared [2, 3].

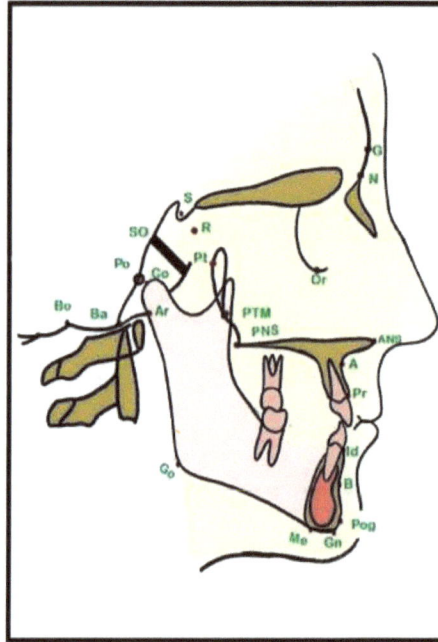

Fig. (5). Lateral cephalometric landmark.

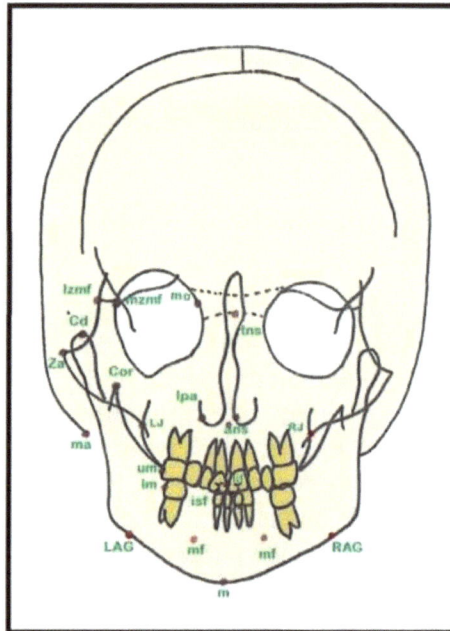

Fig. (6). Postero-anterior (frontal) cephalometric reference points.

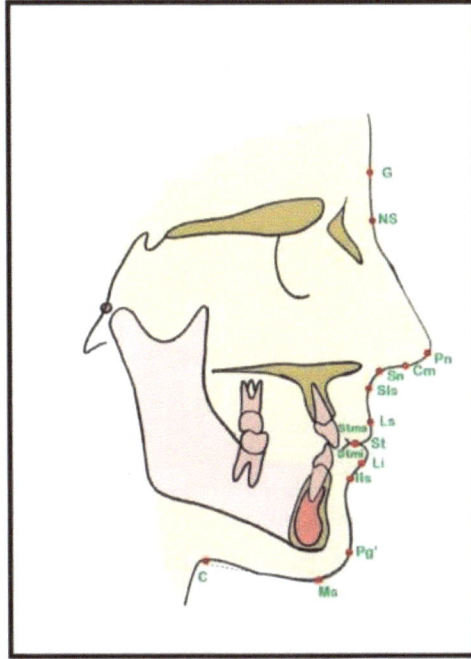

Fig. (7). Soft tissue landmarks.

Table 4. Cephalometric horizontal and vertical planes (Fig. 8).

Reference plane	Description	Symbol
Bolton's plane	A plane that connects the Bolton's point posterior to the occipital condyle and the Nasion.	BP
Occlusal Plane	Plane drawn through the region of the overlapping of the first premolars and first molars	OP
Frankfort Horizontal Plane	Represented by a line connecting the porion and orbitale.	FHP
Mandibular Plane	Plane drawn between the gonion and gnathion.	MP
Palatal Plane	Plane formed between the anterior nasal spine and posterior nasal spine.	PP
Basion-Nasion Plane	Drawn from nasion to basion representing the cranial base.	Ba-Na
Sella-Nasion Plane	Drawn from sella to nasion	S-Na
Sella-Bolton Plane	Drawn from sella to Bolton point.	S-Bo
Pterygoid Vertical Plane	Line drawn perpendicular to Frankfort plane through Pt point.	PTV
Facial Plane	Line drawn through nasion perpendicular to FH plane.	FP
Y-axis	Line drawn through S-Gn line with FH plane.	YX

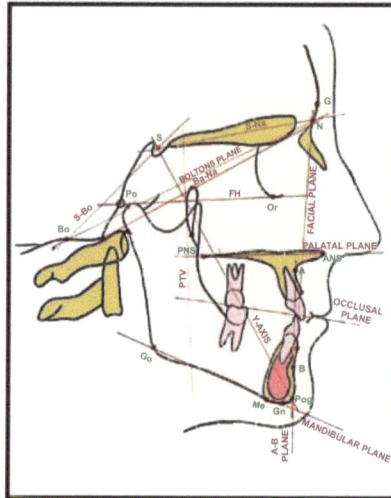

Fig. (8). Cephalometric horizontal and vertical plane.

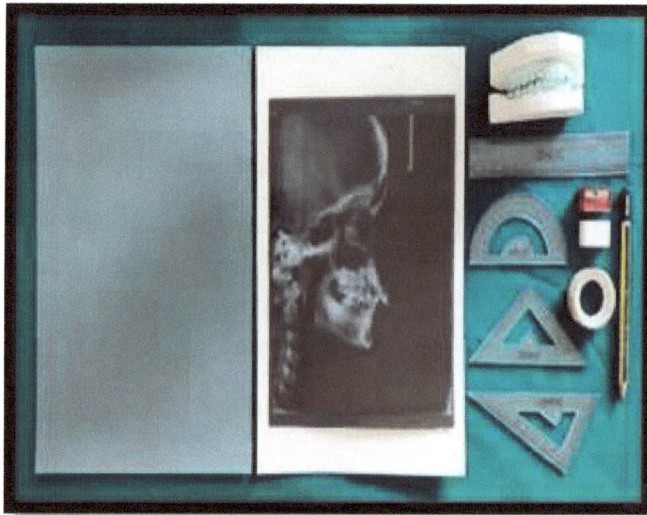

Fig. (9). Armamentarium for cephalometric tracing.

Clinical Applications or Uses of Cephalometrics

- A useful method for identifying and classifying skeletal and dental abnormalities.
- Are useful in estimating the facial type.
- Helps in treatment planning.
- The anatomical, dental, and soft-tissue associations of the craniofacial area are elucidated using this method of orthodontic diagnosis.
- Used in growth prediction.

• Cephalograms are useful for doing functional analysis.
• In surgical orthodontics, it is used to prepare skeletal repositioning.
• It is possible to use it to measure the treatment's effects.

General Considerations for Cephalometric Tracing (Fig. 9)

• Four corners of the radiograph with the tracing paper should be taped to the view box.
• Use Acetate matte tracing paper (0.003 inches thick. 8X10 inches) to trace the landmarks. (Shining side is placed down on the radiograph).
• 311 drawing pencil or fine felt-tipped pencils are used for tracing (image lines are traced without stopping or lifting the pencil).
• Three registration crosses, two in the cranium and one over the cervical vertebrae are drawn. This assists in reorienting the film, if the film gets displaced during tracing.
• Bilateral structures are traced first.
• Keep the lateral head plate on the right side of the operator.

Cephalometric Analysis

The cephalometric analysis aims to ascertain the skeletal and dental associations that occur in a particular patient and lead to his or her malocclusion. The basic idea behind cephalometric analysis is to equate the patient to a standard control group to assess the discrepancies between the patient's real dentofacial relationships. Down's analysis, developed at the University of Illinois and focused on the skeletal and facial proportions of a comparison sample of 25 untreated teenage whites chosen for their perfect dental occlusion, popularised this form of cephalometric analysis after WWII [4].

Down's Analysis

This is the most frequently used cephalometric analysis introduced by W. B. Downs in 1948, after conducting a study on 20 Caucasian subjects, with an age range of 12-17 years belonging equally to both sexes. His analysis consists of 5 skeletal and 5 dental parameters (Tables **5** and **6**).

Table 5. Skeletal parameters in down's analysis (Fig. 10).

Parameters Skeletal Analysis	Description	Normal Values (in Degrees)	Interpretation
Facial angle	Angle formed by the intersection of the FH and the FP (N-Pog). Used to measure the degree of protrusion or retrusion of the lower jaw.	82-95	Increases in class III malocclusion with a prominent chin.
Angle of convexity	Angle formed by the intersection of lines N-A and A-Pog.	8.5 – 10	Decreases in class II malocclusion.
A-B plane angle	Measures convexity or concavity of skeletal profile. Line connecting points A and B and a line joining N-Pog.	-9 to 0	Positive value: convex profile Negative value: concave profile
Mandibular plane angle	Represents maxillomandibular relationship in relation to facial plane.	17 to 28	A large negative value: class II facial pattern.
Y – Axis (Growth Axis)	The angle is formed by the intersection of the FH plane and a tangent to the lower border of the mandible and symphysis. The angle is formed by the intersection of the S-Gn line with the FH plane. Indicates the degree of downward, backward, or forward position of the chin about the upper face.	53 to 6	Increased angle: vertical grower with hyperdivergent facial pattern. Larger angle: class II facial pattern and vertical growth of the mandible. Smaller angle: class III pattern and horizontal growth of the mandible.

Steiner's Analysis

Steiner's analysis was introduced by Cecil Steiner in 1950. It includes three basic components dental, skeletal, and soft-tissue components. The sella-nasion plane is the main reference plane used in this analysis which represents the anterior cranial base and Steiner considered it a stable reference plane. Because according to Steiner, the anterior cranial base completes its growth as early as 8 years of age, later it undergoes slight change (Tables **7-9**).

For two factors, this study can be considered the first of the early cephalometric analyses [1]. It displayed measurements in a way that highlighted not only individual measurements but also their interrelationship in a pattern, and [2] It provided detailed guidelines for using cephalometric measurements for case planning.

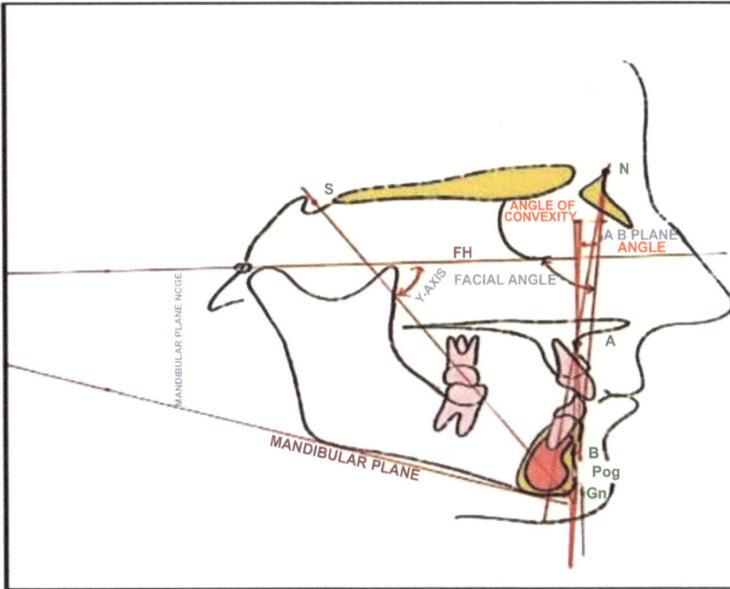

Fig. (10). Skeletal parameters in Down's analysis.

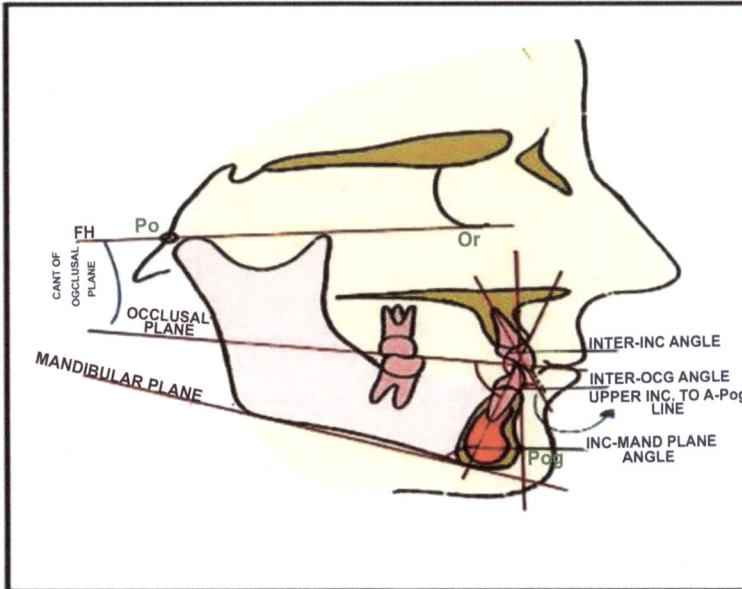

Fig. (11). Dental parameters in Down's analysis.

Table 6. Dental parameters in Down's analysis (Fig. 11).

Parameters Dental Analysis	Description	Normal Values (in Degrees)	Interpretation
Cant of the occlusal plane (OP)	Line bisecting the overlapping cusps of the first molars and the incisal overbite.	1.5 to 14	Measures the slope of the OP to the FH plane.
Interincisal angle	Angle formed by the intersection of the long axes of the maxillary and mandibular central incisors.	130 to 150	Decreased in class II division I and Bimaxillary cases. Increased in class II division II cases.
Lower incisor – occlusal plane angle/Inter-occlusal plane angle	Angle formed by intersection between the long axis of lower central incisor and occlusal plane.	3.5 to 20	Increased angle: lower incisor proclination
Lower incisor -mandibular plane angle	Angle formed by intersection of the long axis of lower incisor and mandibular plane.	8.5 to 7	Increased angle: lower incisor proclination.
Upper incisor to A-Pog line	Linear measurement between incisal edge of maxillary central incisor and the line joining point A to Pog.	1 to 5 mm	Increased angle: lower incisor proclination.

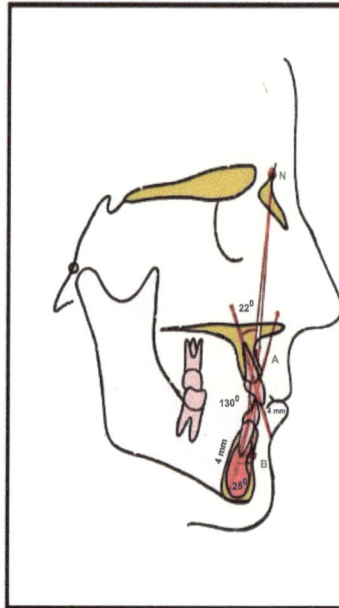

Fig. (12). Dental parameters in Steiner's Analysis.

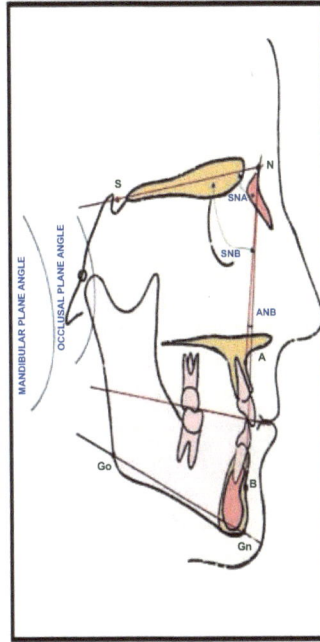

Fig. (13). Skeletal parameters in Steiner's Analysis.

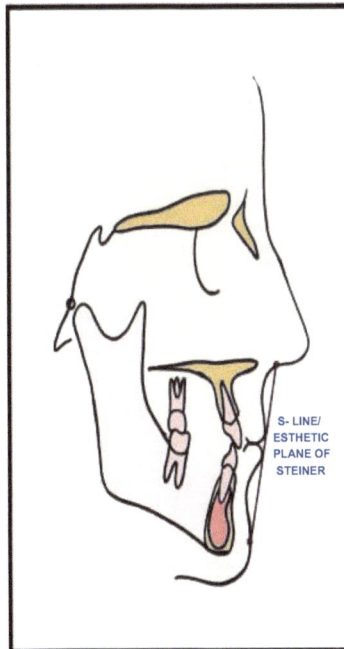

Fig. (14). Soft tissue analysis in Steiner's Analysis.

Table 7. Dental parameters in Steiner's analysis (Fig. 12).

Parameter (Dental)	Description	Normal Range	Interpretation
Maxillary incisor position	The relative location and axial inclination of the maxillary incisors are assessed by relating the teeth to the NA line.	-	-
Upper incisor to NA (angle)	Indicates the relative angular relationship of the upper incisor teeth.	22^0+4	Increased in proclined maxillary incisor.
Upper incisor to NA (linear)	Indicates the relative forward or backward positioning of the upper incisor teeth.	4 mm	Increased in forwardly placed maxillary incisor.
Mandibular incisor position	-	-	-
Lower incisor to NB (angle)	The Relative angulation of the lower incisor is evaluated by the angle between the long axis of the lower incisor and the NB line.	25^0+4	Decreased in retroclined lower incisor.
Lower incisor to NB (linear)	The relative antero-posterior position of the lower incisors by relating the teeth to the NB line.	4 mm	Decreased in posteriorly placed lower incisor.
Lower incisor to the chin (Holdaway ratio)	Relation between the position of the lower incisor edge to NB line and pogonion to NB line.	2mm	Both lines should be equidistant from the NB line for a harmonious facial Profile (Holdaway Ratio).
Interincisal angle	Angle between the long axis of the upper and lower incisors.	132^0	Decreased in proclined upper and lower incisors.

Table 8. Skeletal parameters in Steiner's analysis (Fig. 13).

Skeletal Analysis	Description	Normal Range	Interpretation
Skeletal Analysis	Parameters used: SNA, SNB, ANB, Go-Gn to SN, ANS-PNS to SN, and occlusal plane to SN.	-	Relates the maxilla and mandible to the skull and to each other.
Maxilla to SN (SNA)	Angle formed by intersection of the Sella-nasion line to a line formed by nasion-point A.	82°	Increased in maxillary prognathism.
Mandible to SN (SNB)	Angle between SN and NB line SNB gives the position of the mandible in relation to the cranial base.	80°	Decreased in mandibular retrognathism.
Maxilla-manidbular relation (ANB)	Angle ANB is the difference between SNA and SNB. Represents the sagittal or antero-posterior maxillomandibular relation.	2°	Increased in class II skeletal base Decreased in class III skeletal base.
The mandibular plane (Go-Gn to SN)	Drawn between gonion(Go) and gnathion (Gn).	32°	Increased in vertical growth pattern.

(Table 8) cont.....

	Drawn through the regions of overlapping cusps of the first premolars and molars. Indicates the inclination of occlusal plane to SN.		
Occlusal plane to SN (OCC-SN)	Drawn through the regions of overlapping cusps of the first premolars and molars. Indicates the inclination of occlusal plane to SN.	14°	Increased in steep occlusal plane.
Palatal plane to SN (PAL-SN)	Shows the inclination of the palatal plane (anticlined or retroclined), with respect to the cranial base.	8°	Increased in retroclined palatal plane.

Table 9. Soft tissue parameters of Steiner's analysis (Fig. 14).

Parameter	Description	Normal range	Interpretation
Soft Tissue Analysis (S -line or Esthetic plane of Steiner) (Fig. 16)	Formed by a line extending from soft tissue contour of the chin to the middle of "S" line formed by lower border of the nose.	-	Provides a mean of assessing the balance and harmony of the lower facial profile.
	Upper lip to S line	0 mm	Negative value indicates protrusive lips.
	Lower lip to S line.	+2mm	Increased value indicates protrusive lips.

Tweed's Analysis

This analysis was introduced by CH Tweed in 1946. He proposed a connection between the tilt of the mandibular incisors and the mandibular plane angle. He also claimed that for stabilization and aesthetics, the mandibular incisors should be positioned upright over the basal bone. Frankfort horizontal plane is the basic reference plane used in this analysis. He designed the diagnostic facial triangle which consists of 3 angles and gives the diagnostic information about the patient's vertical skeletal pattern, the relationships of mandibular incisors to basal bone, and the relative amount of protrusion (Table **10**). Tweed used the following 3 angles in this analysis [5, 6].

1. Incisor mandibular plane angle (IMPA)

2. Frankfort mandibular incisor angle (FMIA)

3. Frankfort mandibular plane angle (FMA)

Table 10. Parameters in Tweed's Analysis (Fig. 15).

Angle	Description	Normal values (in degrees)	Interpretation
FMA	Angle formed at the intersection of the Frankfurt horizontal plane with the mandibular plane.	25	Increased in vertical growth pattern
FMIA	Indicates the vertical relation of the mandible to the face.	65	Decreased in proclined lower incisor
IMPA	Indicates the inclination of the lower incisor.	90	Increased in proclined lower incisor

Clinical Applications of Tweed's Analysis

1. Tweed proposed tooth extraction to address alveolo-dental prognathism and to place the lower incisors upright on the basal bone.

2. Tweed's triangle is used in determining the classification, diagnosis, prognosis, and treatment planning.

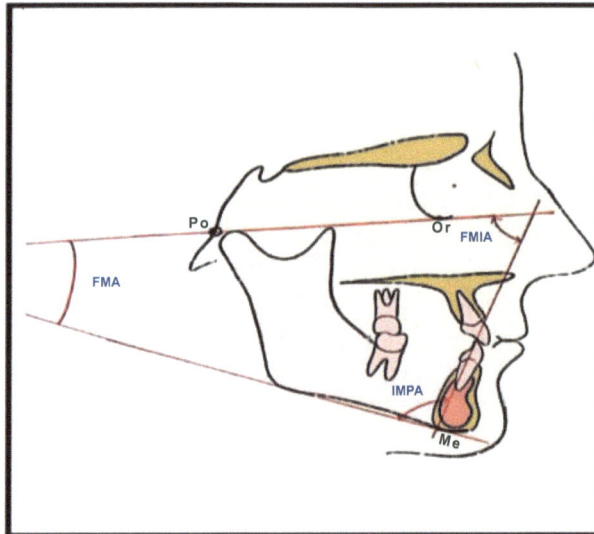

Fig. (15). Parameters in Tweed's analysis.

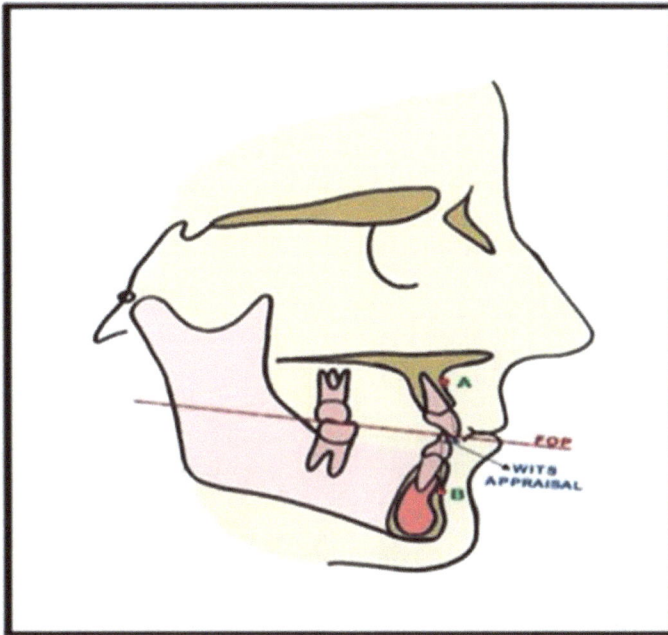

Fig. (16). Parameters in Wits analysis.

Wit's Analysis or Appraisal

Wit's analysis was designed by Jacobson after recognizing the shortcomings of the ANB angle. It expresses the degree to which the maxilla and mandible

are attached to each other in the sagittal or anteroposterior plane. Its application lies in the cases with unreliable ANB angle due to factors like the rotation of jaws and position of nasion. This analysis was created at the University of the Witwatersrand with the primary goal of studying the anteroposterior association of the maxilla and mandible (Table **11**).

Table 11. Parameters in Wit's Analysis or Appraisal (Fig 16).

Reference Plane	Description	Interpretation
Functional Occlusal Plane (FOP)	A line drawn connecting the point of maximum intercuspation of posterior teeth is extended forward.	Males: BO is ahead of AO by 1 mm. Females: both BO and AO coincide
AO point	Obtained by dropping a perpendicular from point A to the occlusal plane.	Calss II malocclusion: AO is well ahead of BO.
BO point	Obtained by dropping a perpendicular from point B to the occlusal plane.	Class III malocclusion: BO is well ahead of AO.

Drawbacks of Wit's Appraisal

• Inclination of occlusal plane changes with growth or treatment. So, wit's appraisal also varies.

• Also influenced by the vertical dimensions of the jaws.

Limitations of Conventional Cephalometrics [7]

1. Cephalometric accuracy is not always reliable.

2. Analytical method standardization is complex.

3. It creates a static image that does not take time into account.

4. It shows a two-dimensional representation of a three-dimensional object.

5. The tracing process can be time-consuming.

6. There can be errors in landmark identification.

7. Technical measurement errors can occur.

Recent Advances in Cephalometrics [8]

With a new era of digitalization, multiple cephalometric programs have been made available to overcome the disadvantages of the pre-existing era of manual tracing. These programs provide a means to digitalize the various cephalometric landmarks.

Advantages of Digitalization

1. Fast due to the usage of the semi-automatic computer-based software

2. Precise

3. Minimization of manual tracing errors

4. Swift execution of the measurements

5. Easy determination of the treatment plan

6. High rate of reproducibility

7. Eradication of the chemical and environmental hazards

8. Easy storage of the images and the subsequent data

9. Cost-effective and rapid superimposition

Disadvantages of Digitalization

1. Limited battery life of mobile devices and tablets

2. Limited memory space of mobile devices

3. Computer viruses including "Spyware," "data leakage," *etc.*

4. The absence of applications on smartphones with different operating systems can hinder their use in daily practice.

With the easy availability and the accessibility of smartphones and tablets, the new trend is the use of various cephalometric applications available on them to mark various linear and angular measurements [9].

Various Computer-Based Software for Cephalometric Analysis [10]

1. QuickCeph 2000 (Sarasota, Florida, USA)

2. NemoCeph (Madrid, Spain)

3. Dolphin (Oakdale, Chatsworth, USA)

4. FACAD (Beilkegaton, Linkoping, Sweden)

5. Vistadent (Woodbridge, Canada)

6. OnyxCeph Software (Neidelwald, Chemnitz, Germany)

Various Smartphone/ Tablets-Based Applications are

1. CephNinja

2. OneCeph (android based)

3. EasyCeph (android based)

4. SmartCeph (i.o.s.)

<u>OneCeph</u> – An Android-based application, has programs for the most commonly used analysis in cephalometric studies such as Down's, Holdway, Jarabak, McNamara, Rickett's, Steiner's, Schwarz, Tweed's, Wit's appraisal, Beta angle, and Yen angle.

CONCLUSION

Cephalometric roentgenography has provided a method of correctly evaluating the interactions of the parts of the face prominent to a picture of the mean or average facial form of normal occlusion. It also shows the range of modifications that may occur. These abilities permit the attempt to classify facial types. This method of study and explanation of the skeletal and dental patterns of an individual at any particular time has been described as a Static Appraisal.

CONSENT FOR PUBLICATION

Not applicable.

CONFLICT OF INTEREST

The authors declare no conflict of interest, financial or otherwise.

ACKNOWLEDGEMENT

Declared none.

REFERENCES

[1]   Giuca MR, Inglese R, Caruso S, Gatto R, Marzo G, Pasini M. Craniofacial morphology in pediatric patients with Prader-Willi syndrome: a retrospective study. Orthod Craniofac Res 2016; 19(4): 216-21.
        [http://dx.doi.org/10.1111/ocr.12131] [PMID: 27717123]

[2]   Min LJ, Soo SJ, Hong-Keun H, Young-Jae K, Jung-Wook K, Ki-Taeg J. Lateral cephalometric measurements of class I malocclusion patients with uncertainty. J Korean Aca Pediatr Dent 2018; 45(1): 65-74.

[3]   Helal NM, Basri OA, Baeshen HA. Significance of cephalometric radiograph in orthodontic treatment plan decision. J Contemp Dent Pract 2019; 20(7): 789-93.
        [http://dx.doi.org/10.5005/jp-journals-10024-2598] [PMID: 31597797]

[4]   Galeotti A, Festa P, Viarani V, *et al*. Correlation between cephalometric variables and obstructive sleep apnoea severity in children. Eur J Paediatr Dent 2019; 20(1): 43-7.
        [PMID: 30919644]

[5]   Gregório L, de Medeiros Alves AC, de Almeida AM, Naveda R, Janson G, Garib D. Cephalometric evaluation of rapid and slow maxillary expansion in patients with BCLP: Secondary data analysis from a randomized clinical trial. Angle Orthod 2019; 89(4): 583-9.
        [http://dx.doi.org/10.2319/081018-589.1] [PMID: 30741579]

[6]   Singh TS, Sridevi E, Kakarla P, Vallabaneni SSK, Sridhar M, Sai Sankar A. Cephalometric assessment of dentoskeletal characteristics in children with digit-sucking habit. Int J Clin Pediatr Dent 2020; 13(3): 221-4.
        [http://dx.doi.org/10.5005/jp-journals-10005-1761] [PMID: 32904107]

[7]   Chae JM, Park JH, Kim SH, Mangal U, Seo HY. Prognostic indicators for anterior mandibular repositioning in adolescents with class II malocclusion: A cross-sectional cephalometric study. J Clin Pediatr Dent 2020; 44(4): 274-82.
        [http://dx.doi.org/10.17796/1053-4625-44.4.10] [PMID: 33167022]

[8]   Khader D, Peedikayil F, Chandru TP, Kottayi S, Namboothiri D. Reliability of One Ceph software in cephalometric tracing: A comparative study. SRM Journal of Research in Dental Sciences 2020; 11(1): 35-9.
[http://dx.doi.org/10.4103/srmjrds.srmjrds_69_19]

[9]   Novruzov ZG, Aliyeva RK, Garayev ZI. Cephalometric analysis of influence of the Frankel-2 appliance in the treatment of distal malocclusion. Stomatologia (Mosk) 2020; 99(1): 49-54.
[http://dx.doi.org/10.17116/stomat20209901149] [PMID: 32125302]

[10]   Alirezaei M, Naghvialhosseini A, Pakkhesal M, Alirezaei M, Behnampour N. Investigating the correlations among Witt's and ANB cephalometric indices and the upper pharyngeal airway width in individuals with Class II malocclusion: A cross-sectional study. IJSRDMS 2020; 239255: 1072.

CHAPTER 5

Infection Control in Pediatric Dentistry

Prachi Goyal[1,*] and **Dhanashree Sakhare**[2]

[1] *Department of Pediatric and Preventive Dentistry, MMCDSR, Mullana, Ambala, India*

[2] *Lavanika Academy, Melbourne, Australia*

Abstract: Centres for disease control and prevention (CDC) has developed a framework for healthcare personnel and healthcare systems for the delivery of non-emergent care. Infection control is important in dentistry because patient saliva may be contaminated with oral commensal and opportunistic pathogens. In addition, it can harbour specific pathogens during infection as well as during the carrier state, including SARS-CoV-2. Due to the nature of the dental procedures, exposure to the blood and saliva aerosols is unavoidable. Direct contact with fluid-contaminated environmental surfaces, instruments and equipment is also a potential source of pathogen transmission. In a dental practice, the dentist, dental assistant, instrument processing and administration staff, as well as the patients, are at risk of transmission of infections. Dental laboratory staff members are also at risk due to the cross-contamination between the clinic and the laboratory. In addition, it can be extended to their families if the infection control measures are not taken correctly. Therefore, historically step by step infection control measures have been recommended by the CDC and countries across the globe have drawn up individual country-specific guidelines.

Keywords: Biodegradable waste management, Infection control, Personal protective equipment.

INTRODUCTION

Infection control is the discipline concerned with preventing nosocomial or healthcare-associated infection, a practical (rather than academic) sub-discipline of epidemiology. It is an essential, though under-recognized and under-supported, part of the important organization of health care. Infection control and hospital epidemiology are parallel to public health practice, practised within the confines of a particular health care delivery system rather than directed at society as a whole. The application of standard precautions regarding infection control during dental treatment is paramount. The Centres for disease control and prevention (CDC) [1, 2] and the occupational safety and health administration (OSHA) [3],

---

*** Corresponding author Prachi Goyal:** Department of Pediatric and Preventive Dentistry, MMCDSR, Mullana, Ambala, India; E-mail: pra21chi@gmail.com

Satyawan Damle, Ritesh Kalaskar & Dhanashree Sakhare (Eds.)

as well as the state and local regulatory boards or agencies and equipment manufacturers, guide patient care, laboratories, and equipment management.

INFECTION CONTROL IN PEDIATRIC DENTISTRY

Definition- Infection Control, also called the "exposure control plan" by OSHA (Occupational Safety and Health Administration), is a required office program that is designed to protect personnel against risks of exposure to infection (Fig. **1**).

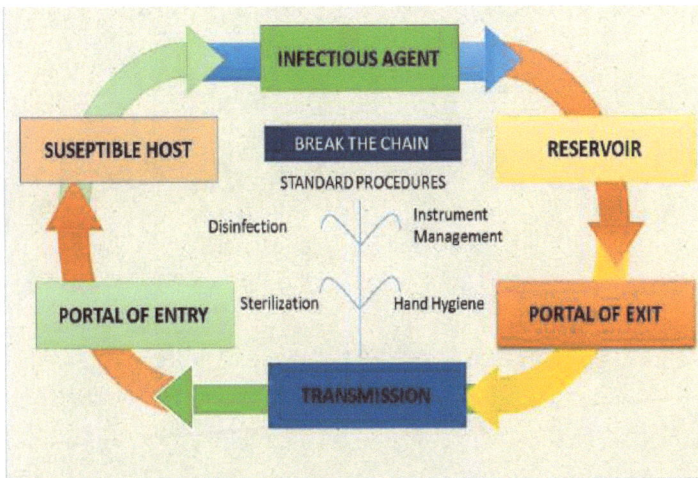

Fig. (1). Modes of transmission of infectious agents.

The recommendations for infection control procedures (Fig. **2**) in routine dental practice are as follows:

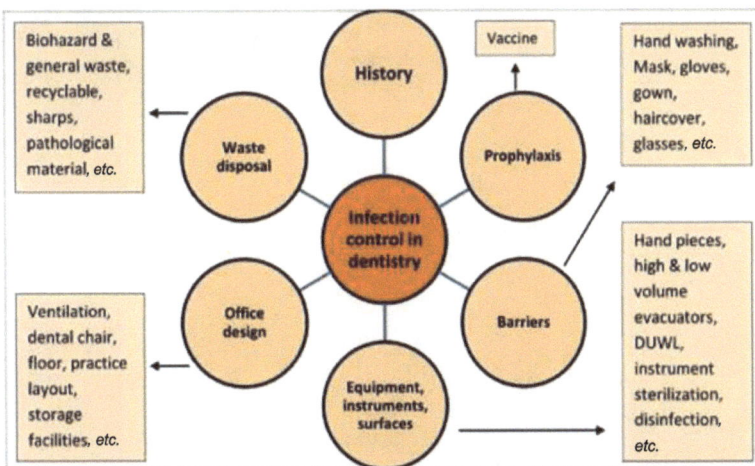

Fig. (2). Infection control in dentistry.

Training in Infection Control

The Dental staff must be aware of the procedures required to prevent the transmission of infection and should understand why these procedures are necessary.

Surgery Design (Figs. 3 and 4)

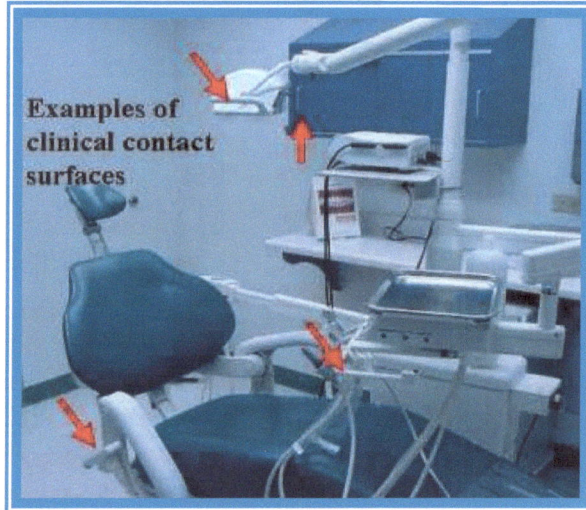

Fig. (3). Clinical contact surfaces.

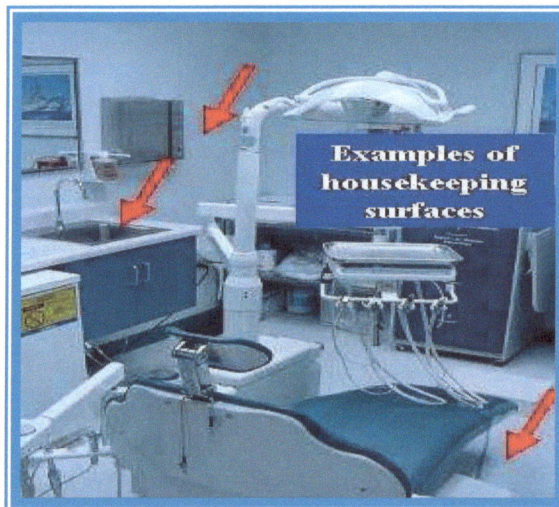

Fig. (4). Housekeeping surfaces in dental clinic.

The layout of the surgery should be simple and uncluttered. There should be two distinct areas: one for the operator and one for the dental nurse, each with a washbasin. The operator's area would have access to the turbines, a three-in-one syringe, a slow handpiece, a bracket table, and operating light. The dental nurse's area would contain the suction lines, perhaps the three-in-one syringe, curing light, all the cabinetry containing dental materials and a designated area for clinical waste disposal and the decontamination of instruments. Clean and dirty areas within the surgery should be clearly defined [3].

Instruments should be decontaminated away from the surgery in a room containing the autoclave(s), ultrasonic bath(s), instrument washer(s) and sinks and a separate hand wash basin.

Ventilation

The surgery should be well ventilated. Ventilation systems should exhaust to the outside of the building without risk to the public or re-circulation into any public building. Mechanical ventilation systems must be regularly cleaned, tested, and maintained according to the manufacturer's recommendations to ensure they are free from pathogens that may contaminate the air recycling air conditioning systems are not recommended.

Floor Covering

The floor covering should be impervious and non-slip. Carpeting must be avoided. The floor covering should be seamless (one piece); where seams are present, they should be sealed properly. The junctions between the floor and wall and the floor and cabinetry should cover or sealed to prevent inaccessible areas where cleaning might be difficult.

Work Surfaces

Work surfaces should be impervious and easy to clean and disinfect – needs to check with manufacturers on suitable products for decontamination.

Water Supplies

Water from the dental operatory units is subject to the standard for safe drinking water set by the Environmental Protection Agency, the American Public Health Association, and the American Water Works Association [4]. A water management plan that includes routine maintenance procedures for dental unit waterlines and monitoring water quality can help keep bacterial counts low [5]. The CDC states that "conventional dental units cannot reliably deliver sterile water even when equipped with independent water reservoirs containing sterile water because the water-bearing pathway cannot be reliably sterilized" [6]. Sterile water and sterile saline have been recommended for use as coolant irrigants during oral surgical procedures [4, 5, 7]. When a pulp exposure occurs and pulp therapy is indicated, irrigants should not come from dental unit water lines. A single-use disposal syringe should be used to dispense irrigants for pulpal therapy. All water lines and airlines should be fitted with anti-retraction valves to help to prevent contamination of the lines, but these valves cannot be relied upon to prevent infected material from being aspirated back into the tubing (Fig. **5**).

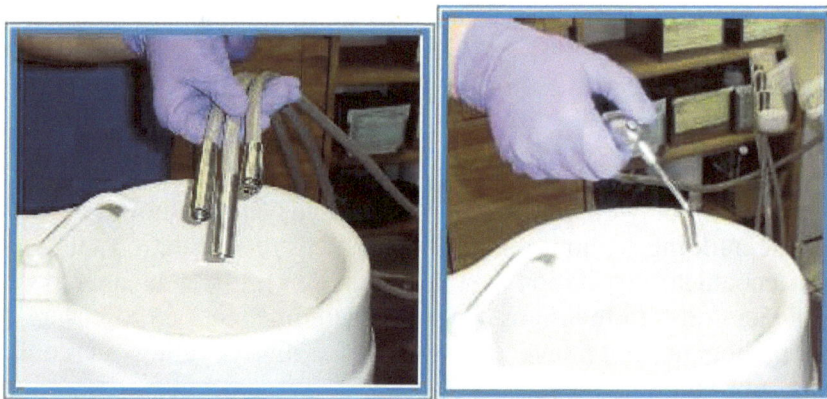

Fig. (5). Anti-retraction valves in the three-way syringe.

Most dental unit waterlines generally may harbour biofilm, which acts as a reservoir of microbial contamination and may be a source of known pathogens (*Legionella* spp.) A bottled water system can help to control microbial contamination – disinfectants can be introduced into the water supply to reduce the microbial load. The design of dental equipment requiring a water supply should be designed in such a way that the entry of microbe contaminants is restricted or minimized for contaminated water to be drawn back through the waterlines to the mains water supply (backflow/ back siphonage).

Decontamination of Instruments and Equipment

All instruments contaminated with oral and other body fluids must be thoroughly cleaned and sterilised after use. However, instruments selected for a treatment session not used must be regarded as contaminated. There are three stages to the decontamination process: pre-sterilisation cleaning, sterilisation, and storage. A systematic approach to the decontamination of instruments after use will ensure that dirty instruments are segregated from clean. The flow diagram depicts a possible approach (Fig. **6**).

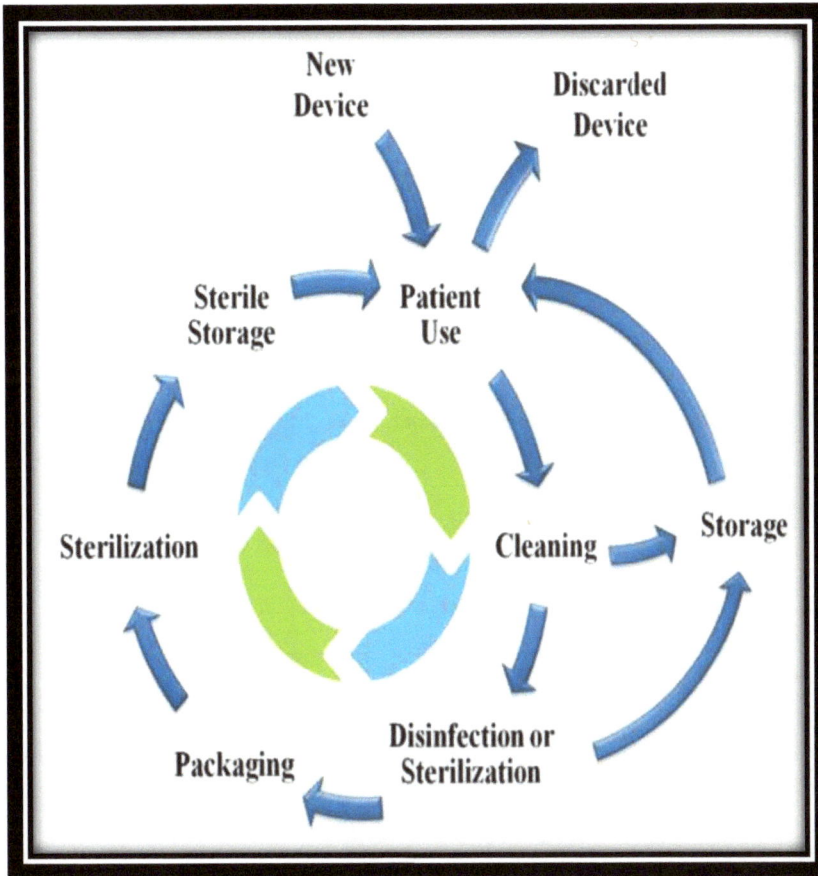

Fig. (6). Decontamination of instruments.

Sterilization

The method of choice for the sterilisation of all dental instruments is autoclaving (Fig. **7**). Sterilisation should be performed at the highest temperature compatible with the instruments in the load. For dental instruments and equipment, autoclaves should reach a temperature of 134-137 ℃ for three minutes. Hot air ovens, ultraviolet light, boiling water and chemiclaves are not recommended for sterilising dental instruments and equipment (Table **1**).

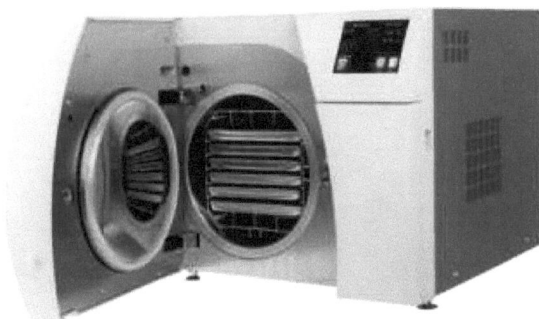

Fig. (7). Autoclave.

Table 1. Sterilization temperature ranges, holding times and pressure for autoclaves with high-temperature steam.

Option	Sterilization Temperature Range (°C)			Approx. Pressure (bar)	Minimum Hold (min)
-	Normal	Minimum	Maximum	-	-
A	136	134	137	2.25	3
B	127.5	126	129	1.50	10
C	122.5	121	124	1.15	1

Effective sterilisation depends on steam condensing on all surfaces of the instruments in the load to be autoclaved, so it is essential that instruments be placed to allow free circulation of steam; the autoclave chamber must not be overloaded.

Chemical and Biological Indicators do not demonstrate the sterility of the load. Chemical indicators serve only to distinguish loads that have been processed in an autoclave from those that have not. **Biological indicators** are of limited value in moist heat sterilisation and can only be regarded as additional to the measurement of physical parameters. Hand pieces must be cleaned and autoclaved after each patient. Pre-sterilisation cleaning machines are recommended. Those using an alcohol/disinfectant combination or a washing cycle must only be used disinfect handpieces on the manufacturer's advice [8].

Glass Bead Sterilizer (Fig. 8)

This method employs a heat transfer device. The media used are glass beads, molten metal, and salt. The temperature achieved is 220°C (425-475°F). Instruments are submerged at least a quarter-inch below the salt surface – in the peripheral area:

a. Broaches, files, and reamers – 5 sec
b. Absorbent points and pellets – 10 sec.

However, this method is not commonly used these days as only the tip of the instrument is sterilized, and the handle remains infected. Also, high heat melts the glass beads in the sterilizer which get attached to the endodontic files resulting in clogging of the pulp canals while performing the pulp therapy.

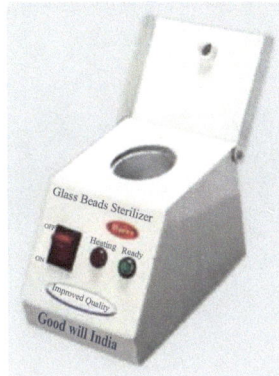

Fig. (8). Glass bead sterilizer.

Decontamination of Handpieces [6 - 8]

If a cleaning machine is not used, the following protocol should be adopted for the pre-sterilisation cleaning of handpieces:

− Leave the bur in place during cleaning to prevent contamination of the handpiece bearing.
− clean the outside of the handpiece with detergent and water – never clean or immerse the handpiece in disinfectant
− remove the bur
− if recommended by the manufacturer, lubricate the handpiece with pressurised oil until clean oil appears out of the chuck and clean off excess oil, sterilise in an autoclave
− lubricate the handpiece after sterilisation and run it briefly before use to clear excess lubricant
− The oil used for pre-sterilisation cleaning/lubrication should not be the same as used for post sterilisation lubrication; either two canisters should be used, or the nozzle changed between applications.
  ○ Instrument Storage (Fig. **9**)

− Sterilised instruments should be stored in dry, covered conditions – trays with

lids are now readily available. Sterilised instruments should not be stored in a disinfectant or antiseptic solution.
– Pouches can be useful for storing infrequently used instruments such as extraction forceps and elevators. Pouches with a clear side allow instruments to be easily identified before opening.

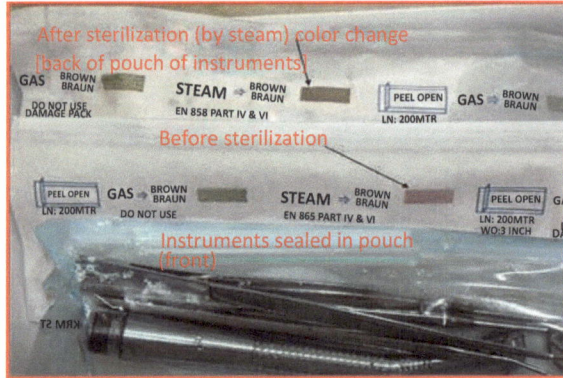

Fig. (9). Packaging of instruments.

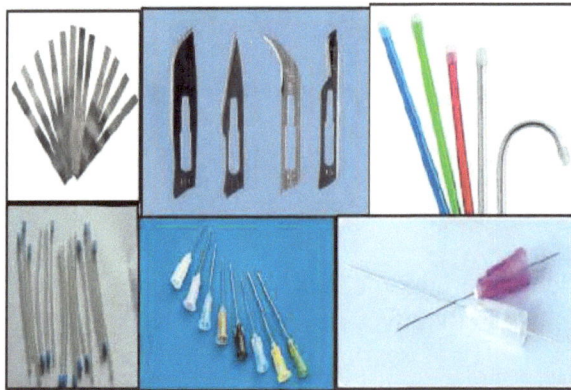

Fig. (10). Single-use items.

Single-Use (Disposable) Items (Fig. 10)

'Single use' means a device can be used on a patient during one treatment session and then discarded and never to be reused. These items include local anaesthetic needles and cartridges, scalpel blades, saliva ejectors, matrix bands, and impression trays.

Standard Principles of Infection Control

Universal Precautions

It is not always possible to identify people who may spread the infection to others, therefore precautions to prevent the spread of infection must be followed at all times. These routine procedures are called Standard Principles of Infection Control (or Universal Precautions). These include Hand Hygiene and Skin Care, Protective Clothing, Safe Handling of Sharps and Spillage Management. All blood and body fluids are potentially infectious, and precautions are necessary to prevent exposure to them. A disposable apron and latex or vinyl gloves should always be worn when dealing with excreta, blood, and body fluids. Everyone involved in providing care in dental practice should know and apply the standard principles of hand decontamination, the use of protective clothing ng, and the safe disposal of sharps and body fluid spillages.

Hand Hygiene and Skin Care (Fig. 11) (Table 2)

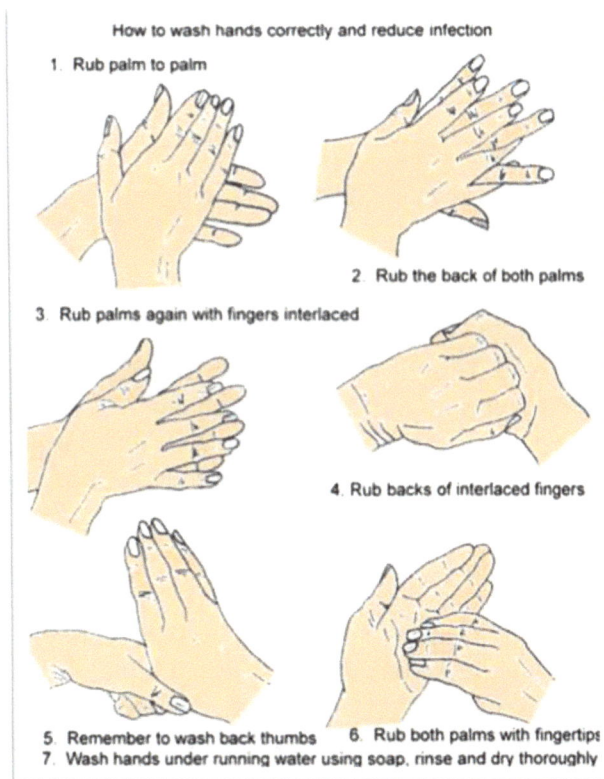

How to wash hands correctly and reduce infection

1. Rub palm to palm
2. Rub the back of both palms
3. Rub palms again with fingers interlaced
4. Rub backs of interlaced fingers
5. Remember to wash back thumbs
6. Rub both palms with fingertips
7. Wash hands under running water using soap, rinse and dry thoroughly

Fig. (11). Step by step procedure of correct hand washing.

Table 2. Key recommendations for HAND HYGIENE in Dental Settings.

1. Perform hand hygiene-
    a. When hands are visibly soiled.
    b. After barehanded touching of instruments, equipment, materials, and other objects likely to be contaminated by blood, saliva, or respiratory secretions.
    c. Before and after treating each patient.
    d. Before putting on gloves and again immediately after removing gloves.
2. Use soap and water when hands are visibly soiled (*e.g.*, blood, body fluids) otherwise an alcohol-based rub may be used.

Hand washing is recognized as the single most effective method of controlling the infection.

An effective hand washing technique involves three stages [5 - 8]:

Preparation

Before washing hands, all wrists and, ideally, hand jewellery should be removed. Cuts and abrasions must be covered with waterproof dressings. Fingernails should be kept short, clear, and free from nail polish. Hands should be wet under tepid running water before applying liquid soap or an antimicrobial preparation.

Washing and Rinsing

Wet the hands under running water. Apply the hand wash solution, ensuring that it comes into contact with all of the surfaces of the hand. The hands must be rubbed together vigorously for a minimum of 10-15 seconds, giving particular attention to the tips of the fingers, the thumbs, and the areas between the fingers. Hands should be rinsed thoroughly. When decontaminating hands use an alcohol hand rub, hands should be free from dirt and organic material. The hand rub solution must come into contact with all surfaces of the hand. The hands must be rubbed together vigorously, paying particular attention to the tips of the fingers, the thumbs, and the areas between the fingers, until the solution has evaporated, and the hands are dry.

Drying

Dry hands using good-quality paper towels. In clinical settings, disposable paper towels are the method of choice because communal towels are a source of cross-contamination. Store paper towels in a wall-mounted dispenser next to the washbasin and throw them away in a pedal-operated domestic waste bin. Do not use your hands to lift the lid or they will become re-contaminated. Hot air dryers are not recommended in clinical settings.

Surgical Scrub

Surgical hand washing destroys transient organisms and reduces resident flora before surgical or invasive procedures. Oral surgical procedures are those that involve the incision, excision or reflection of tissue that exposes sterile areas of the oral cavity. At the start of a session, an aqueous antiseptic detergent solution is applied to moistened hands and forearms for approximately 2 minutes. The nails are scrubbed, and a manicure stick can be used to remove dirt from beneath the nail. The disinfection process must be thorough and systematic, covering all aspects of the hands and forearms. The procedure should take 3 to 5 minutes.

Hand Creams

An emollient hand cream should be applied regularly to protect skin from the drying effects of regular hand decontamination. If a particular soap, antimicrobial hand wash or alcohol product causes skin irritation, and OH team or general practitioner (GP or a dermatologist) should be consulted.

Hand Washing Facilities

Facilities should be adequate and conveniently located. Hand washbasins must be placed in areas where needed and where client consultations take place. They should have elbow- or foot-operated mixer taps. Separate sinks should be available for other cleaning and rinsing purposes - such as cleaning and rinsing of instruments:

- Use wall-mounted liquid soap dispensers with disposable soap cartridges - keep them clean and replenished
- Place disposable paper towels next to the basins - soft towels will help to avoid skin abrasions
- Position foot-operated pedal bins near the hand washbasin - make sure they are the right size [9].

Personal Protective Equipment (PPE) (Table 3)

Table 3. Key recommendations for personal protective equipment in dental settings.

1. Provide sufficient and appropriate PPE and ensure it is accessible to DHCP.
2. Educate all DHCP on proper selection and use of PPE.
3. Wear gloves whenever there is potential for contact with blood, body fluids, mucous membranes, non-intact skin, or contaminated equipment.
a. A Do not wear the same pair of gloves for the care of more than one patient.
b. Do not wash gloves. Gloves cannot be reused.
c. Perform hand hygiene immediately after removing gloves.
4. Wear protective clothing that covers the skin and personal clothing during procedures or activities where contact with blood, saliva or OPIM is anticipated.
5. Wear mouth, nose and eye protection during procedures that are likely to generate splashes or spattering of blood or other body fluids.
6. Remove PPE before leaving the work area.

OSHA requires the employer to provide employees with appropriate personal protective equipment.

Respiratory Hygiene (Table 4)

Table 4. Key Recommendations for respiratory hygiene/ cough etiquette in dental settings.

1. Implement measures to contain respiratory secretions in patients and accompanying individuals who have signs and symptoms of a respiratory infection, beginning at the point of entry to the facility and continuing throughout the visit.
a. Post signs at the entrance with instructions to patients with symptoms of respiratory infection to-
i. Cover their mouth/ nose when coughing or sneezing.
ii. Use and dispose of tissues.
iii. Perform hand hygiene after hands have been in contact with respiratory secretions.
b. Provide tissues and no-touch receptacles for disposal of tissues.
c. Provide resources for performing hand hygiene in or near waiting areas.
d. Offer masks to coughing patients and other symptomatic persons when they enter the dental setting.
e. Provide space and encourage persons with symptoms of respiratory infections to sit as far away from others as possible. If available, facilities may wish to place these patients in a separate area while waiting for care.
2. Educate DHCP on the importance of infection prevention measures to contain respiratory secretions to prevent the spread of respiratory pathogens when examining and caring for patients with signs and symptoms of a respiratory infection.

Protective Clothing

Disposable Gloves (Figs. 12 and 13)

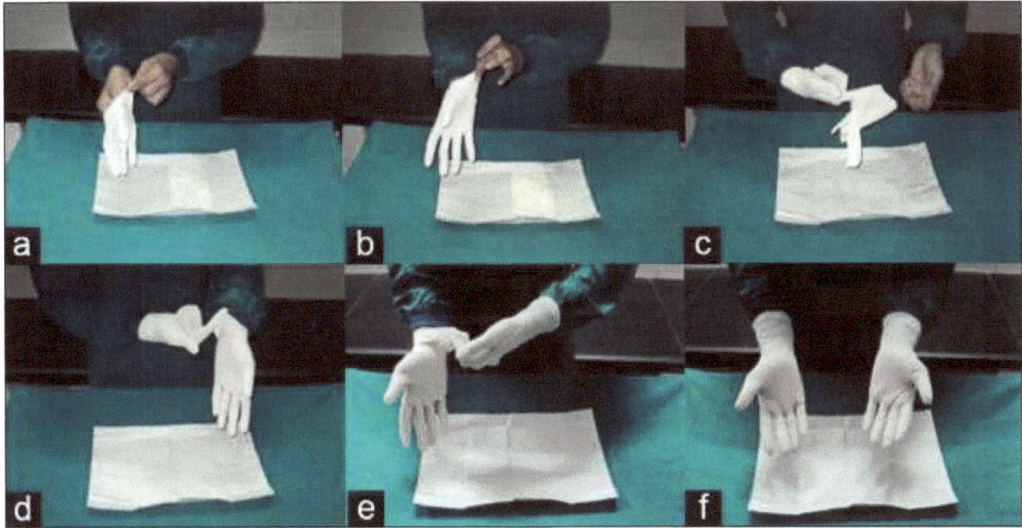

Fig. (12). Step-by-step diagrammatic representation of wearing gloves.

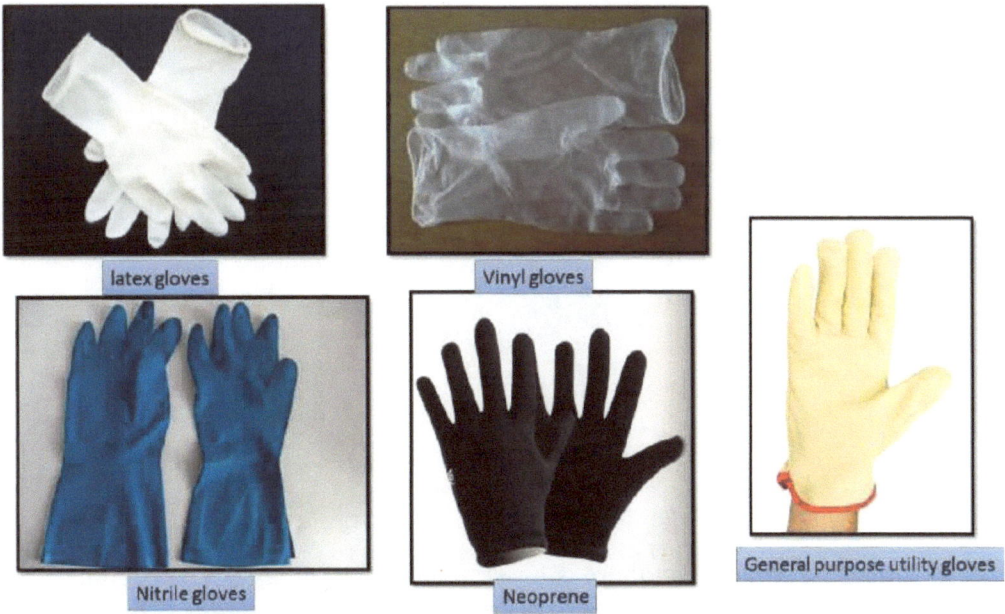

Fig. (13). Types of disposable gloves (Do not wash, disinfect, or sterilize gloves for reuse).

Gloves must be worn for invasive procedures, contact with sterile sites and non-intact skin or mucous membranes, and all activities that have been assessed as carrying a risk of exposure to blood, body fluids, secretions, or excretions, or to sharp or contaminated instruments.

DO NOT USE powdered latex gloves as it exacerbates the risk of latex allergy through increased exposure to the allergens present in the powder. Polythene gloves do not provide any barrier protection and do not have a place in the clinical setting. Gloves must be worn as single-use items. They must be put on immediately before an episode of patient contact or treatment and removed as soon as the activity is completed. Gloves must be changed between caring for different patients, and between different care or treatment activities for the same patient, and do not substitute for hand washing. Gloves must be disposed of as clinical waste and hands decontaminated after the gloves have been removed. Sensitivity to natural rubber latex in patients, caretakers and healthcare personnel must be documented. Alternatives to natural rubber latex gloves must be available, *e.g.*, nitrile. To prevent transmission of infection, gloves must be discarded after each procedure. Gloves should not be washed between patients as the gloves may be damaged by the soap solution and, if punctured unknowingly, may cause body fluid to remain in direct contact with the skin for prolonged periods [8, 9].

Disposable Plastic Aprons (Fig. 14)

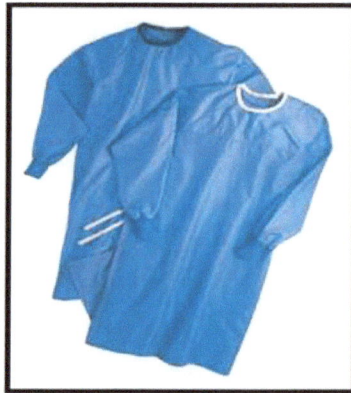

Fig. (14). Disposable aprons.

These should be worn when there is a risk that clothing may be exposed to blood, body fluids, secretions, or excretions, except sweat. Plastic aprons should be worn as single-use items, for one procedure or episode of patient care, and then discarded and disposed of as clinical waste.

Visors or Face Masks and Goggles (Fig. 15)

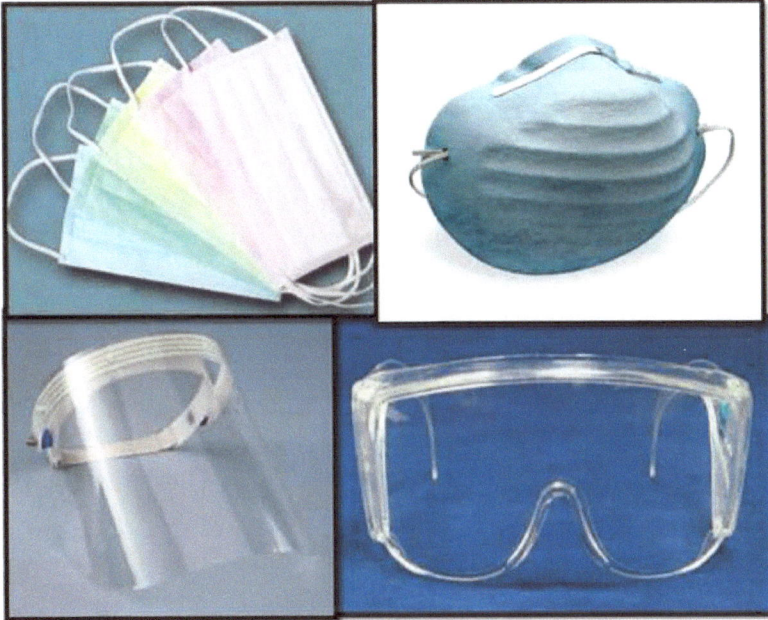

Fig. (15). Face masks, eyewear, and face shield.

These must be worn where there is a risk of blood, body fluids, secretions or excretions splashing into the face or eyes.

Respirator (Fig. 16)

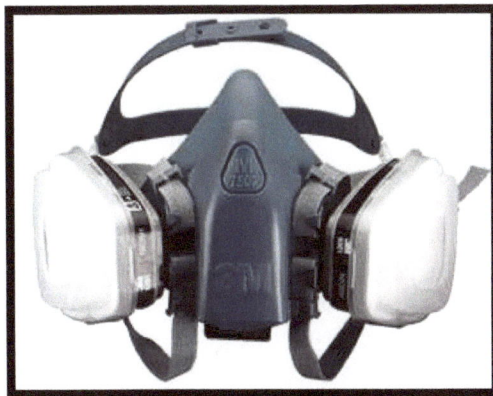

Fig. (16). Respirator.

It is a personal protective device worn on the face, covers at least the nose and mouth, and is used to reduce the wearer's risk of inhaling hazardous airborne particles (including dust particles and infectious agents), gases, or vapours. Respirators are certified by CDC/National Institute for Occupational Safety and Health (NIOSH), including those intended for use in healthcare. Respirator use must be in the context of a complete respiratory protection program by OSHA Respiratory Protection standard. DHCP should be medically cleared and fit tested if using respirators with tight-fitting facepieces (*e.g.*, a NIOSH-approved N95 respirator) and trained in the proper use of respirators, safe removal and disposal, and medical contraindications to respirator use.

Aerosol and Saliva/Blood Splatter (Table 5)

Table 5. Centres for disease control and prevention (CDC) classification.

Category	Definition	Dental Instrument or Item
Critical	Penetrates soft tissue, contacts bone, enters into or contacts the bloodstream or other normally sterile tissue.	Surgical instruments, periodontal scalers, scalpel blades, surgical dental burs
Semi critical	Contacts mucous membranes or Non-intact skin; will not penetrate soft tissue, contact bone, enter into or contact the bloodstream or other normally sterile tissue.	Dental mouth mirror, amalgam condenser, reusable dental impression trays, dental handpieces
Noncritical	Contacts intact skin.	Radiograph head/cone, blood pressure cuff, face bow, pulse oximeter

Good surgery ventilation and efficient high-volume aspirators, which exhaust externally from the premises, will reduce the risk of infection by dispersing and eliminating aerosols. External vents should discharge without risk to the public or re-circulation into any building. Rubber dam isolation of teeth also offers substantial advantages and should be used whenever practicable. When working without a rubber dam, the use of high-volume aspiration is essential.

Inoculation Injuries

Inoculation injuries are the most likely route for transmission of blood-borne viral infections in dentistry. It includes all incidents where a contaminated object or substance breaches the integrity of the skin or mucous membranes or comes into contact with the eyes, *e.g.*, sticking or stabbing with a used needle or other instrument, splashes with a contaminated substance to the eye or other open lesion, cuts with contaminated equipment, Bites or scratches inflicted by patients.

Management of Sharps and Splash Injuries (Figs. 17 & 18) (Table 6)

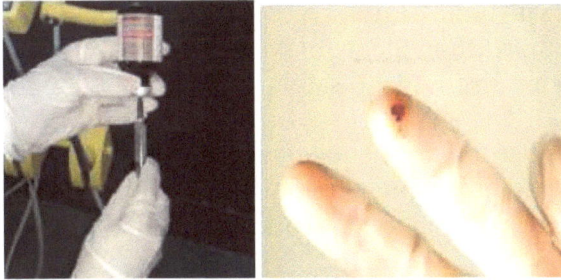

Fig. (17). Needle prick injury.

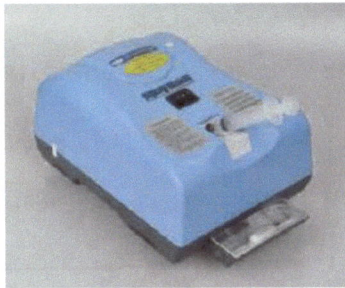

Fig. (18). Needle destroyer.

Table 6. Key recommendation for sharps safety in dental settings.

1. **Consider sharp items (*e.g.*, needles, scalers, burs, lab knives and wires) that are contaminated with patient blood and saliva as potentially infective and establish engineering controls and work practices to prevent injuries.**
2. **Do not recap used needles by using both hands and any other technique that involves directing the point of a needle toward any part of the body.**
3. **Use either a one-handed scoop technique or a mechanical device designed for holding the needle cap when recapping (*e.g.*, between multiple injections and before removing from a non-disposable aspirating syringe).**
4. **Place used disposable syringes and needles, scalpel blades and other sharp items in appropriate puncture-resistant containers located as close as possible to the area where the items are used.**

Sharps include needles, scalpels, root canal reamers, stitch cutters, glass ampoules, sharp instruments and broken crockery and glass. Sharps must be handled and disposed of safely to reduce the risk of needle stick injury and possible exposure to blood-borne viruses.

In the event of a sharp's injury/contamination incident during working hours, these guidelines should be followed:

- Encourage bleeding from the wound
- Wash the wound in soap and warm running water (do not scrub)
- Cover the wound with a dressing
- Skin, eyes or mouth, wash in plenty of water
- Ensure the sharp is disposed of safely, *i.e.*, using a non-touch method in a sharp's container
- Report the incident to the immediate supervisor. An incident form should be completed as soon as the recipient of the injury is able
- The incident should be reported to the recipient's General Practitioner/OH department
- Attempt to identify the source of the needle/sharp. Depending on the degree of exposure and the knowledge of the source patient/client, it may be necessary to take further immediate action.

Environmental Infection Prevention and Control in Dental Settings (Table 7)

Table 7. Key recommendations for environmental infection prevention and control in dental settings.

1. Establish policies and procedures for routine cleaning and disinfection of environmental surfaces in dental health care settings.
   a. Use surface barriers to protect clinical contact surfaces, particularly those that are difficult to clean (*e.g.*, switches on dental chairs, computer equipment) and change surface barriers between patients.
   b. Clean and disinfect clinical contact surfaces that are not barrier protected with an EPA-registered hospital disinfectant after each patient. Use an intermediate-level disinfectant (*i.e.*, tuberculocidal claim) if visibly contaminated with blood.
2. Select EPA-registered disinfectants or detergents/disinfectants with label claims for use in health care settings.
3. Follow manufacturer instructions for use of cleaners and EPA-registered disinfectants (*e.g*, amount, dilution, contact time, safe use, disposal).

Dental Unit Water Quality (Table 8)

Table 8. Key recommendations for dental unit water quality in dental settings.

1. Use water that meets EPA regulatory standards for drinking water (*i.e.*,$\leq$ 500 CFU/ml of heterotrophic water bacteria) for routine dental treatment output water.
2. Consult with the dental unit manufacturer for appropriate methods and equipment to maintain the quality of dental water.
3. Follow recommendations for monitoring water quality provided by the manufacturer of the unit or waterline treatment product.
4. Use sterile saline or sterile water as a coolant/ irrigant when performing surgical procedures.

Control Measures

Any staff working in a healthcare facility that handles sharps or clinical waste should receive a full course of Hepatitis B vaccine and have their antibody level checked.

Bio-Medical Waste Management

Wastes may be of various types:

- Solid, liquid, gaseous
- Radioactive, bioactive (containing bacteria, fungi, viruses, parasites, and other infectious agents), chemical (inflammable, explosive, corrosive, *etc.*), physically injurious (sharp, abrasive, *etc.*), thermal (hot, cold).

"Bio-medical waste" means any waste, which is generated during the diagnosis, treatment or immunization of human beings or animals or research activities pertaining thereto or in the production or testing of biological substances or health camps. Internationally, biomedical waste is symbolized as shown in Fig. (**19**) below:

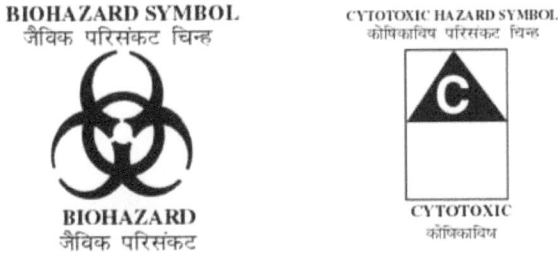

Fig. (**19**). Symbols used.

What Risks are Posed by Biomedical Waste?

- Infections and infestations communicated by contact, ingestion, or inoculation (bacterial, fungal, viral, or parasitic).
- Toxicity leads to physiological, biochemical, cytological, or even genetic disruptions, including risks to fetuses.
- Physical injury from prick (puncture), cut (incision) or scratch (abrasion).
- Chemical injury.

Sources of Biomedical Waste (Fig. 20)

MAJOR SOURCES	MINOR SOURCES
• Hospitals	• Clinics
• Labs	• Dental clinics
• Research centres	• Home care
• Animal research	• Cosmetic clinics
• Blood banks	• Paramedics
• Nursing homes	• Funeral services
• Mortuaries	• Institutions
• Autopsy centres	

Fig. (20). Sources of biomedical waste.

Process of Biomedical Waste Management (Fig. 21)

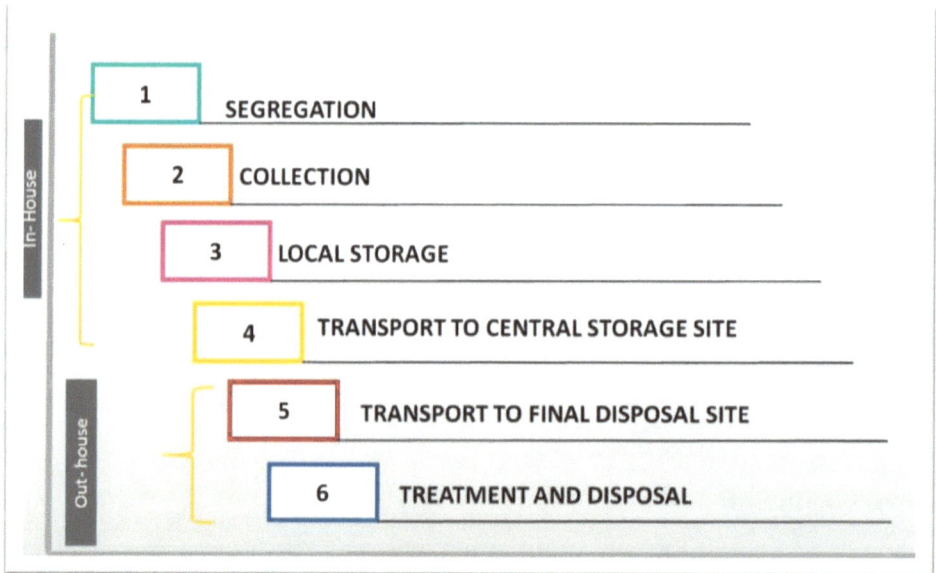

Fig. (21). Process of biomedical waste management.

Steps in Biomedical Waste Management (Tables 9 and 10)

Table 9. Biomedical waste segregation in a dental unit.

Bin Colour	Red	Yellow	Blue	Green Or Black
Contents	Gloves Syringes Drains Catheters Rubber- Tubes Impression Materials Fluid Bottles All Plastic & Rubber Items	Cotton Gauze Dressings Plaster-Of-Paris Tissue- Pieces Teeth Bone Calculus Blood- Clot Pus Hair	Glass Items Glass Pieces Needles Knife-Blades Saw-Blades Sharp Items	Civil Waste Paper Envelopes Plastic Bags Match Sticks Food- Remnants Wrappers

Table 10. Waste disposal and treatment.

Category	Waste Category	Treatment and Disposal
1	Human anatomical waste(human tissue, organs, body parts)	Incineration, deep burial
2	Animal waste (animal tissue, organs, body parts, fluids, discharge from research labs and animal houses)	Incineration, deep burial
3	Microbiology and biotechnology waste (waste from lab culture, stocks and specimens of micro organisms, live or attenuated vaccines, wastes from production of biological toxins, dishes and devices and transfer of cultures)	Local autoclaving, microwaving/ incineration
4	Waste sharps (needles, syringes, scalpels, blades, glass *etc.* that may puncture and cut)	Disinfection (chemical treatment, autoclaving/ microwaving and mutilation/ shredding)
5	Discarded medicines and cytotoxic drugs	Incineration, destruction and drugs disposal in solid landfills
6	Solid waste (items contaminated with blood, and fluids, including cotton, dressings, soiled plaster casts, linen, and beddings)	Incineration; autoclaving/ microvaing
7	Solid waste (tubings, catheters, intravenous sets *etc.*)	Disinfection by chemical treatment and autoclaving/ microwaving and mutilation/ shredding
8	Liquid waste (waste from labs and washing, cleaning, housekeeping and disinfecting activities)	Disinfection by chemical treatment and discharge into drain
9	Incineration ash	Disposal in municipal landfill

(Table 10) cont.....

Category	Waste Category	Treatment and Disposal
10	Chemicals used in the production of biological, chemicals used in disinfection, as insecticides *etc.*	Chemical treatment and discharge into drains for liquids and secured landfill for solids.

Generation

Authorized healthcare personnel and facilities, named "occupiers" generate biomedical waste as a result of their activities. These are clinics, hospitals, nursing homes, *etc*. Each healthcare unit (occupier) has to get authorization from the state pollution control board to work as a waste generator.

Segregation

This should be the responsibility of all staff members and should be done at the source of generation itself (Figs. **22 - 25**, Table **9**).

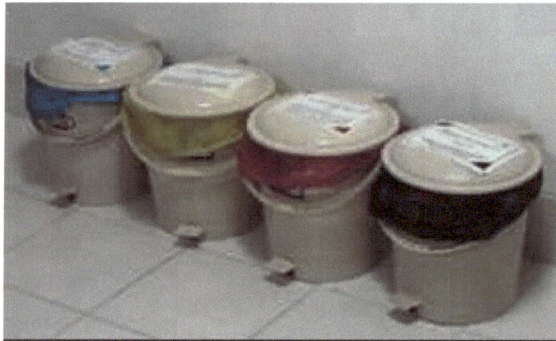

Fig. (22). Colour-coded bins.

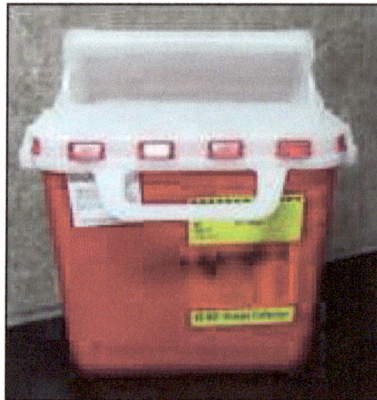

Fig. (23). Sharp collector.

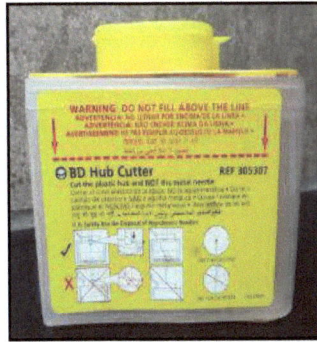

Fig. (24). Hub Cutter.

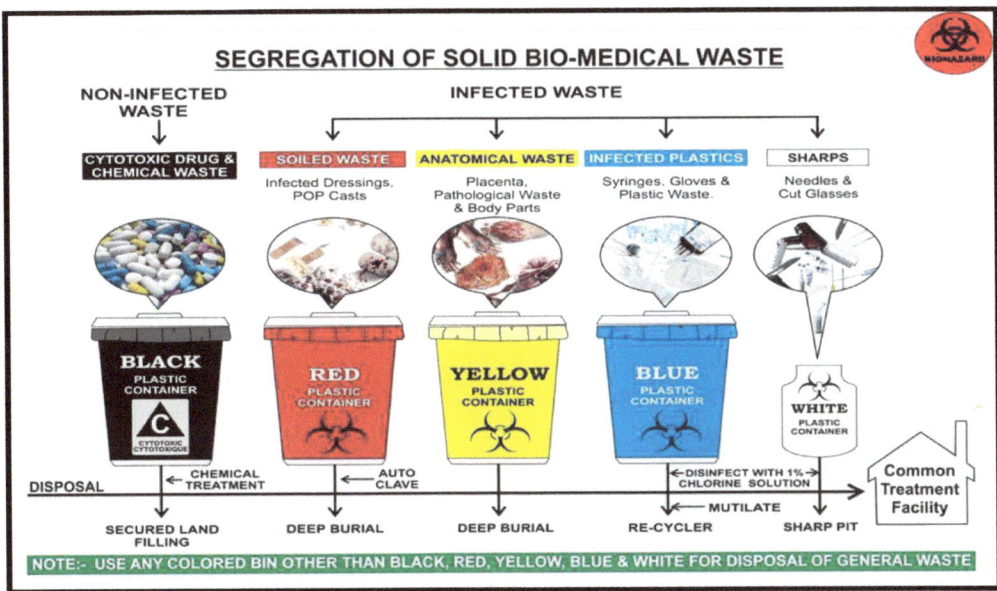

Fig. (25). Segregation of solid biomedical waste.

- Allow to fill the bag/bin up to 3/4th level.
- Hub cutters for needles.
- Proper segregation facilitates the further collection, handling, storage & disposal of waste.

Collection and Transportation

"Operators" of biomedical waste disposal units collect and safely transport the waste. Scheduled collection by Housekeeping Staff.

- 2 hourlies in ICUs

• 4 hourlies inwards/other clinical areas

Temporary Storage

• Colour-coded containers/big polythene bags
• Labelling
• Local collection points (closed dirty utility rooms)
• Away from patient areas
    ◦ No mixing of infectious and non-infectious waste.

From Local Storage areas to Central Storage Areas

• Closed air-tight colour-coded container trolleys
• Scheduled time interval
• Pre-defined waste route
• Well demarcated dirty utility lift
• Scheduling & separate routes for waste trolleys & food trolleys.
• Regular washing & disinfection of container trolleys. Checklist for washing/disinfection.
• Use of PPE while transporting waste.

Transportation to Final Disposal Site

• Daily.
• Outsourced to Government-authorized CBWTF (Common Biomedical Waste Treatment Facility).
• In a closed cart/vehicle with smooth & impermeable surfaces.

Thumb Rule

No waste should be kept stored in the hospital beyond the period of 48 hours.

Disposal

"Operators" of biomedical waste disposal units dispose of the categorized biomedical waste in a manner appropriate to each category.

Other Hazardous Waste in Dental Healthcare Units [10]

In addition to infectious waste, several other hazardous wastes, not essentially biomedical waste, are generated in dental clinics, *e.g.*, amalgam, free mercury, x-ray films, lead foils, x-ray developer and fixer solutions. These also need to be stored and disposed of appropriately.

Spillage Management [11]

Deal with blood and body fluid spills quickly and effectively. A blood spillage kit should be readily available to deal with the spillage of blood. Commercial blood spillage kits (Fig. **26**) can be purchased, or the practice can put together a kit as described below. The kit should be kept in a designated place (depending on the size of the establishment, there may be more than one kit).

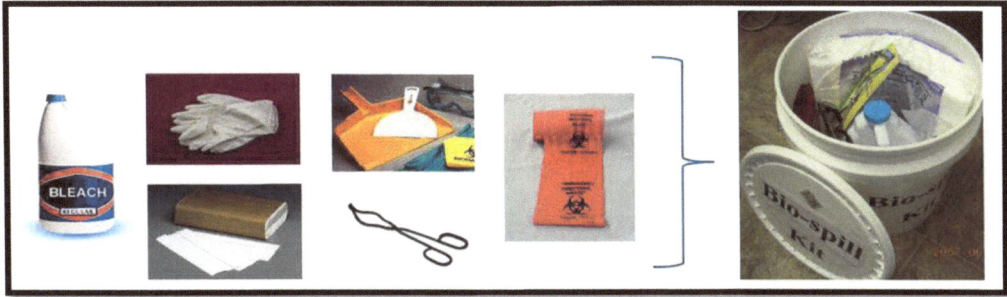

Fig. (26). Bio spill kit.

The Kit Should Comprise

- 'Nappy' type bucket with a lid
- Non-sterile, unpowdered latex gloves or vinyl gloves
- Disposable plastic apron (Safety glasses, Biohazardous waste autoclave bags)
- Dustpan and scoop or tongs for broken glass
- Disposable paper towels and Disposable cloths
- Small container of general-purpose detergent
- Hypochlorite solution (*e.g.*, Household bleach or Milton) or sodium dichloroisocyanurate compound (*e.g.*, Precept, Sanichlor) – to comply with COSHH 1988 – this compound should be stored in a lockable cupboard.

The kit should be immediately replenished after use. For spillage of high-risk body fluids such as blood, method 1 (below) is recommended. For spillage of low-risk body fluids (non-blood containing excreta) such as excreta, vomit *etc* use method 2.

Hypochlorite / Sodium Dichloroisocyanurates (NaDCC) Method (for blood spillages on a hard surface) [10, 11]

- Prevent access to the area containing the spillage until it has been safely dealt with
- Open the windows to ventilate the room if possible
- Wear protective clothing

- Soak up excess fluid using disposable paper towels and/or absorbent powder, *e.g.*, vernal
- Cover area with NaDCC granules (*e.g.*, Precept, Sanichlor).

Or

- Cover the area with towels soaked in 10,000 parts per million of available chlorine (1% hypochlorite solution = 1 part household bleach to 10 parts water), *e.g.*, household bleach, Milton, and leave for at least two minutes
- Remove organic matter using the towels and discard it as clinical waste
- Clean area with detergent and hot water, and dry thoroughly
- Clean the bucket/bowl in fresh soapy water and dry
- Discard protective clothing as clinical waste
- Wash hands.

Detergent and Water Method (for all other body fluids and blood on carpeted areas)

- Prevent access to the area until spillage has been safely dealt with
- Wear protective clothing
- Mop up the organic matter with paper towels or disposable cloths and/or absorbent powder, *e.g.*, vernagel
- Clean the surface thoroughly using a solution of detergent and hot water and paper towels or disposable cloths.
- Rinse the surface and dry thoroughly
- Dispose of materials as clinical waste
- Clean the bucket/bowl in fresh hot, soapy water and dry
- Discard protective clothing as clinical waste
- Wash hands
- Ideally, once dry, go over the area with a mechanical suction cleaner.

CONCLUSION

Most postoperative infection results from faulty surgical technique, inadequate asepsis, and disinfection. The success of prevention and control of infection in healthcare areas is largely dependent on the aseptic technique of all personnel, who perform the invasive procedures, the sterility of all items directly concerned in such procedure and the disinfection of all surfaces.

CONSENT FOR PUBLICATION

Not applicable.

CONFLICT OF INTEREST

The authors declare no conflict of interest, financial or otherwise.

ACKNOWLEDGEMENT

Declared none.

REFERENCES

[1] Centres for disease control and prevention. Summary of infection prevention practices in dental settings. http://www.cdc.gov/oralhealth/infectioncontrol/pdf/safe-care2pdf

[2] Centres for disease control and prevention. Guidance for dental settings. Interim infection prevention and control guidance for dental settings during the coronavirus disease 2019 (COVID-19) Pandemic 2019.

[3] U.S. Department of labour occupational safety and health administration. Covid -19 control and prevention/dentistry workers and employers. http://www.osha.gov/SLTC/covid-19/dentistry.html

[4] U.S. Food and Drug Administration. Dental unit waterlines 2018. http://www.fda.gov /medicaldevices/dentaldevices/dental

[5] Boretti VS, Corrêa RN, dos Santos SS, Leão MV, Gonçalves e Silva CR. Sensitivity profile of *Staphylococcus spp.* and *Streptococcus spp.* isolated from toys used in a teaching hospital playroom. Rev Paul Pediatr 2014; 32(3): 151-6.
[http://dx.doi.org/10.1590/0103-0582201432301] [PMID: 25479842]

[6] Infection control. Centre for scientific information. ADA Science institute;updated from the ADA Statement on infection control in dentistry, adopted by the council on scientific affairs. March 29, 2016.

[7] Infection prevention and control guidelines and recommendations. 2016.

[8] Marhofer P, Schebesta K, Marhofer D. Hygiene aspects in ultrasound-guided regional anesthesia. Anaesthesist 2016; 65(7): 492-8.
[http://dx.doi.org/10.1007/s00101-016-0168-1] [PMID: 27142364]

[9] Seavey R. Taking the chaos out of accreditation surveys in sterile processing: High-level disinfection, sterilization, and antisepsis. Am J Infect Control 2016; 44(5) (Suppl.): e35-9.
[http://dx.doi.org/10.1016/j.ajic.2016.03.002] [PMID: 27131133]

[10] Wallace CA. New developments in disinfection and sterilization. Am J Infect Control 2016; 44(5) (Suppl.): e23-7.
[http://dx.doi.org/10.1016/j.ajic.2016.02.022] [PMID: 27131131]

[11] Rutala WA, Weber DJ. Disinfection, sterilization, and antisepsis: An overview. Am J Infect Control 2016; 44(5) (Suppl.): e1-6.
[http://dx.doi.org/10.1016/j.ajic.2015.10.038] [PMID: 27131128]

CHAPTER 6

Isolation Techniques in Pediatric Dentistry

Dhanashree Sakhare[1] and **Prachi Goyal**[2,*]

[1] *Lavanika Dental Academy, Melbourne, Australia*

[2] *Department of Pediatric and Preventive Dentistry, MMCDSR, Mullana, Ambala, India*

Abstract: Isolation of the operating field is a fundamental aspect of pediatric dentistry. The complexity of the oral environment presents many obstacles to performing dental treatment procedures. To minimize them, proper isolation is required to control the operating field as well as provide safe and quality treatment [1]. A rubber dam is considered the optimum isolation technique due to several advantages, such as providing an aseptic environment, minimizing the potential risk of transferring infective microbes between the operator and the patient, and preventing any ingestion or aspiration of dental instruments during a dental procedure [2]. Children may feel that the treatment takes place outside of their mouth. Nevertheless, children indeed tolerate longer treatments once the rubber dam has been applied. Other techniques such as cotton rolls and saliva ejectors are routinely used in paediatric dentistry besides rubber dams due to their ease of usage.

Keywords: Clamps, Cotton Rolls, Isolation, Retraction Cords, Rubber Dam, Throat Shields.

INTRODUCTION

Isolation of the operating field is a fundamental aspect of pediatric dentistry. The complexity of the oral environment presents many obstacles to performing dental treatment procedures. To minimize them, proper isolation is required to control the operating field as well as provide safe and quality treatment [1]. A rubber dam is considered the optimum isolation technique due to several advantages, such as providing an aseptic environment, minimizing the potential risk of transferring infective microbes between the operator and the patient, and preventing any ingestion or aspiration of dental instruments during a dental procedure [2]. Children may feel that the treatment takes place outside of their mouth. Nevertheless, children indeed tolerate longer treatments once the rubber dam has been applied. Other techniques such as cotton rolls and saliva ejectors are rout-

---

* **Corresponding author Prachi Goyal:** Department of Pediatric and Preventive Dentistry, MMCDSR, Mullana Ambala, India; E-mail: pra21chi@gmail.comm

inely used in paediatric dentistry besides rubber dams due to their ease of usage.

SIGNIFICANCE OF ISOLATION

Isolation is more significant in the case of pediatric dentistry as children have higher levels of anxiety that causes excessive salivation. Inappropriate or undesirable movements of the tongue, chances of aspiration or swallowing of restorative materials or broken instruments or fluids such as root canal irrigants or aerotor coolants are more common in the case of children.

METHODS FOR ISOLATION

Direct methods: Rubber dam, cotton rolls and cotton roll holder, gauze pieces, absorbent wafers, suction devices, gingival retraction cord and mouth props

Indirect methods: Comfortable position of patient and relaxed surroundings, local anaesthesia and drugs like anti-sialogogues, anti-anxiety, and a Muscle relaxant.

DIRECT METHODS OF ISOLATION

Absorbent Systems

Absorbents such as cotton rolls, cellulose wafers, gauze pads and throat shields can be used for isolation. They are placed in the first maxillary molar region at the opening of the parotid gland duct and in the anterior lingual sulcus at the opening of the submandibular or sublingual salivary gland ducts to absorb the secretions from the major salivary glands.

Cotton Rolls and Wafers (Fig. 1)

They absorb moisture and retract the soft tissues. They can be placed in the mouth where the salivary gland duct exits. It is either rolled manually or prefabricated (available in three sizes-small, medium, and large) cotton rolls are available. They act by absorption and therefore must be replaced frequently when saturated. Cellulose wafers may be used to retract the cheek and provide additional absorbency.

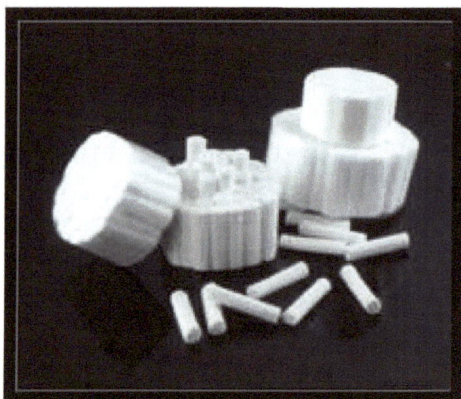

Fig. (1). Cotton rolls.

If removed improperly, a dry cotton roll may stick to the oral mucosa and can injure it, causing cotton roll burn/cotton roll stomatitis. Therefore, removing cotton rolls necessitates moistening them using an air-water syringe to prevent inadvertent removal of the epithelium from cheeks, the floor of the mouth or lips.

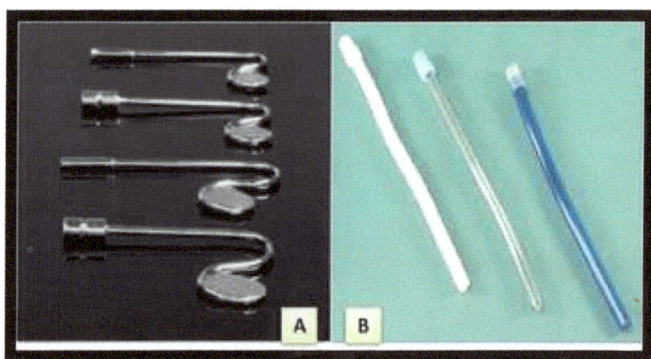

Fig. (2). A. Metallic saliva ejectors. **B.** Plastic saliva ejectors.

Throat Shields

Throat shields are indicated when there is a danger of aspirating or swallowing small objects, especially in the maxillary arch. A gauze sponge (2 x 2 inches) unfolded and spread over the tongue, and the posterior part of the mouth helps recover a small object, such as fillings, parts of teeth, parts of dental equipment, *etc.*, from falling into a patient's throat.

High Volume Evacuators & Saliva Ejectors (Figs. 2a and 2b)

Saliva ejectors prevent the pooling of saliva on the floor of the mouth, which help in maintaining a dry operative field. They are of two types: Metallic saliva ejectors (autoclavable) and Plastic saliva ejectors (disposable and inexpensive). Its tip should always be moulded to face backward with a slight upward curvature. The floor of the mouth under the tip should be covered with gauze to prevent injury to soft tissues and should not interfere with instrumentation.

Other Types of Saliva Ejectors (Figs. 3a , b, c)

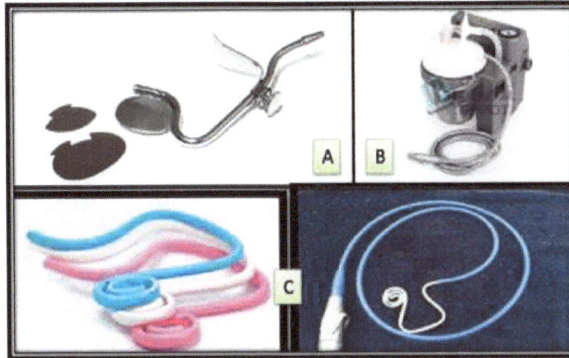

Fig. (3). **A.** Svedopter; **B:** Hygroformic saliva ejector; **C:** vac-ejector.

a. **Svedopter**: This is the most used tongue retraction device. It serves as a saliva ejector & tongue retractor. This is extremely useful for the preparation & cementation of fixed prostheses. It has a mirror-like vertical blade which holds the tongue away from the field of operation.

b. **Hygroformic saliva ejector:** This is a combination of saliva ejector and tongue retractor. It has a unique coil design which can be adjusted for maximum patient comfort. It has smooth edges that eliminate irritation and is ideal for patients with sensitive tissues.

c. **Vac-ejector**: It is used for the isolation of posterior teeth. It incorporates **a** bite block, tongue retractor for mandibular areas & high-speed suction attachment. It comes with three flexible deflectors; one when operating in mandibular areas, and one universal deflector or operating on either side in the maxillary arch. The bite block is adjustable by rotation for large or small arches.

Retraction Cord (Figs. 4a, b)

These can be used while restoring cervical lesions, tooth preparations and impressions. The cord should extend 1mm beyond the gingival width of the cavity or extends around the whole circumference of the tooth. The ideal location for the ends of the cord is at the axial angles of the tooth.

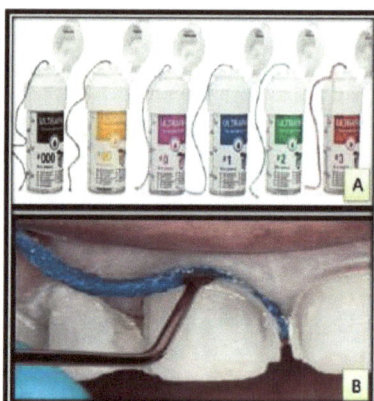

Fig. (4). A. Types of Retraction cord. **B.** Placement of retraction cord.

Classification of Gingival Retraction Cords

a. **Surface texture:** Wet and Dry
b. **Configuration:** Knitted, Braided and Twisted
c. **Material used:** Synthetic and Cotton
d. **Chemical treatment:** Plain and Impregnated
e. **Number of strands:** Single and Multiple

RUBBER DAM

The rubber dam was introduced in dental practice by Dr. Sanford Barnum in 1864 [3]. It is still the ideal means of isolation to date. It provides better control of cross-infection and improves treatment efficiency. It provides an aseptic field that isolates the tooth from salivary contamination and improves access and visibility to the operating field by retracting soft tissues. It prevents aspiration or swallowing of instruments, drugs, irrigating solutions, and tooth/material debris. The disadvantages of a rubber dam are it takes time to be applied and sometimes makes communication with the patient difficult.

Contraindications of rubber dam are as follows

• Patients Allergic to latex (non-latex rubber dam sheets can be used in such cases).
• Asthmatic individuals and Mouth breathers.
• Teeth with short clinical crowns making retention of the clamp difficult.
• Partially erupted teeth and extremely mal-positioned teeth.

The Armamentarium of Rubber Dam: Rubber dam instruments include the rubber dam material (sheet), rubber dam template, rubber dam punch, clamps, clamp holding forceps and rubber dam frame (Fig. **5**).

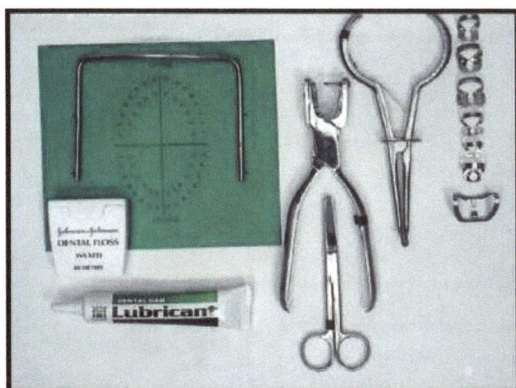

Fig. (5). Armamentarium of rubber dam.

Rubber dam sheet: The rubber dam sheet has a dull and shiny surface. The dull surface is placed facing the oral cavity as it reflects less light. It is available in varied sizes, colours, and thicknesses (Table 1).

Table 1. Varied sizes, colours, and thicknesses of rubber dam sheets.

Rubber Dam Sheets Size	Rubber Dam Colour	Rubber Dam Thickness
Pediatric sheets -5" x 5" inches (12.5 X 12.5 cms)	Light blue	Thin – 0.006" (0.15mm)
Adult sheets- 6" x 6" inches (15 X 15 cms)	Gray	Medium – 0.008" (0.20mm)
-	Green	Heavy – 0.010" (0.25mm)
-	-	Extra heavy – 0.012" (0.30mm)
-	-	Special heavy – 0.014" (0.35mm)

Newer Advances in Rubber Dam Sheets (Fig. 6A, B, C, D)

Hygienic Dental Dam

Is a non-latex rubber dam for patients with latex allergies. It is a powder-free, synthetic dam and comes in just one size, *i.e.*, 6 X 6 inches. It has a shelf life of 3 years and has the same tensile strength as that of a latex dam.

Derma Dam (Ultradent Products. Inc, USA)

Derma dam is also a non-latex dam that removes the possibility of latex reactions. It has a low content of surface proteins and has the advantage of having low dermatitis potential, reduced allergic reactions and greater tear resistance.

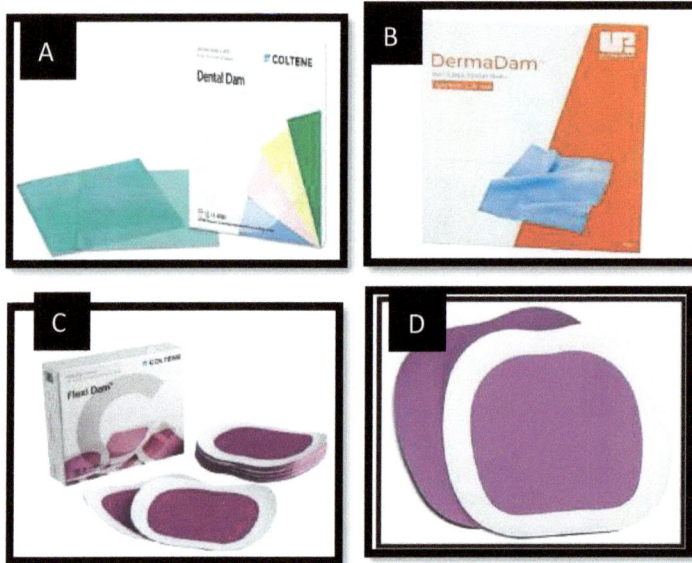

Fig. (6). A- Hygienic dental dam, B-Derma dam, C- Flexi dam, D- Preframed rubber dam sheets.

Flexi Dam (Coltene/Whaledent)

Flexi dam is an elastic non-latex dental dam made from an elastic plastomer. It can be elongated more than 1000% before tearing. It is more tenacious than a latex dam and is simple to place. The punched hole is smaller than normally used for latex dam and it needs to be stretched before use.

Pre-framed Rubber Dam Sheets

They have been introduced recently in which individual rubber dam sheets are attached to modified frames. They are easy to use and remove as the rubber dam and holder are applied as a single unit, are comfortable for the patient, and are less time-consuming.

Rubber Dam Template

It serves as a guide for marking the correct location of the tooth/teeth to be isolated on the am sheet (Fig. 7).

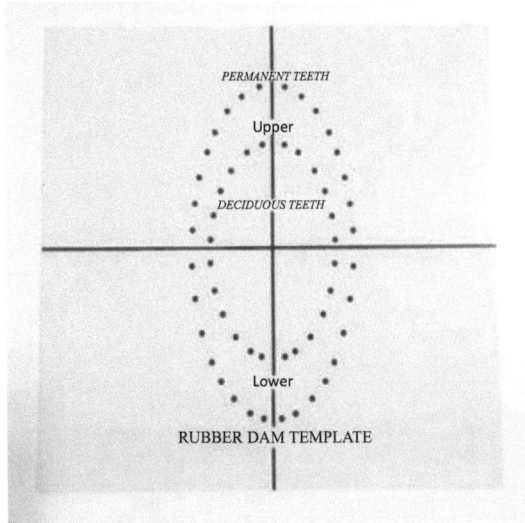

Fig. (7). Rubber dam template.

Rubber Dam Punch (Fig. 8)

The rubber dam punch usually consists of a rotating punch plate that consists of five or six holes of varied sizes and a metal point (punch) that creates the holes. The larger holes are used for posterior teeth, smaller holes for premolars and canines and the smallest holes for incisors. Rubber dam punch is of three types:

Ainsworth Type Punch (Fig. 8a)

It has two jaws. Lower jaw incorporates a rotating metal wheel with six holes, which allows selection of different hole sizes whereas the upper jaw has a tapered, sharp-pointed plunger.

Ivory Type Punch (Fig. 8b

It has a self- cantered coned piston /punch point that prevents partially punched holes. It has a hole plate with six openings ranging in size from 1-2 mm.

Ash Pattern Punch (Fig. 8c)

It has only one hole and is usually adequate for most situations. In ash pattern punch jaw can be removed and replaced at minimal cost if they are damaged.

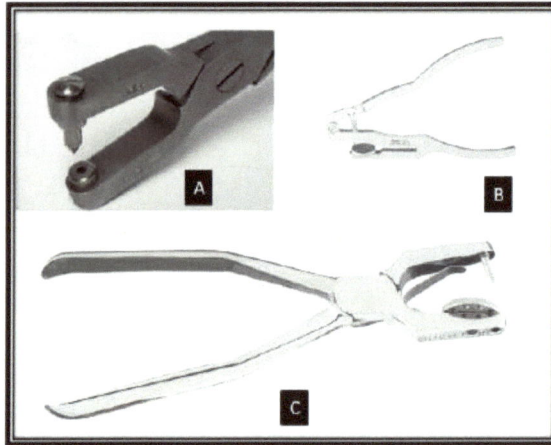

Fig. (8). Different types of rubber dam punch.

Rubber dam clamps: It is used to maintain a snug fit of the rubber dam around the neck of the tooth. These clamps are made of spring steel and are available in various sizes to fit the contours of different teeth. Clamps commonly used in paediatric dentistry are the #2, #4, #8A and #14A.

Parts of a clamp/retainer: Bow, Jaw, Prongs, and wings.

Clamps are of two types (Fig. **9**): wingless (Fig. **9A**) and Winged (Fig. 9B **9B**).

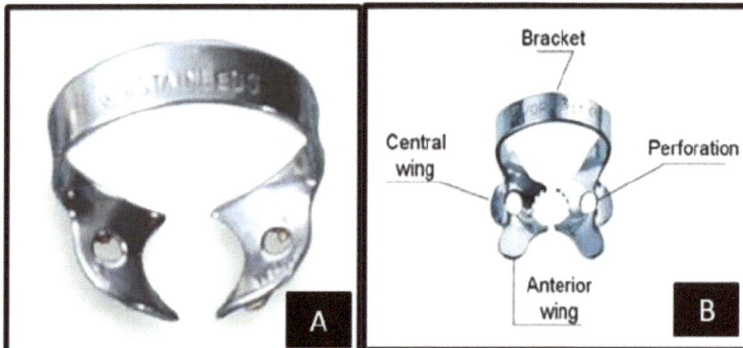

Fig. (9). Type of clamps; **A**- Wingless clamp, **B**- Winged clamp.

Wingless clamps are the clamps having 'W' prefixes, such as the #W8A or W3; which indicate that the clamps are without wings on the outer portions opposite the holes.

The most used clamps (Fig. **10**) are:

- Front teeth - IVORY # 6, IVORY # 9, IVORY # 90N, IVORY # 212S, IVORY # 15
- Premolars - IVORY # 1, IVORY # 2, IVORY # 2A
- Molars that are incompletely erupted or already prepared for the full crown-IVORY # 7, IVORY # 14
- Asymmetrical molars, in particular the second and third IVORY # 10, IVORY # 11 IVORY # 12A, IVORY # 13A
- Wingless, to be used when the wings obstruct the working field -IVORY # W8AIVORY # 26N

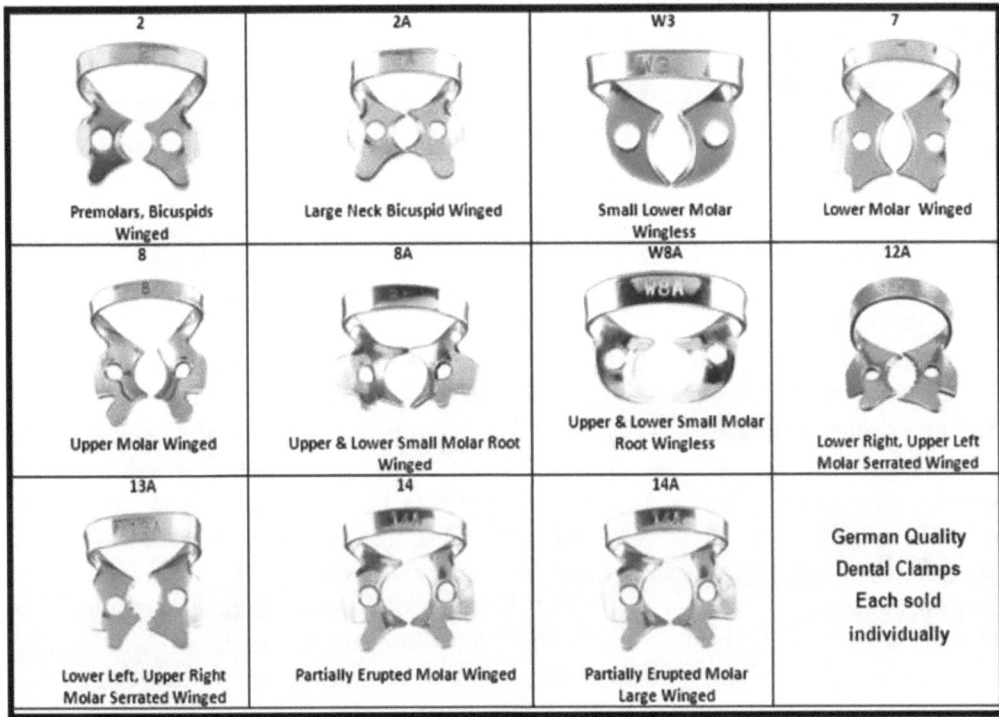

2	2A	W3	7
Premolars, Bicuspids Winged	Large Neck Bicuspid Winged	Small Lower Molar Wingless	Lower Molar Winged
8	**8A**	**W8A**	**12A**
Upper Molar Winged	Upper & Lower Small Molar Root Winged	Upper & Lower Small Molar Root Wingless	Lower Right, Upper Left Molar Serrated Winged
13A	**14**	**14A**	
Lower Left, Upper Right Molar Serrated Winged	Partially Erupted Molar Winged	Partially Erupted Molar Large Winged	German Quality Dental Clamps Each sold individually

Fig. (10). Different sizes of clamps used in Pediatric dentistry.

The clamps are secured with 18" dental floss to prevent accidental slipping and swallowing of the clamp. The space between the gripping edges of the clamp is narrower than the diameter of the corresponding tooth. Thus, to place the clamp around the tooth, it is necessary to spread the gripping edges wider than the tooth's diameter with a rubber dam clamp forceps.

Newer Advances in Rubber Dam Clamps (Fig. 11)

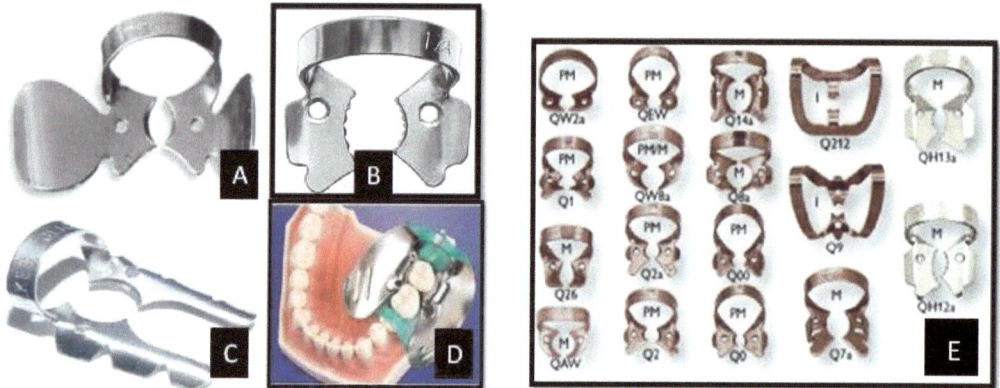

Fig. (11). A-Clamp with long guard extension, **B-** Tiger clamps, **C-** Silker-Glickman clamp, **D-**Super clamp, **E-**Gold coloured clamps.

- **Clamp with a long guard extension** has a larger wing which is used for retraction of the tongue. These clamps retract and protect the cheek and tongue along with isolation.
- **Tiger clamps** are clamps with serrated jaws. These serrations increase the stabilization of the clamp on the partially erupted or broken-down teeth.
- **Silker-Glickman clamp (S-G clamp)** is a clamp with an anterior extension that allows for retraction of the dam around a severely broken-down tooth. It is usually placed on a tooth proximal to the one being treated. It is made from durable cast stainless steel, which is autoclavable, corrosion-resistant, flexible, and long-lasting. It is an ideal clamp for molar isolation.
- **Super clamp** comes with a pre-cut rubber dam material designed to fit the clamp. It is very simple to use, quick and easy to place. It allows for easy evacuation of oral fluids with a saliva ejector or a high-volume evacuator, and also can be used without the rubber dam to protect the tongue and soft tissues. The clamp is made from thin, flexible stainless steel. It can be sterilized by autoclave, chemical ve or even dry heat. However, it has one disadvantage it cannot be used for anterior teeth. It comes in three sizes: L- large clamp for molars, M- medium clamp, which can also be used for molars and S- small clamp, which can be used for premolars.
- **Gold-coloured clamps** have diamond grit on their jaw to improve the retention of the clamp.

Rubber Dam Forceps (Fig. 12) [4]

They are designed in such a way that the two working ends of the forceps spread apart when the handles are closed. The working ends have small projections that fit into two corresponding holes on the rubber dam clamps. The area between the working end and the handle has a sliding lock device. This sliding lock device locks the handles in position while the operator places a rubber dam clamp.

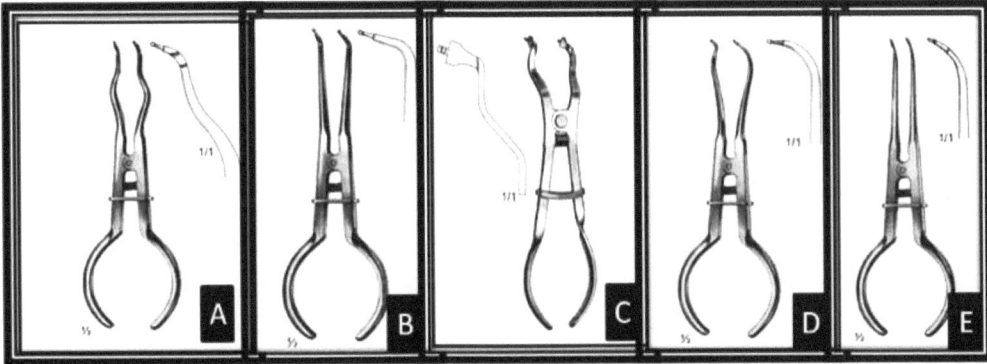

Fig. (12). Type of rubber dam forceps; **A**- Brewer 246-046, **B**-Stockes 246-047, **C**- Ivory 246-048, **D**-White 045-051, **E**- Plamer 046-052.

Rubber Dam Frame (Fig. 13)

It is used to secure the loose outer edges of the rubber dam sheet to have visibility and access to the tooth being treated [4].

Types of Rubber Dam Frame

- **Plastic frame:** Star visiframe and Nygard Ostby frame
- **Metallic frame**: Young rames
- **Pre-attached frames**: Handidam frames and Quick dam

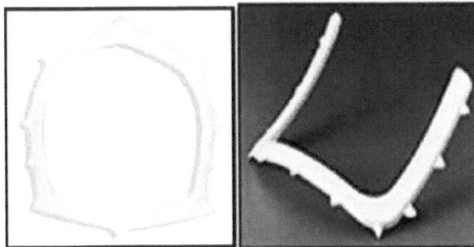

Fig. (13). Rubber dam frame.

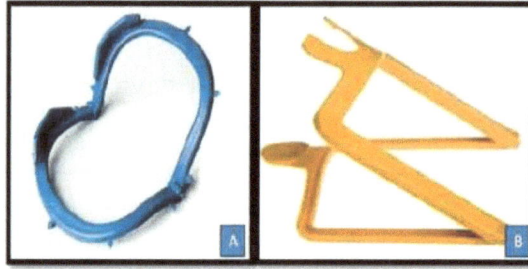

Fig. (14). A- Articulated frame, **B-** Safe T frame.

Modifications of Rubber Dam Frames

The Articulated Frame (Fig. 14a)

The articulated rubber dam frame (IRED, France) is made of non-irritant plastic material (polysulfone) currently used in the agro alimentary industry. A double hinge is situated in the vertical axis of the frame, which allows it to be folded in half in the vertical direction. A brace is situated at the bottom of the frame, allowing turning the dam sheet back on itself, creating a reservoir into which compresses, or an aspiration device may be placed. It has an advantage in providing access to the buccal half of the cavity. This accessibility facilitates proper positioning of the radiographic film, administration of additional local anaesthetic and evacuation of therapeutic liquids, which may have accidentally entered the buccal cavity. In addition to this, it has a reservoir at the bottom of the frame that allows the placement of gauze to compress and an aspiration cannula to avoid leakage of fluids such as sodium hypochlorite onto the patient's clothing.

Safe T- frame (Fig. 14b)

The Safe-T-frame (Sigma Dental Systems) is composed of two hinged frame members whose snap-shut locking mechanism securely clamps the rubber dam sheet in place. This concept also makes it possible to retain the traditional U-formed frame geometry and dimensions and offers a secure fit without stretching the rubber dam sheet. It also has a further advantage of raised edges of the frame, which provide a barrier around the sheet preventing fluids from escaping onto the patient. This contributes to greater patient comfort [4, 5].

Rubber Dam Placement and Removal (Figs. 15 and 16)

Before positioning the dam, it is advisable to lubricate the inner surfaces well with Vaseline so that the sheet will slide better over the contours of the teeth, easily overcome the contact areas, and close tightly around the cervix of the tooth. A rubber dam napkin **(Fig. 17)** is placed between the rubber sheet and the patient's cheek to absorb the saliva that accumulates beneath the dam. Their use is not mandatory; however, they are particularly indicated in cases of allergy to the rubber of the dam.

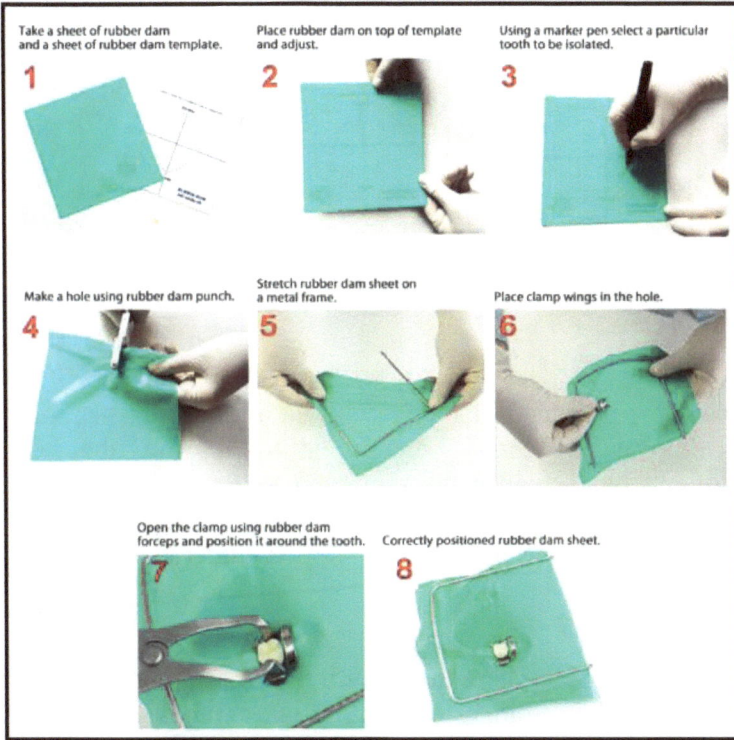

Fig. 15. Steps in rubber dam placement.

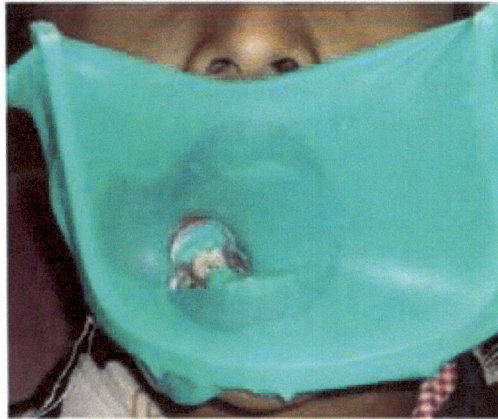

Fig. 16. Rubber dam in place.

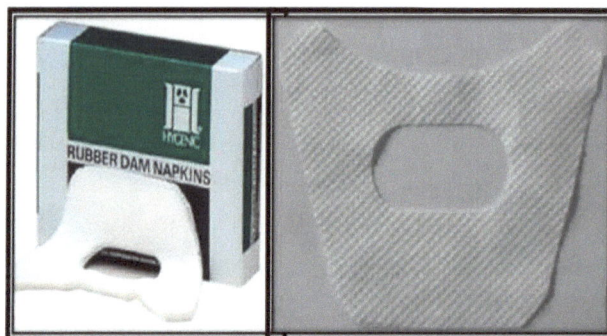

Fig. 17. Rubber dam napkin.

Recent Advances in Rubber Dam Isolation

Hat Dam

It is a clear plastic form shaped like a hat without a top; this is trimmed and fitted around a clinical crown that cannot be clamped, to hold the rubber dam in place. The cylinder of the hat replaces the damaged walls and the rim rests on the occlusal surface of the adjacent tooth. Once the 'hat' is cemented with glass ionomer, the rubber dam is punched and slipped under the rim of the hat.

In Dam (Zirc) (Fig. 18a)

Insti dam has an in-built flexible radiolucent nylon frame eliminating the need for a separate one. It is made of translucent natural latex that is very stretchable, tear-resistant and provides easy visibility. There is an off-centre pre-punched hole which customizes fit to any quadrant. More holes can be added if desired. Its compact design is just the right size to fit outside the patient 's lips.

Handi Dam (Fig. 18b)

Is a pre-framed rubber dam which eliminates the need for traditional frames. It is quick and easy to place. It allows easy access to the oral cavity during the root canal procedure.

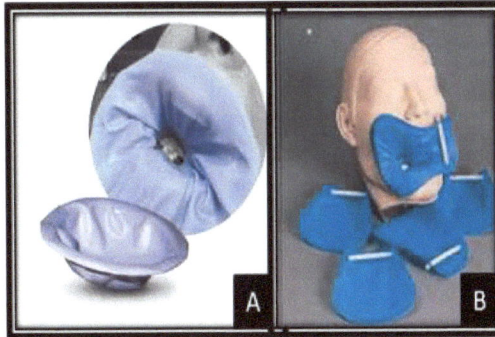

Fig. (18). A- Insti dam, B- Handi dam.

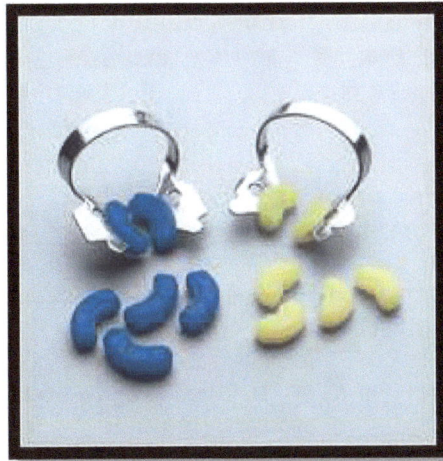

Fig. (19). Cushees.

Cushees (Fig. 19)

Cushees are soft thermoplastic cashew-shaped nodules which are grooved on their inner surface and function as rubber dam clamp cushions. It is slipped over the tooth attachment blade of the clamp before clamp application. It increases patient comfort through the elimination of contact of steel clamp with gingiva or tooth enamel and thus helps to protect the natural tooth structure and costly restorations. It also enhances the rubber dam seal to limit leaking from above or below the dam and reduces clamp slippage. They are sterilizable and reusable. They are available in two sizes: yellow for anterior and bicuspid clamps and blue for molar clamps.

Fibre Optic Clamps

In the illuminator system, the high-intensity light transilluminates the pulp chamber and canal orifices. Fibre optic plastic clamps are used with this system.

Liquid Dam

It is a resinous material applied on the gingival aspect of the tooth surface before power bleaching, sandblasting or other procedures requiring intraoral protection. It is also used to block out undercuts before taking an impression. Kool dam is the first heatless liquid dam uniquely formulated to eliminate the problems associated with paint on dam material. This does not produce heat when cured and remains flexible after curing [5 - 8].

Cleaning of Clamps [9]

Clamps should be rinsed and cleaned immediately after the procedure. Failure to clean will decrease the life of the clamp & can result in staining & corroding. It is important to remove excess restorative material from the clamp before sterilization as it may damage the clamp. The clamps should be autoclaved for 15 min at *130*130 °C/266 °F. Inspect the clamp for wear, distortion, or damage. Discard if distorted. Do not bend or distort the clamp. Do not let clamps get scratched by other clamps or instruments. When using obturation techniques involving sodium hypochlorite, immediately rinse clamps with water after the clamp is removed.

Errors In Application and Removal of Rubber Dam

- **Inappropriate retainer**: An appropriate retainer should maintain stable four-point contact with the anchor tooth. Retainer, if too small, results in an occasional breakage when the jaws are overspread.
  - **Retainer pinched tissue**: Jaws & prongs of the retainer usually slightly depress the tissues but should never pinch or impinge on them.
- **Shredded or torn dam**: Care should be taken to prevent tearing the dam during hole punching or passing the septa through contact.

INDIRECT METHODS OF ISOLATION

The above-described measures are either helpful in eliminating the collected moisture and saliva directly or aid in restricting the flow of saliva to the operating site. However, indirect methods are the ones that reduce the amount of salivation and thus aid indirectly in isolation.

Relaxed and Comfortable Position of the Patient

The patient should be comfortably seated in the dental chair. Care should be taken to keep the surroundings pleasant and relaxing. They should not be tensed at any time. All these aspects and the comforting attitude of the dental staff reduce the anxiety levels of the patient and aid in reducing salivation.

Local Anaesthesia

Local anaesthetics containing a vasoconstrictor such as Adrenaline reduces the procedural pain and salivation. It also reduces the discomfort associated with the treatment making the patient comfortable and less anxious. Another advantage is vasoconstriction which reduces haemorrhage at the operating site [10, 11].

Drugs

Drugs can reduce salivation but are rarely indicated. These drugs include:

Antisialogogoues

These are the drugs that reduce oral secretions. Premedication may be indicated using ant-cholinergic agents such as Atropine.

Anti-Anxiety Agents and Sedatives

Premedication with these drugs is quite helpful in apprehensive patients. Avoid psychological dependence on these drugs; they should be given only for short periods and to selected patients [8 - 12].

CONCLUSION

Thorough knowledge of the preliminary procedures reduces the physical strain on the dental team associated with the daily dental treatment, reduces patient anxiety associated with dental procedures & enhances moisture control, thereby improving the quality of operative dentistry. The time it takes to achieve good isolation will pay itself forward exponentially in time as well as in the quality of treatment and reduction of stress. Good isolation will preserve tooth structure, prevent contamination of the field, provide better visibility, and prevent iatrogenic misadventures

CONSENT FOR PUBLICATION

Not applicable.

CONFLICT OF INTEREST

The authors declare no conflict of interest, financial or otherwise.

ACKNOWLEDGEMENT

Declared none.

REFERENCES

[1]   Ammann P, Kolb A, Lussi A, Seemann R. Influence of rubber dam on objective and subjective parameters of stress during dental treatment of children and adolescents - a randomized controlled clinical pilot study. Int J Paediatr Dent 2013; 23(2): 110-5.
[http://dx.doi.org/10.1111/j.1365-263X.2012.01232.x] [PMID: 22404253]

[2]   Alhareky MS, Mermelstein D, Finkelman M, Alhumaid J, Loo C. Efficiency and patient satisfaction with the Isolite system versus rubber dam for sealant placement in pediatric patients. Pediatr Dent 2014; 36(5): 400-4.
[PMID: 25303507]

[3]   Abrams RA, Drake CW, Segal MS, Alhareky H. Barnum and the invention of the rubber dam. Gen Dent 1982; 30: 320-2.

[4]   Alqarni MA, Mathew VB, Alsalhi IY, *et al.* Rubber dam isolation in clinical adhesive dentistry: The prevalence and assessment of associated radiolucencies. J Dent Res Rev 2019; 6: 97-101.
[http://dx.doi.org/10.4103/jdrr.jdrr_81_19]

[5]   Terry DA. An essential component of adhesive dentistry. The Rubber Dam. Pract Proced Aesthet Dent 2005; 17: 106-8.

[6]   Al-Sabri FA, Elmarakby AM, Hassan AM. Attitude and knowledge of isolation in operative field among undergraduate dental students. Eur J Dent 2017; 11(1): 083-8.
[http://dx.doi.org/10.4103/ejd.ejd_191_16] [PMID: 28435371]

[7]   Hill EE, Rubel BS. Do dental educators need to improve their approach to teaching rubber dam use? J Dent Educ 2008; 72(10): 1177-81.
[http://dx.doi.org/10.1002/j.0022-0337.2008.72.10.tb04596.x] [PMID: 18923098]

[8]   Anabtawi MF, Gilbert GH, Bauer MR, *et al.* Rubber dam use during root canal treatment. J Am Dent Assoc 2013; 144(2): 179-86.
[http://dx.doi.org/10.14219/jada.archive.2013.0097] [PMID: 23372134]

[9]   Barros de Campos PR, Maia RR, Rodrigues de Menezes L, Barbosa IF, Carneiro da Cunha A, da Silveira Pereira GD. Rubber dam isolation-key to success in diastema closure technique with direct composite resin. Int J Esthet Dent 2015; 10(4): 564-74.
[PMID: 26794052]

[10]   Csinszka KIA, Monica M, Mihai P, Aurita A-S, Angela B, Angela B. Prevalence of rubber dam usage among dental practitioners and final year students in Tirgu Mures: A questionnaire survey. Acta Med Marisiensis 2015; 61(3): 188-91.
[http://dx.doi.org/10.1515/amma-2015-0059]

[11]   Awooda E, Alwan M. Knowledge, attitudes and practice of rubber dam use among dentists working in private clinics in Khartoum city. Saudi J Oral Dent Res 2016; 1: 19-23.

[12]   Zou H, Li Y, Lian X, Yan Y, Dai X, Wang G. frequency and influencing factors of rubber dam usage in Tianjin: a questionnaire survey. Int J Dent 2016; 2016: 1-7.
[http://dx.doi.org/10.1155/2016/7383212] [PMID: 27555870]

CHAPTER 7

Space Management

M.H. Raghunath Reddy[1,*], H. Sharath Chandra[2] and Clins Thankachan[3]

[1] *Professor and Head, Department of Paediatric and Preventive Dentistry, SJM Dental College and Hospital, Chitradurga, Karnataka, India*

[2] *Reader, Department of Paediatric and Preventive Dentistry, SJM Dental College and Hospital, Chitradurga, Karnataka, India.*

[3] *Research Officer, Royal Dental College, Chalissery, Kerala, India*

Abstract: Deciduous teeth play a significant role in the normal development of occlusion, as a guide for the eruption of permanent successors. Early loss of deciduous teeth in the primary and mixed dentition stage alters the integrity of dental arches and is one of the main causes of malocclusion in permanent dentition. Management of space created by early loss of the deciduous tooth is important to prevent or intercept malocclusion, either by eliminating the need for orthodontic correction in future or to reduce the complexity of correction in permanent dentition. Hence, the role of paediatric dentistry is immense in space management as a part of managing developing dentition and occlusion in comprehensive oral health care of children.

Keywords: Deciduous teeth, Malocclusion, Space maintainers, Space management, Space regainers.

INTRODUCTION

In the growth and development of a child, primary dentition plays a pivotal role as it aids in mastication, speech, and prevention of deleterious oral habits and also guides the eruption of succedaneous teeth. It is imperative to preserve the primary dentition till its normal physiological exfoliation time by preventive measures, restorative or endodontic treatments since they act as natural space maintainers. But the proximal carious or premature loss of primary teeth leads to arch length reduction by migration of adjacent teeth resulting in malocclusion in the permanent dentition. This malocclusion can be seen as crowding, rotation, ectopic eruption or impaction of the succedaneous tooth, supra eruption of opposing tooth and dental midline shift [1, 2] (**Figs. 1** and **2 a, b**).

---

* **Corresponding author M.H. Raghunath Reddy:** Department of Paediatric and Preventive Dentistry, SJM Dental College and Hospital, Chitradurga, Karnataka, India; E-mail: pedoreddy@gmail.com

Satyawan Damle, Ritesh Kalaskar & Dhanashree Sakhare (Eds.)
All rights reserved-© 2023 Bentham Science Publishers

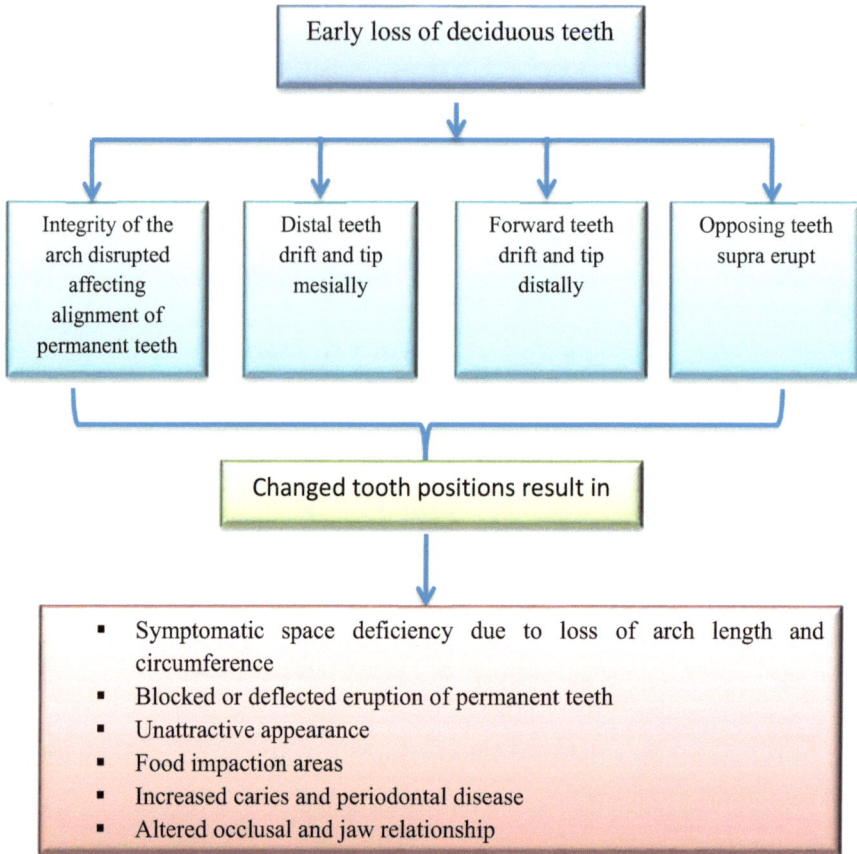

Fig. (1). Sequelae of early loss of the deciduous tooth.

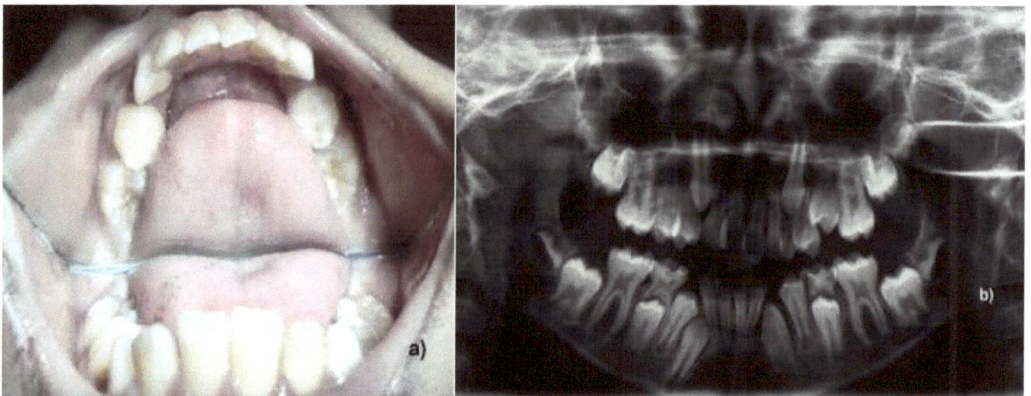

Fig. (2). a. Early bilateral loss of the deciduous first molar leads to space loss and a decrease in arch length. **b.** OPG of mixed dentition stage with a decrease in arch length resulting in inadequate space for the first premolar in the fourth quadrant.

Reasons for Premature Loss of Deciduous Teeth

- Early childhood caries
- Trauma
- Failure of endodontic treatment of deciduous tooth

Consequences of Early Loss of Deciduous Teeth

Space management of developing dentition is an important consideration in planning comprehensive paediatric oral care, thus preventing loss of arch length and obviating complex orthodontic corrections in the future. According to the American Academy of Paediatric Dentistry guidelines, the main aim of space management is to prevent arch length, arch perimeter and arch width by maintaining relative positions of existing dentition [2].

Definition: Space management is defined as the measures that diagnose and prevent or intercept situations, so as to guide the development of dentition and occlusion.

Space management includes four sub-stages (Fig. **3**).

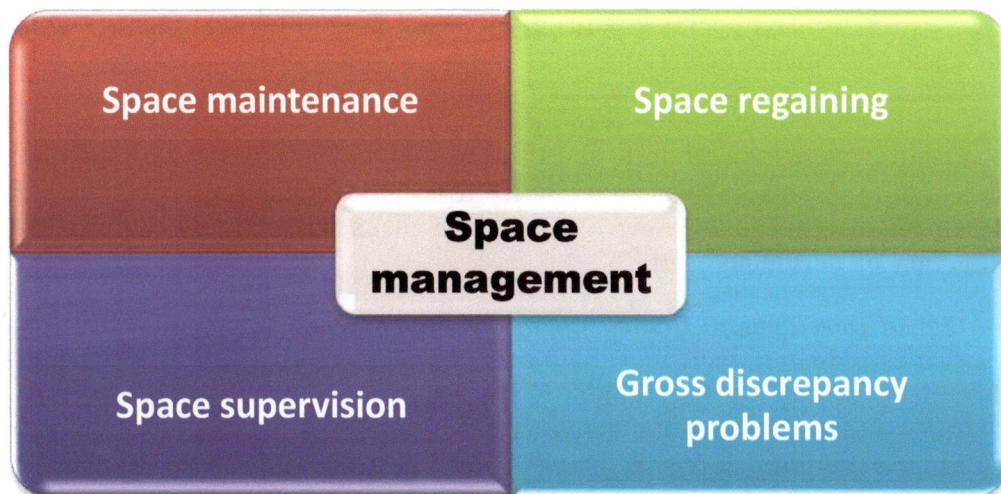

Fig. (3). Sub stages of Space management.

Objectives of Space Management

- a. Maintain the integrity of dental arches
- b. Maintain primate spaces
- c. Maintain normal occlusal plane
- d. Proper phonetics and esthetics in case of anterior space management

Space Maintenance

It is defined as the provision of an appliance (active or passive) which is concerned only with the control of space loss without taking into consideration, measures to supervise the development of the dentition.

Space Maintainers

It can be defined as appliances used to maintain space or regain a minor amount of space lost, so as to guide the unerupted tooth into a proper position in the arch.

The most effective way to prevent space loss occurring by early loss of the deciduous tooth is to give space maintainer, which is a kind of passive occlusal guidance, thus aiding in normal exchange of primary to the permanent dentition in their proper positions [4].

OWEN put forth certain factors for consideration before planning space maintainers after the early loss of deciduous tooth

1) Incidence of space loss: Arch length decreases with premature loss of deciduous molars, and the loss depends on the tooth involved and the time taken. Arch length decrease occurs as a result of mesial migration of permanent molars and distal movement of anterior teeth.

2) Time elapsed since space loss: Maximum space loss occurs in the first 6 months of deciduous tooth loss, and this tendency is more in the maxillary arch compared to the mandibular arch. Hence if a clinical situation necessitates the placement of space maintainer, it should be placed as early as possible post extraction of deciduous teeth.

3) Stage of Development/Dental Age of the Patient: Significant amount of space is lost if early loss of deciduous tooth occurs before or during the active eruption of the permanent first molar. Similarly, space loss occurs due to distal movements of primary canines during the active eruption of the permanent lateral incisors resulting in midline shift and lingual collapse of the anterior segment in the mandibular arch, thereby increasing overbite.

4) Amount of space closure: Severity of space loss is high if the primary tooth is lost during the active eruption stage of the permanent first molar, irrespective of which primary molar is lost or arch of loss. After the permanent molar has erupted and occlusion is established, the amount of space loss is more for deciduous second molar loss compared to the first molar (Fig. **4**).

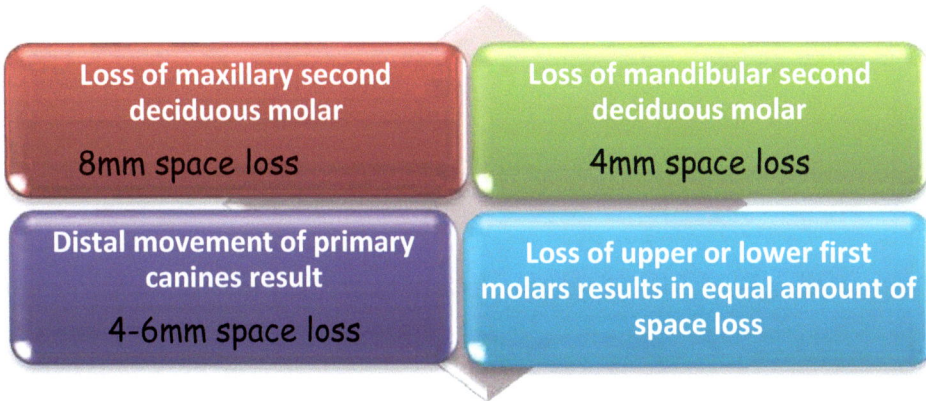

Loss of maxillary second deciduous molar	Loss of mandibular second deciduous molar
8mm space loss	4mm space loss
Distal movement of primary canines result	Loss of upper or lower first molars results in equal amount of space loss
4-6mm space loss	

Fig. (4). Amount of space closure.

5) Direction of Space Closure: In the maxillary posterior region, space closure occurs mainly by mesial bodily movement and mesiolingual rotation of the permanent first molar. In the mandibular arch, space closure occurs by mesial tipping of the permanent first molar along with retroclination and distal movement of teeth anterior to edentulous space (Figs. **5 a,b**).

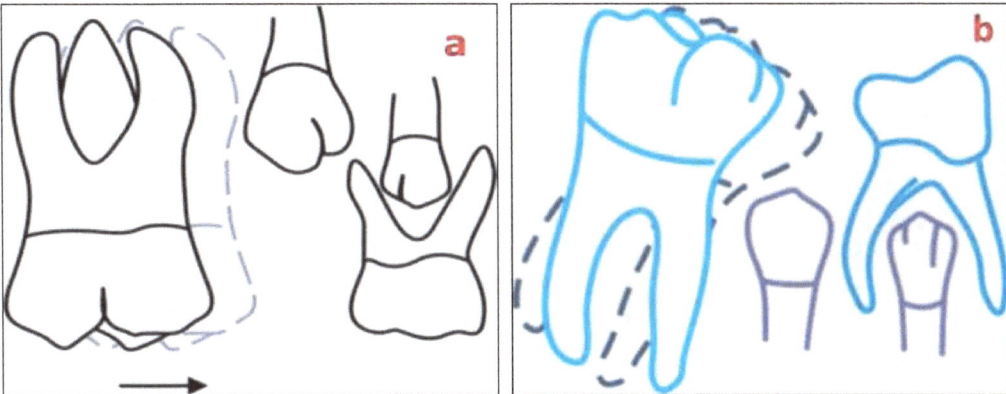

Fig. (5). a. Dotted lines indicate bodily movement of the permanent first molar in maxilla after early loss of deciduous tooth; **b.** Dotted lines indicate mesial tipping of the permanent first molar in mandible after early loss of deciduous tooth.

6) Eruption timing of permanent successors: Irrespective of the child's chronological age, permanent teeth usually erupt when three fourth of the root formation is completed. Timing of the eruption might alter based on developmental status, bone density in the area of eruption and the nature of early tooth loss.

> **Mickey mantle rule:**
>
> If the primary tooth is lost before 7 years of age, eruption of permanent successors might be delayed whereas if it is lost after 7 years of age, eruption of permanent successors is accelerated.

The magnitude of delay in eruption depends on the age at which the deciduous tooth is lost.

> If the loss occurs at 4 years of age, eruption of successor might be delayed by around 1 year with emergence at root completion and if the loss occurs at 6 years of age, eruption might be delayed by around 6 months with emergence at nearing root completion.

Eruption of permanent successor is accelerated if the deciduous tooth is lost within 6-12 months of normal exfoliation time. If the succedaneous tooth is impacted or deviated from the path of eruption, a delay in eruption occurs.

7) Amount of Bone Covering the Non-erupted Tooth: As a guide, to move through 1mm of bone as measured in bitewing radiograph, the erupting premolar would take 4-6 months. But if the bone covering is destroyed by infection, the eruption of the tooth is accelerated.

8) Abnormal Oral Musculature: After the early loss of deciduous teeth, distal drifting of anterior dental segment and collapse of the lower dental arch occurs as a result of strong mentalis activity and also by oral habits like thumb or digit sucking.

9) Congenital Absence of Permanent Teeth: The presence of permanent teeth must be ensured before planning space maintainer treatment. If in case of congenitally missing permanent tooth, based on the clinical situation, the paediatric dentist should decide whether to maintain the space till the permanent prosthesis is placed or to orthodontically close the space.

Ideal Requirements of Space Maintainers

a. Maintain mesiodistal dimension of prematurely lost deciduous teeth.
b. Prevent mesial migration of buccal segment and lingual collapse of anterior segments.

c. It should not interfere with masticatory function.
d. Easy to maintain and cleanable without causing soft tissue irritation or dental caries.
e. It should be easy to construct and durable, strong, and stable.
f. Should not deflect or inhibit normal changes in growth.
g. Prevent supra eruption of opposing tooth.
h. Improve esthetics and should aid in a speech in the case of anterior space maintainers.
i. It should not exert any force on the remaining tooth causing orthodontic movement, hence it should be passive [3].

Indications

- After the early loss of the deciduous tooth, the space shows signs of closing.
- If space analysis indicates positive arch length or space deficiency of 1-2mm per quadrant, holding space by maintainers would prevent malocclusion.

Contraindications

- Absence of succedaneous tooth.
- When two-thirds of the root formation of the succedaneous tooth is formed.
- Space left after premature loss of the deciduous tooth is more than the space required for a succedaneous tooth.
- Radiographically, no alveolar bone covering above the succedaneous tooth, but it should be non-pathologic.

CLASSIFICATION OF SPACE MAINTAINERS

Space maintainers are classified in different ways (Figs. **6a, b, c**).

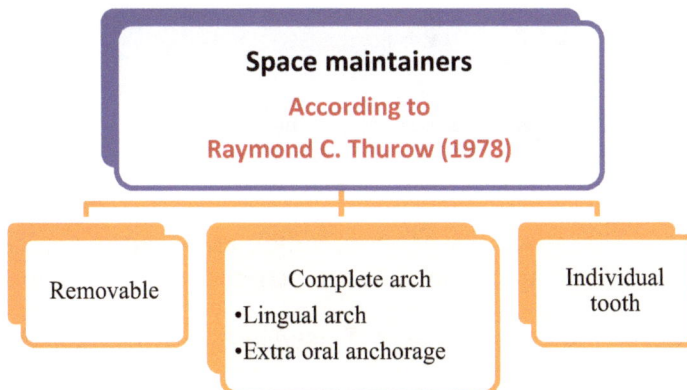

Fig. (6a). Classification Space maintainers according to Raymond C. Thurow.

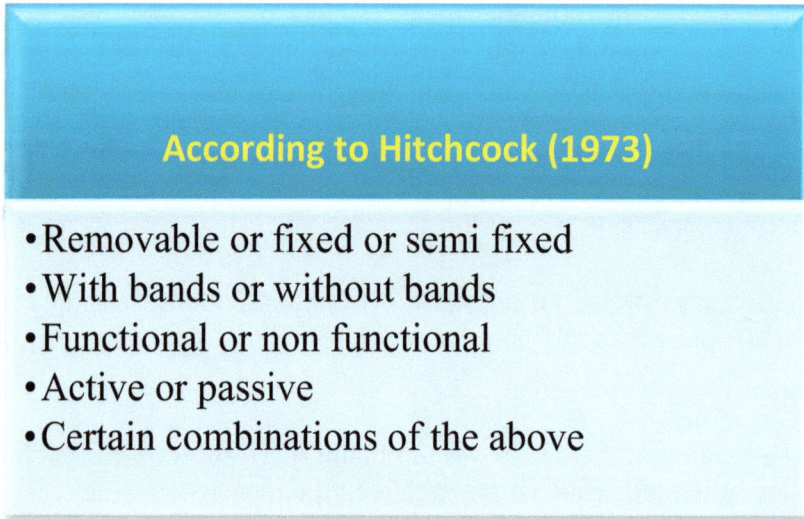

According to Hitchcock (1973)

- Removable or fixed or semi fixed
- With bands or without bands
- Functional or non functional
- Active or passive
- Certain combinations of the above

Fig. (6b). Classification Space maintainers according to Hitchcock.

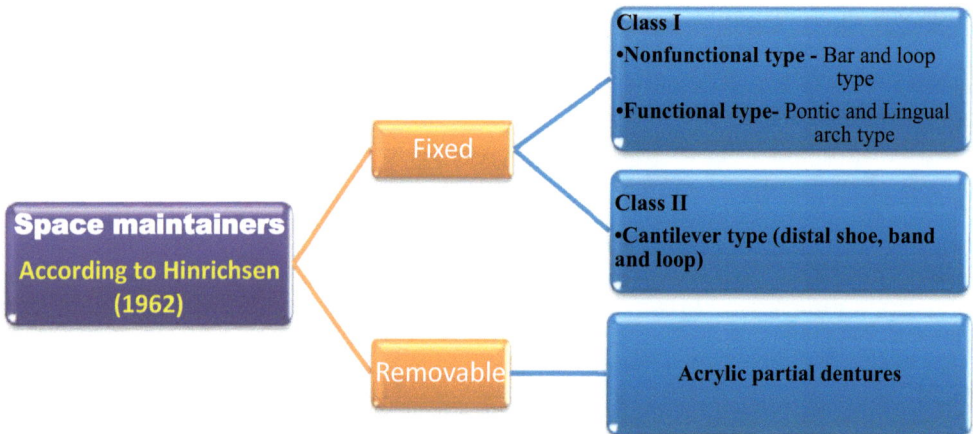

Fig. (6c). Classification of Space maintainers according to Hinrichsen.

Fixed Space Maintainers

These are the kind of space maintainers which are fixed to the abutment tooth with bands or crown and are not intended to be removed by the patient.

Various advantages and disadvantages of fixed space maintainers (Fig. **7**) [2].

Advantages

- Best suited for uncooperative patient.
- Jaw growth is not effected.
- Succedaneous tooth can be guided to its position.
- If pontic is placed it can restore function.
- Does not interfere with passive eruption of abutment tooth.
- Bands placed do not require any tooth preparation.
- Minimum preparation.

Disadvantages

- Decalcification of tooth under the band.
- Caries of tooth at the line of tooth.
- Plaque accumulation.
- Supra erution of opposing tooth.
- Extensive instrumentation and labraotary procedure requiring high amount of skill.

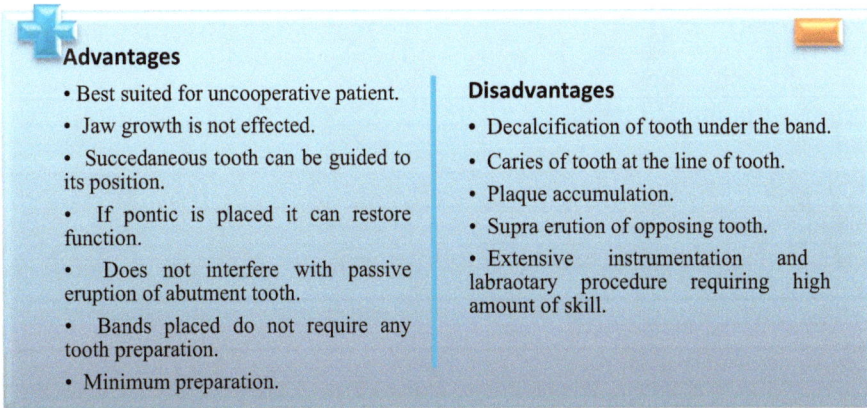

Fig. (7). Advantages and disadvantages of fixed space maintainers.

Fabrication of Fixed Space Maintainers

It involves the following steps

a. Banding procedure
b. Recording impression and preparing working model
c. Loop/archwire fabrication
d. Soldering procedure
e. Finishing and polishing
f. Cementation of the appliance
g. Patients follow up

Banding Procedure

In the fabrication of a fixed space maintainer, the band is an important part that should be strong, well contoured and properly fitting. Various types of bands include Loop bands, Custom made bands and Prefabricated seamless bands; made of chrome alloy or precious metal.

Ideal Requirements of the Band

- No occlusal interference.
- Should not extend more than 0.5-1mm subgingivally.
- Resist deformation under stress.
- Fit contours of the tooth closely.
- Tarnish resistance.
- Armamentarium Required.

- Separator placement plier
- Band material (Table **1**).
- Johnson contouring plier
- Howe pliers straight and curved
- Peak pliers
- Double beak pliers
- Band crimping pliers
- Oliver jones posterior band removing plier
- Band cutting scissors
- Mershon Band pusher
- Nylon band seater (Fig. **8**)
- Heatless stone and finishing burs
- Spot welder unit

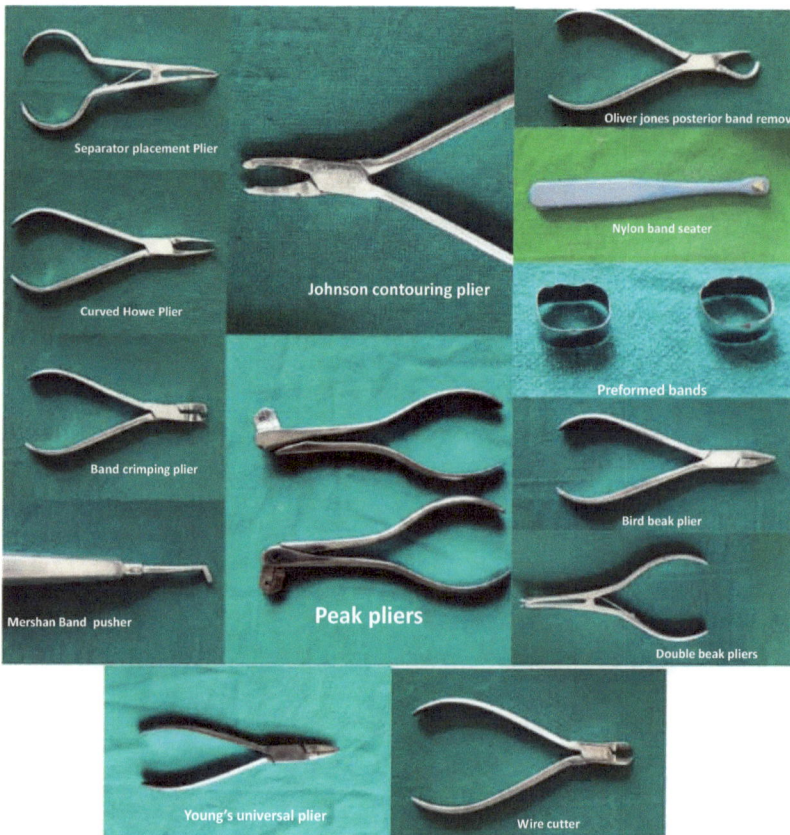

Fig. (8). Armamentarium for fabrication of fixed space maintainers.

Table 1. Different thicknesses of bands used for teeth.

Tooth	Thickness	Width	Length
Anterior	0.003 inches	0.125 inches	2 inches
Bicuspids	0.004 inches	0.150 inches	2 inches
Primary molars	0.005 inches	0.180 inches	2 inches
Permanent molars	0.006 inches	0.180 inches	2 inches

Recommended Thickness of Band Material for Different Teeth

Steps in Banding: Direct Method

1. Separators are placed interdentally if the contact of the tooth to be banded is too tight with the adjacent tooth.
2. Suitable band material is selected, and the required length is cut with band cutting scissors. Dull surface of the band should face the tooth side, and the shiny surface should be outside.
3. Two free ends of the band are formed into a loop and spot welded. Sharp edges at the joint should be rounded to prevent hurting the soft tissues.
4. Band is contoured at incisogingival and occlusogingival ends using Johnsons contouring plier. Then the band is placed on the tooth and trial pinched at the cuspal area rather than the groove area, as it will be difficult to adapt double thickness band to the grooves later.
5. Excess band should be marked on the buccal and lingual part and is trimmed, tried again in the mouth. Mesially and distally, it should be just below the marginal ridge (1mm) and just above the contact area.
6. With Howe plier, the band is placed on the tooth as far as possible till it goes comfortably with tails of the band in the plier. Seam of the bands is now closer and is spot welded at 3 or 4 spots.
7. Festooning of bands is done on the cervical area proximally. Level of the band at the marginal ridge is also adjusted. Proximal festooning is blended with buccal and lingual cervical parts of the band by trimming burs.
8. Final pinching is done with peak piers or double beak pier by holding the band firmly in its position with finger pressure on the buccal side.
9. Band is removed and the new contact that is formed is spot welded, cutting the excess off leaving a small remnant.
10. ***Folded flap method:*** Band is placed on the tooth and the remnant band is folded against the lingual surface of the tooth distally. Then this seam is spot welded together. Sharp edges are trimmed and the band is polished.
11. Band is refitted on the tooth. Extensions of the band should be

○ Occlusally, band margins should be slightly below the proximal ridges (1mm).

○ Gingival, band margins should extend 0.5 to 1mm into the gingival sulcus. It can be checked by signs of blanching and can be relieved if seen.

○ Buccally, band margins position should be just below the level where the opposing cusps touch the grooves.

○ Lingually, the position should be just below the deepest portion of the lingual developmental groove.

Indirect Method

Banding is done on the cast providing faster and more efficient results.

b) Recording impression and preparing working model:

Pinched and adapted band is placed on the tooth and the impression is recorded. Band is removed from the tooth with band remover, transferred to the impression and stabilised.

Stabilisation is done by various methods:

a. Orthodontic wires
b. Sticky wax
c. L shape orthodontic wire
d. Stapler pins
e. Superglue
f. Bobby pins
g. Greenstick compound

After stabilisation working model is prepared with dental stone.

c) Loop/archwire fabrication

- Stainless steel wire (0.036 to 0.040 inches)
- Wire cutter
- Three prong plier
- Bird beak plier/ universal plier
- Each space maintainer requires a different design which can be fabricated with the above armamentarium.

d) Soldering:

Quick setting plaster or asbestos putty is used to stabilise the wire component over the band on the working model. Borax flux is applied above and below the solder joint, heated to melt and increase the flow of the flux. Once flux melts 3-4 mm length, solder is placed at the solder joint and flame is directed at solder. It should flow smoothly, covering the wire forming a solid union with band and wire. Soldering flame in the reducing zone should be used which is 3mm beyond the blue zone. After soldering is completed, appliance is quenched.

e) Finishing and polishing:

Heating process decreases the hardness of the stone and the appliance can be easily removed from the stone. Remnants of stone are removed, solder joint is contoured to the band, surface roughness is reduced with rubber wheels and polishing is done with cold rouge on rag wheel. The acrylic button of the Nance appliance is trimmed, smoothened and polished.

ESSENTIAL STEPS IN PLANNING SPACE MANAGEMENT

a. Complete clinical examination
b. Diagnostic data from IOPA radiographs, OPG, clinical pictures, diagnostic models
c. Determining of tooth development stage
d. Determining tooth size and available space
e. Growth prediction and future occlusal relationship.

Mixed Dentition Analysis

Dental diagnostic models are important aids in planning space management which helps to visualize dentition in all three dimensions. It also helps in taking necessary measurements of teeth, dental arches and basal bone to do model analysis.

Mixed dentition analysis helps to determine space available for permanent dentition and space required for its eruption and determine whether to plan for active or passive occlusal guidance space maintenance.

In mixed dentition analysis, it is imperative to know the mesiodistal width of teeth anterior to the first molar, arch perimeter and changes that occur during growth and development. Mesiodistal dimensions of mandibular incisors are considered as a standard index to determine the size of an unerupted tooth as they have the least morphological variations [5].

Various Mixed Dentition Analyses Include

a. Moyers analysis

b. Huckaba analysis
c. Hixon and Old father analysis
d. Staley Kerber analysis
e. Tanaka Johnson analysis
f. Nance method
g. Iowa prediction method for both arches
h. Ballard and Wylies analysis
i. Boston university prediction
j. Total space analysis.

Moyer's Mixed Dentition Analysis

It is a widely used mixed dentition analysis with less systemic error. This analysis is based on the fact that there is a significant correlation between different teeth in an individual, which helps in the prediction of the size of unerupted teeth based on teeth clinically present [5].

Procedure

It involves calculating the space available and space required from the probability chart based on mandibular permanent incisors. (Fig. **9**)

Greatest mesiodistal width of all four mandibular incisors is determined

Determine the amount of space required for alignment of maxillary and mandibulalr incisors

Space available for erupting cuspids and bicuspids is determined by measuring distance from distal aspect of aligned lateral inciosrs to mesial aspect of 1st permanent molar in maxillary and mandibular arches

Space required for erupting cuspids and bicuspids is deterimend by a probability chart using combined mesiodistal width of mandibular incisors. Probability chart is different for maxilla and mandible, males and females.

Fig. (9). Procedure for Moyers analysis.

Based on the combined mesiodistal width of mandibular incisors 21/12 and considering 75% probability, the space required for cuspids and bicuspids is determined from the probability chart (Tables **2a, b, c, d**). In maxillary arch, allowance for overjet correction should be considered when calculating space required for aligned incisors. If the available space is lesser than that of the predicted value, crowding can be expected.

Probability Chart for Predicting Unerupted Cuspids and Bicuspids

Table 2a. Probability chart for males for the mandibular arch.

21/12 %	19.5	20	20.5	21	21.5	22	22.5	23	23.5	24	24.5	25	25.5
95	21.6	21.8	22.0	22.2	22.4	22.6	22.8	23.0	23.2	23.5	23.7	23.9	24.2
85	20.8	21.0	21.2	21.4	21.6	21.9	22.1	22.3	22.5	22.7	23.0	23.2	23.4
75	20.4	20.6	20.8	21.0	21.2	21.4	21.6	21.9	22.1	22.3	22.5	22.8	23.0
65	20.0	20.2	20.4	20.6	20.9	21.1	21.3	21.5	21.8	22.0	22.2	22.4	22.7
50	19.5	19.7	20.0	20.2	20.4	20.6	20.9	21.1	21.3	21.5	21.7	22.0	22.2
35	19.0	19.3	19.5	19.7	20.0	20.2	20.4	20.67	20.9	21.1	21.3	21.5	21.7
25	18.7	18.9	19.1	19.4	19.6	19.8	20.1	20.3	20.5	20.7	21.0	21.2	21.4
15	18.2	18.5	18.7	18.9	19.2	19.4	19.6	19.9	20.1	20.3	20.5	20.7	20.9
5	17.5	17.7	18.0	18.2	18.5	18.7	18.9	19.2	19.4	19.6	19.8	20.0	20.2

Table 2b. Probability chart for females for the mandibular arch.

21/12 %	19.5	20	20.5	21	21.5	22	22.5	23	23.5	24	24.5	25	25.5
95	20.8	21.0	21.2	21.5	21.7	22.0	22.2	22.5	22.7	23.0	23.3	23.6	23.9
85	20.0	20.3	20.5	20.7	21.0	21.2	21.5	21.8	22.0	22.3	22.6	22.8	23.1
75	19.6	19.8	20.7	20.3	20.6	20.8	21.1	21.3	21.6	21.9	22.1	22.4	22.7
65	19.2	19.5	19.7	20.0	20.2	20.5	20.7	21.0	21.3	21.5	21.8	22.1	22.3
50	18.7	19.0	19.2	19.5	19.8	20.0	20.3	20.5	20.8	21.1	21.3	21.6	21.8
35	18.2	18.5	18.8	19.0	19.3	19.6	19.8	20.1	20.3	20.6	20.9	21.1	21.4
25	17.9	18.1	18.4	18.7	19.0	19.2	19.5	19.7	20.0	20.3	20.5	20.8	21.0
15	17.4	17.7	18.0	18.3	18.5	18.8	19.1	19.3	19.6	19.8	20.1	20.3	20.6
5	16.7	17.0	17.2	17.5	17.8	18.1	18.3	18.6	18.9	19.1	19.3	19.6	19.8

Table 2c. Probability chart for males for the maxillary arch.

21/12 %	19.5	20.0	20.5	21.0	21.5	22.0	22.5	23.0	23.5	24.0	24.5	25.0	25.5
95	21.2	21.4	21.6	21.9	22.1	22.3	22.6	22.8	23.1	23.4	23.6	23.9	24.1
85	20.6	20.9	21.1	21.3	21.6	21.8	22.1	22.3	22.6	22.8	23.1	23.3	23.6
75	20.3	20.5	20.8	21.0	21.3	21.5	21.8	22.0	22.3	22.5	22.8	23.0	23.3
65	20.0	20.3	20.5	20.8	21.0	21.3	21.5	21.8	22.0	22.3	22.5	22.8	23.0
50	19.7	19.9	20.2	20.4	20.7	20.9	21.2	21.5	21.7	22.0	22.0	22.5	22.7
35	19.3	19.5	19.9	20.1	20.4	20.6	20.9	21.1	21.4	21.6	21.9	22.1	22.4
25	19.1	19.3	19.6	19.9	20.1	20.4	20.6	20.9	21.1	21.4	21.6	21.9	22.1
15	18.8	19.0	19.3	19.6	19.8	20.1	20.3	20.6	20.8	21.1	21.3	21.6	21.8
5	18.2	18.5	18.8	19.0	19.3	19.6	19.8	20.1	20.3	20.6	20.8	21.0	21.3

Table 2d. Probability chart for females for the maxillary arch.

21/12 %	19.5	20.0	20.5	21.0	21.5	22.0	22.5	23.0	23.5	24.0	24.5	25.0	25.5
95	21.4	21.6	21.7	21.8	21.9	22.0	22.2	22.3	22.5	22.6	22.8	22.9	23.1
85	20.8	20.9	21.0	21.1	21.3	21.4	21.5	21.7	21.8	22.0	22.1	22.3	22.4
75	20.4	20.5	20.6	20.8	20.9	21.0	21.2	21.3	21.5	21.6	21.8	21.9	22.1
65	20.1	20.2	20.3	20.5	20.6	20.7	20.9	21.0	21.2	21.3	21.4	21.6	21.7
50	19.6	19.3	19.9	20.1	20.2	20.3	20.5	20.6	20.8	20.9	21.0	21.2	21.3
35	19.2	19.4	19.5	19.7	19.8	19.9	20.1	20.2	20.4	20.5	20.6	20.8	20.9
25	18.9	19.1	19.2	19.4	19.5	19.6	19.8	19.9	20.1	20.2	20.3	20.5	20.6
15	18.5	18.7	18.8	19.0	19.1	19.3	19.4	19.6	19.7	19.8	20.0	20.1	20.2
5	17.8	18.0	18.2	18.3	18.5	18.6	18.8	18.9	19.1	19.2	19.3	19.4	19.5

* Uppermost row indicates combined mesiodistal width of mandibular incisors (21/12). First column on the left side indicates the percentage of probability and rest of the column indicate the estimated value for a combined width of erupting cuspids and bicuspids. Generally, 75% probability is used for the determination of estimated value calculation.

b). Huckaba Analysis

- The width of unerupted cuspids and bicuspids is determined by the use of both radiographs as well as a study cast.
- As there will be a necessity to compensate for the enlargement produced in the radiographic image, measuring the teeth which are present both on the radiograph and cast for example primary molars, thus helping us to predict the

amount of enlargement in radiograph, in turn, helping us to measure the unerupted teeth.

• The accuracy of this method is fair and can be used on both arches.

Calculation: Y1=(X1×Y2)÷X2

X1 = Actual width of primary molar

X2 = Apparent width of primary molar

Y1 = Actual width of an unerupted premolar

Y2 = Apparent width of an unerupted premolar

c). Hixon and Old Father Method

Hixon and Old father in 1958 put forward a method to determine mesiodistal widths of mandibular canine and premolars in mixed dentition from participants in the Iowa facial growth study.

Method

• Measurement of mesiodistal width of mandibular central and lateral incisors is taken.
• Intraoral periapical radiograph is taken for premolars with paralleling technique, and the width of premolars is measured
• The sum of mesiodistal width of unerupted premolars is added to the already calculated mesiodistal width of the anterior teeth.
• Estimated value of the mesiodistal width of cuspids and bicuspids can be obtained from the standard chart.
• The measured sum must be correlated with the standard sum of the mesiodistal width in the chart. (Table 3) [5].

Table 3. Hixon and Old father standard chart to predict the width of canine and premolar.

Sum of mesiodistal width of mandibular incisors and sum of mesiodistal width of first and second premolar on the radiograph in the same quadrant	Predicted sum of mesiodistal widths of erupting canine and premolars (mm)
23	18.4
24	19.0
25	19.7
26	20.3
27	21.0

(Table 3) cont.....

Sum of mesiodistal width of mandibular incisors and sum of mesiodistal width of first and second premolar on the radiograph in the same quadrant	Predicted sum of mesiodistal widths of erupting canine and premolars (mm)
28	21.6
29	22.3
30	22.9

d). Staley and Kerber Analysis

It is a modification of the Hixon and Old Father method, in which separate equations were given for males and females to improve the results (Fig. **10**).

e). Tanaka and Johnston Analysis (1974)

This analysis is similar to Moyer's analysis but without a probability chart. It uses the mesiodistal width of erupted anterior teeth to predict the mesiodistal width of unerupted cuspids and bicuspids [5].

> *Estimated width of mandibular canine and premolars on one quadrant= Half the sum of mandibular incisors + 10.5 mm*
>
> *Estimated width of maxillary canine and premolars in one quadrant= Half the sum of mandibular incisors + 11 mm*

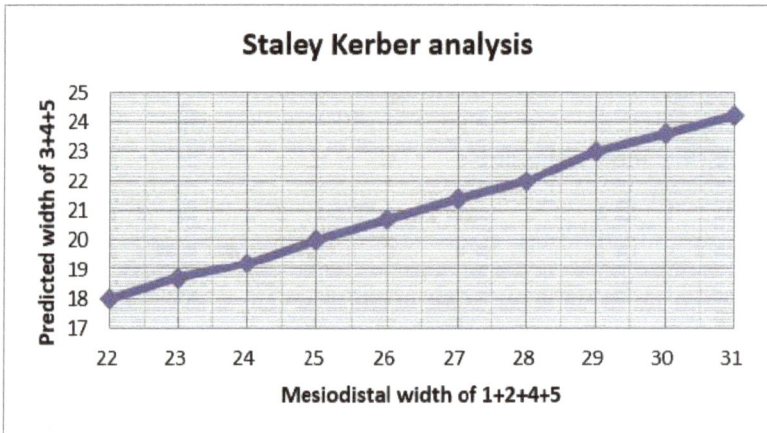

Fig. (10). Prediction graph of Staley Kerber analysis.

f). Nance Method

It is similar to arch perimeter analysis of permanent teeth.

The difference between space required and available will give arch length discrepancy (Fig. **11**).

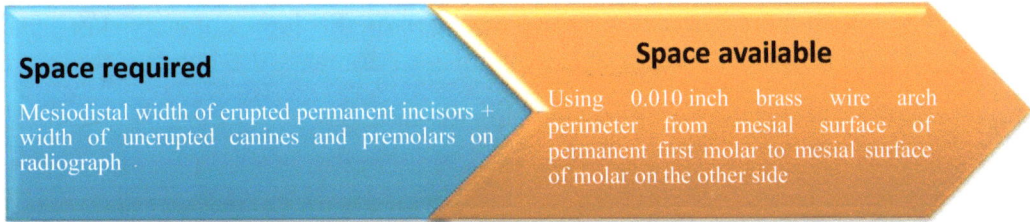

Space required	Space available
Mesiodistal width of erupted permanent incisors + width of unerupted canines and premolars on radiograph ·	Using 0.010 inch brass wire arch perimeter from mesial surface of permanent first molar to mesial surface of molar on the other side

Fig. (11). Nance analysis.

BAND AND LOOP SPACE MAINTAINER

It is the most common and widely used space maintainer, which is a fixed, unilateral, banded and non-functional space maintainer. With a simple cantilever design, it is best suited for maintaining space after unilateral posterior tooth loss [6].

Indications

• Premature loss of the first deciduous molar before or after the eruption of the first permanent molar.
• Premature loss of second deciduous molar after the eruption of the permanent first molar.
• Bilateral early loss of deciduous molar before the eruption of permanent incisors.
• The Period of space maintenance is short with the abutment tooth intact.
• Premature loss of canines.

Contraindications

• Crowded dental arches with already signs of space loss.
• Multiple tooth loss maintenance.
• Children with high caries risk.
• Premature loss of deciduous second molar without or partial eruption of the permanent first molar.

Construction

a) Banding and impression: Appropriate size of the band is selected or a custom fabricated band is pinched on tooth distal to edentulous space. Impression is taken and a working model is prepared with bands on the abutment tooth.

b) Design of the loop: Stainless steel wire of 0.036inch or 19-gauge wire is used to make the loop adapted parallel to the edentulous ridge but is 1mm away from the tissue. The buccolingual diameter of the loop should be more than the buccolingual dimension of the erupting tooth, approximately 8mm allowing succedaneous teeth to erupt freely. Mesial part of the loop contacts the distal surface of the primary canine and the distal part contacts the banded abutment tooth (Fig. **12**).

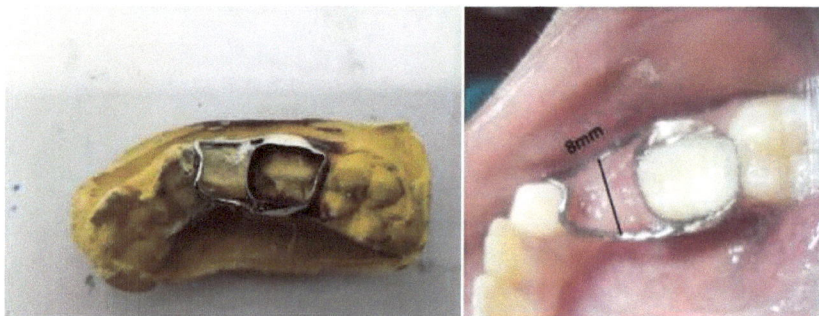

Fig. (12). Band and loop space maintainer.

c) Soldering, finishing and polishing of the appliance are done.

d) Cementation: Appliance is placed and checked for any impingement or occlusal interference. Cementation is done with luting cement, and periodic follow-up is done to examine for the eruption of the succedaneous tooth or any impingement of appliance on the soft tissue (Figs. **13 a, b**).

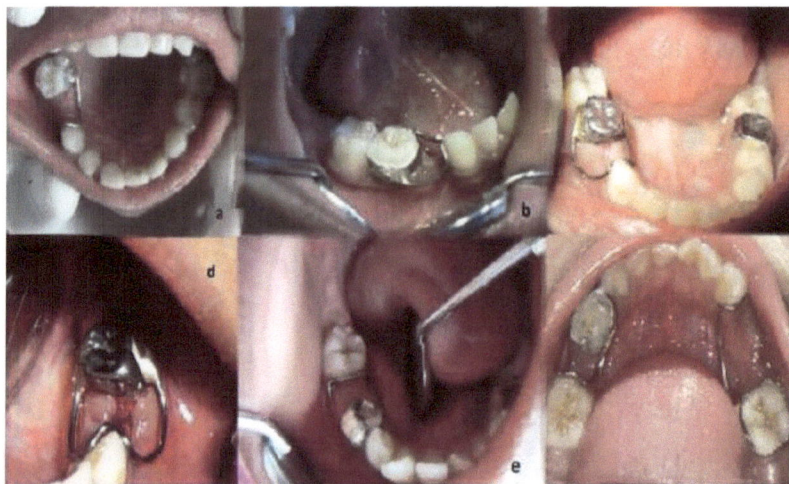

Fig. (13). a, **b**. Band and loop space maintainer, **c**. Crown band and loop, **d**. Crown and loop, **e**. Reverse crown and loop, **f**. Long band and loop on right side and reverse band and loop space maintainer on left side.

Modifications

a) Crown and loop space maintainer: It is similar to band and loop except that crown is placed on the abutment tooth due to various reasons like a hypoplastic tooth or multisurface caries or endodontically treated [7] (Figs. **13c, d**).

b) Mayne's space maintainer: It is similar to band and loop space maintainer, but the loop is made only on one side, which prevents hindrance to permanent successors eruption, but the stability of the appliance is less.

c) Band and bar: Tooth mesial and distal to edentulous space is banded; the bar is connected to both the bands instead of loop. This makes the appliance sturdier, but the bar might interfere with the eruption of the successor.

d) Reverse band and loop: If the tooth distal to the edentulous space cannot be banded due to partial eruption, the mesial tooth is banded and used as an abutment. Loop will extend distally from the mesial abutment. (Figs. **13e, f**)

e) Band and loop with occlusal rest: Band and loop appliance might sometimes slip gingivally, hence to prevent this, occlusal rest is given on the tooth mesial to edentulous space.

f) Long band and loop space maintainer: Used in case of unilateral early loss of deciduous first and second molar (Figs. **13f**).

g) Preformed loops: Different sizes of loops are available, which are selected according to the clinical situation. Minor changes are done and soldered to the band on the abutment tooth. It saves time as it is a single-sitting direct procedure.

Various advantages and disadvantages include (Fig. **14**) [4, 7].

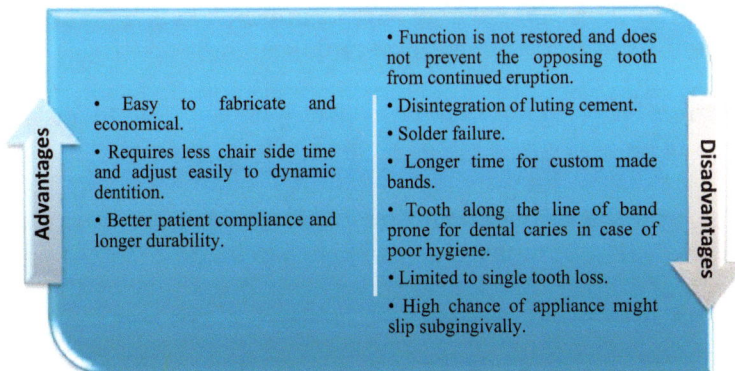

Advantages
- Easy to fabricate and economical.
- Requires less chair side time and adjust easily to dynamic dentition.
- Better patient compliance and longer durability.

Disadvantages
- Function is not restored and does not prevent the opposing tooth from continued eruption.
- Disintegration of luting cement.
- Solder failure.
- Longer time for custom made bands.
- Tooth along the line of band prone for dental caries in case of poor hygiene.
- Limited to single tooth loss.
- High chance of appliance might slip subgingivally.

Fig. (14). Advantages and disadvantages of band and loop space maintainers.

LINGUAL ARCH SPACE MAINTAINER

It is a fixed, bilateral, passive and non-functional space maintainer used in the mandibular arch. Lingual arch was popularised by Burstone as a simple custom-made appliance consisting of heavy gauge wire which is adapted on the lingual surface of the mandibular arch attached to the bands on permanent first molars [6].

Indications

- Used in mixed dentition with premature loss of multiple posterior primary teeth unilaterally or bilaterally after the eruption of mandibular incisors.
- Used in preventive and interceptive orthodontics as it gives critical anchorage for treatment of mandibular arch.
- Used in conjunction with space management, planned by timed extraction of deciduous teeth.
- When there is no possibility of using removable appliances due to poor cooperation and non-compliant patient.
- When minor tooth movements are required in the mandibular arch.

Contraindications

In primary dentition where the tooth buds of anterior permanent teeth are located somewhat lingually, and the eruption will be interfered with by the resting wire lingually adjacent to the primary incisors.

Construction of Appliance

a) Banding and Impression Appropriate band size for the first permanent molar is selected or custom fabricated and an impression is taken and a working model prepared with bands on the permanent first molar

b) Archwire Design Heavy gauge stainless steel wire of 0.036 inches or 0.9 cm in diameter is used. The archwire is bent such that it is in contact at the cingulum level of erupted permanent incisors and is placed 1-2 mm away lingually from the posterior teeth so that the succedaneous teeth can erupt easily in the buccolingual plane and avoid soft tissue impingement. Arch wire should be 1-2mm below the marginal gingiva and edentulous arch to prevent distortion of the lingual arch under load (Fig. **15a**).

c) Soldering, finishing and polishing are done.

d) Try-in and Cementation While try-in the appliance there should be no soft tissue impingement or occlusal interference, and the appliance should be passive.

Cementation should be done using luting GIC with proper isolation.

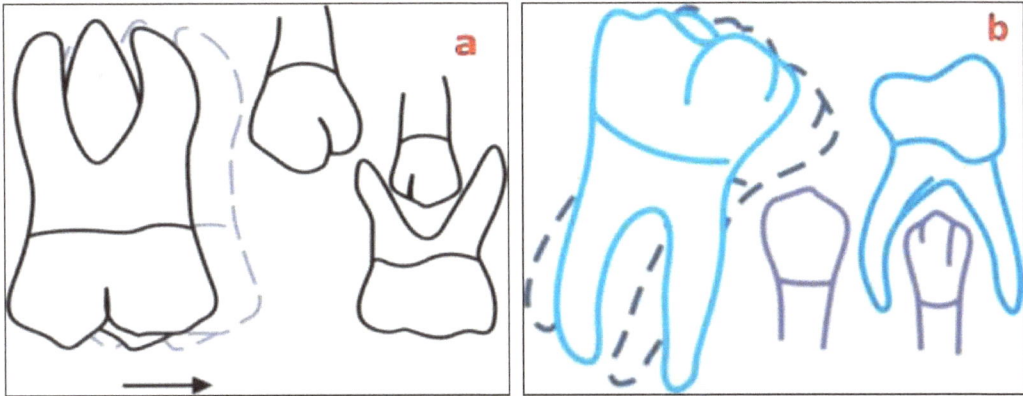

Fig. (15). a. Lingual arch space maintainer, **b.** Holtz lingual arch, **c.** Lingual arch with spurs, **d.** Lingual arch with anterior bend to guide incisor to required position

Modifications

• Lingual holding arch with U loop for space regaining also called Hotz lingual arch (Figs. **15b**).
• Lingual arch with canine spurs (Figs. **15c**).
• *Semi fixed lingual arch:* Archwire is seated into the molar tube on the lingual side of the first permanent molar and stabilised with ligature wire
• Removable lingual arch
• Omega bends in the canine region to prevent interference.
• For erupting incisors, the anterior part of the wire is bent so that the erupting incisors are guided to the required position (Figs. **15d**).

Various advantages and disadvantages of lingual arch include (Fig. **16**) [7].

DISTAL SHOE SPACE MAINTAINER

It is one of the oldest space maintainers which guide the first molar in eruption. *Willet* in 1929 first presented this kind of appliance with distal intra alveolar extension. Generally distal root surface of deciduous second molar helps in guiding the permanent first molar to erupt in its place. If that tooth is lost prematurely, the distal shoe space maintainer is used to guide the eruption pathway of the permanent first molar. It is also known an Intra-alveolar appliance since it has intra alveolar extension which acts as a guiding plane [6].

Indications: If a deciduous second molar is lost before the eruption of the first permanent molar and first deciduous molar can act as an abutment.

Advantages

• It acts as a great source of anchorage due to incorporation of resistance of multiple teeth.

• It helps in maintaining the arch perimeter well which also includes prevention of mesial and lingual drift of molar teeth which may cause severe arch deficiency.

• There is free individual movement of teeth as there will be clearance for the posterior teeth for their eruption.

• Can be used to as a space regainer.

• Space maintainer for multiple tooth.

• Less inconvience to the patient and is less bulky.

Disadvantages

• Prolonged period of usage may lead to decalcification of the teeth which is usual in other fixed banded appliances.

• In patients having poor oral hygiene the wire may get embedded in soft tissue.

• There may be distortion of wire due to masticatory forces and cause unwanted tooth movements.

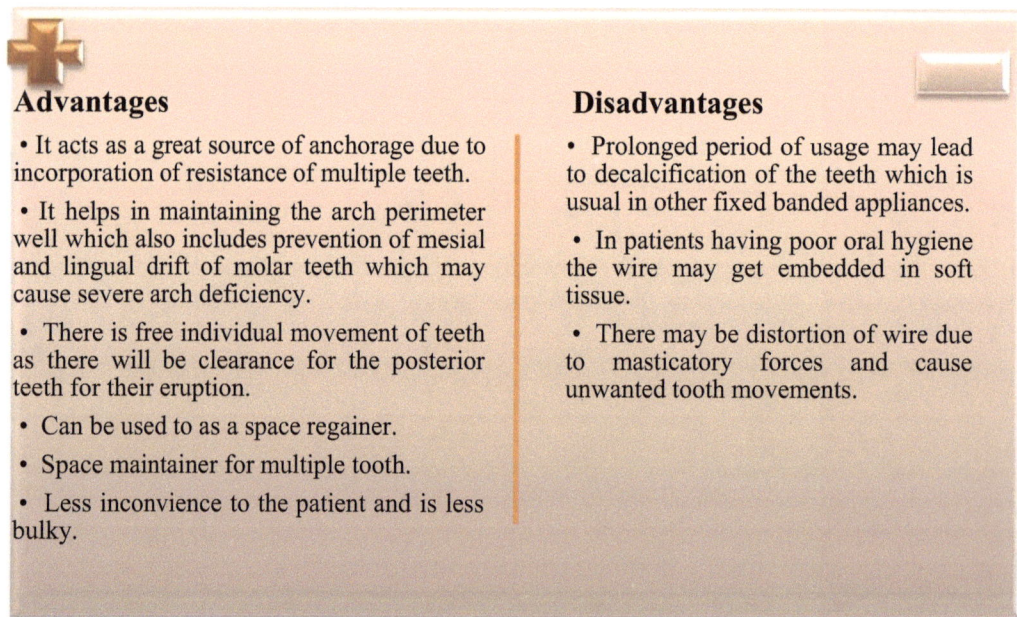

Fig. (16). Advantages and disadvantages of lingual arch space maintainer.

Contraindications

• Absence of multiple teeth and inadequate support for abutment teeth.
• Poor oral hygiene and compliance by the patient.
• Children with systemic conditions like congenital heart disease, hematologic disorders, history of rheumatic fever, juvenile diabetes, kidney disorders, immunosuppression, and generalised debilitation.

Fabrication of Appliance

a) Placement of band: Banding is done on the deciduous first molar, which acts as an abutment, but if the anatomy of the tooth does not permit banding, then tooth preparation is done to place stainless steel crown and banding is done on the crown. The impression is made, and a working model is prepared with the band on the crown of the first deciduous molar.

b) Radiograph: Intraoral periapical radiograph of the region is taken to determine the length of the horizontal and vertical arm of the appliance. Length of the horizontal arm is equal to the maximum mesiodistal width of the second deciduous molar and the vertical arm should be 1mm below the mesial contour of the unerupted first permanent molar or at its emergence from the alveolar, bone as measured on the radiograph (Fig. **17a**).

c) Preparation of working model: Measurements are marked on the working model, and the corresponding part of plaster is removed to attain space for fabrication of the loop or bar.

d) Construction of metal guide plane: Loop is constructed by using 0.040-inch wire based on measurements made on radiograph and the free end is soldered to the band on the first deciduous molar. A preformed cobalt-chromium alloy palatal bar of 3.8 mm width and 3mm height is also available which is bent based on required measurements and soldered to the band.

e) Soldering: Free ends of the wire or bar are soldered to the band or crown on the abutment tooth, finished and polished.

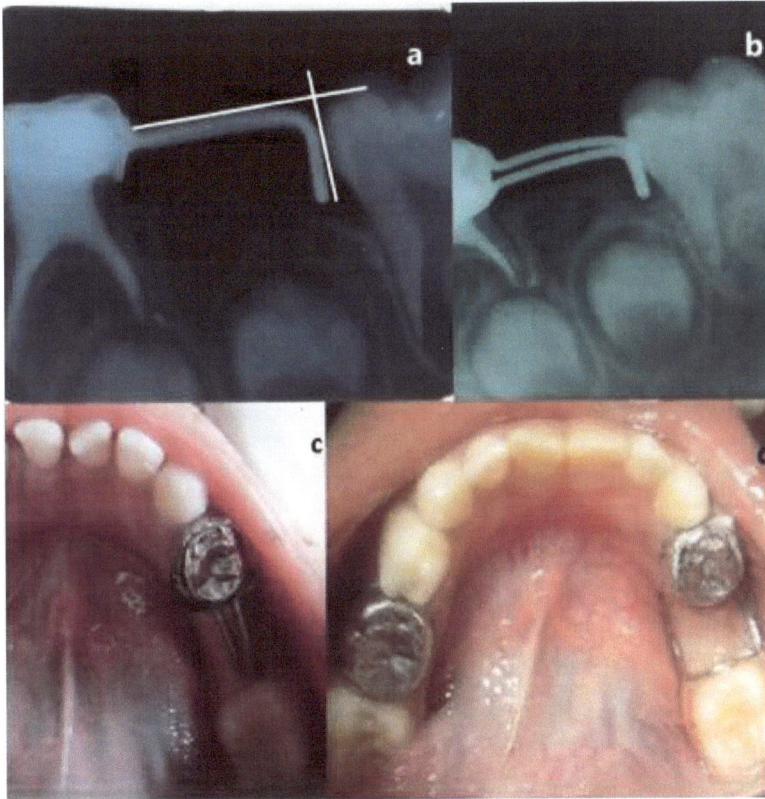

Fig. (17). a. Radiograph of crown distal shoe appliance before cementation to confirm the intra alveolar extension, **b.** Radiograph before removal of appliance after molar erupted clinically, **c.** Intra oral occlusal view after eruption of molar, **d.** Distal shoe replaced with crown reverse band and loop space maintainer.

f) Seating of appliance: Extraction and placement of the appliance are done in the same visit. After extraction of the second deciduous molar, once haemostasis is achieved, appliance is placed in its position and an IOPA radiograph is taken to confirm the intra alveolar position of distal extension (Fig. **17a**). Any adjustments required in length and contour should be. Appliance is cemented with luting cement on the abutment tooth. In case extraction has been done previously, an incision is made in the gingival tissue near the permanent first molar to place the appliance in the tissue and is cemented. Patient should be followed up regularly till the permanent molar erupts. Once permanent molar erupts, distal shoe should be removed followed by band and loop or reverse band and loop space maintainer should be given (Figs. **17b, c, d**).

Various advantages and disadvantages include (Figs. **17e**) [7]:

Advantages	Disadvantages
• Effective in guiding first permanent molar eruption. • Fabrication can be by direct or indirect methods. • Prevents supraeruption of opposing teeth	• Fabrication is highly technique sensitive • Good oral hygiene maintainance is mandatory • Once permanent molar is erupted, distal shoe should be replaced with other space maintainer, number of appointments are increased • Small metallic tattoo may be seen in the gingival tissue • Complete epithelization might not always occur.

Fig. (17e). Advantages and disadvantages of distal shoe space maintainer.

NANCE PALATAL ARCH APPLIANCE

It is a fixed, bilateral, passive and non-functional maxillary appliance. It proximates with the maxillary anterior teeth but does not come in contact with them. This space maintainer was developed by H. N. Nance in 1947 as a modification of the maxillary lingual arch by adding acrylic button to it, hence the name Nance palatal arch space maintainer and an acrylic button is called Nance button. It provides effective space maintenance, preventing mesial movement of the teeth which are distal to edentulous space due to the acrylic button which rests on the most anterior and superior portion of the palatal vault [6].

Construction

• Maxillary molar teeth distal to edentulous space are fitted with the bands, impression is taken and working cast with banded molars is prepared.

- Heavy-gauge stainless steel wire of 0.036 inches (0.9mm) or higher is used and moulded into U shape which passes from palatal aspect of banded molar to anterior part of palatal vault.
- Near the rugae area, a small U shaped bend is given to improve retention of the appliance and is 1-2mm away from the soft tissue. Archwire is soldered to the molar bands on both sides.
- An acrylic button of about 0.5 cm in diameter is placed on the anterior part of the wire which prevents the wire from being buried (Figs. **18a**).

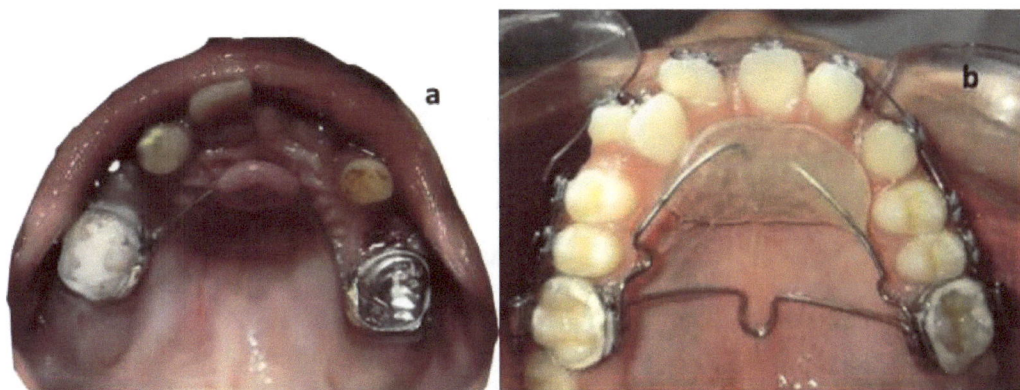

Fig. (**18a, b**). Nance palatal arch.

Indications

- Used in case of bilateral loss of maxillary deciduous molars has occurred, or in case there is a need for reinforced anchorage.
- Also used as a habit breaking appliance by incorporating spikes in the acrylic button.

Modifications:

- Nance button can be modified in case of missing anterior teeth as additional wire components can be soldered to the arch and it can hold pontic teeth for esthetic reasons.
- Can be used in unilateral molar distalization and it takes the support of the palatal vault (Figs. **18b**).
- It can be used as a habit-breaking appliance by incorporating spikes into the acrylic button.

Various advantages and disadvantages include (Fig. **19**) [4, 7]:

Advantages

- Most suitable appliance for maxillary bilateral loss of deciduous molars as it is effective in maintaining the total arch circumference.
- It can be also used in primary dentition.
- It gains additional anchorage from palatal vault.

Disadvantages

- Nance button can get incorporated into the tissue in case of palatal tissue hypertrophy due to poor oral hygiene.
- Palatal tissue inflammation due to deposition of bacteria and debris resulting in pain.
- Palatal tissue hyperplasia due to irritation by acrylic button.
- Should be avoided in patients having allergy to acrylic.

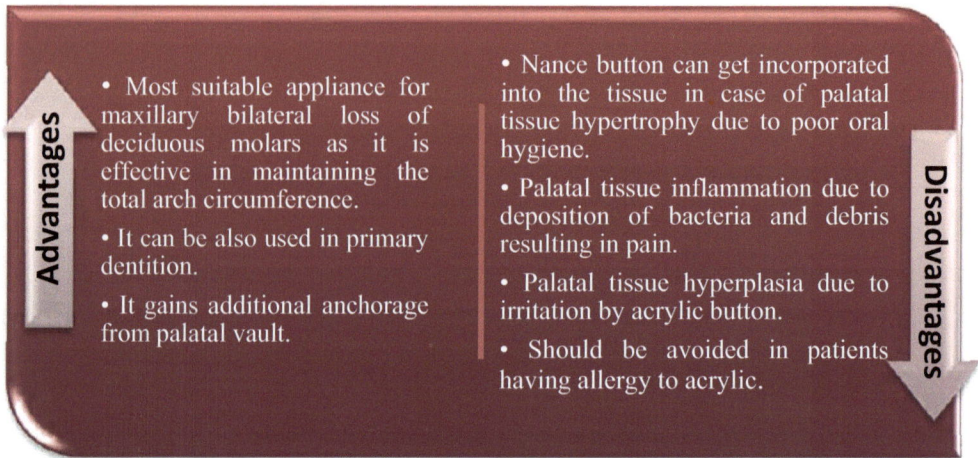

Fig. (19). Advantages and disadvantages of Nance palatal arch space maintainer.

TRANS PALATAL ARCH APPLIANCE

It is a fixed maxillary appliance that is bilateral, passive and was first described by Robert Goshgarian in 1972, also called as Goshgarian appliance. Transpalatal arch space maintainer extends from one maxillary first permanent molar along the palatal contour to the contralateral molar. It is adapted to the palatal curvature and is 2-3 mm away from the palatal tissue with an omega loop in the middle of the palate [6].

Indications

As a space maintainer, it is used in the early loss of deciduous teeth on one side with the other side teeth intact.

Other indications include

- As an arch expansion appliance as it can be adapted to produce a range of forces and couple force in all three planes.
- To prevent molars from rotation around the palatal root.
- Control upper molar eruption.
- To establish arch width and to maintain it (Figs. **20a**).
- Correction of unilateral crossbites.

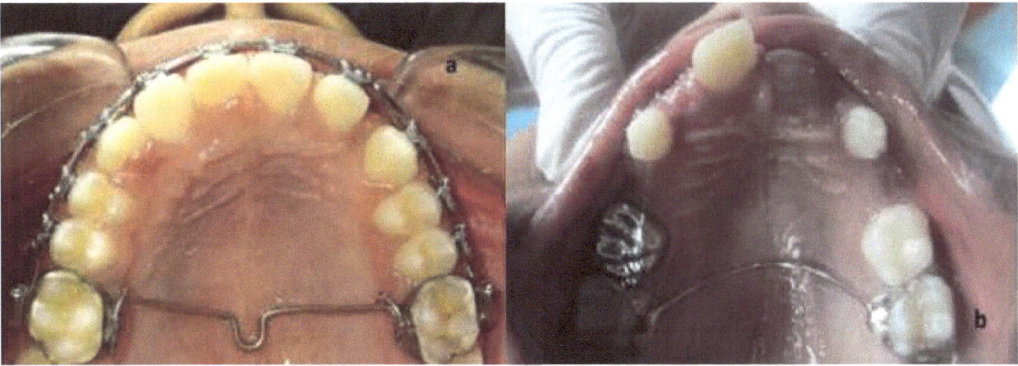

Fig. (20). a. Transpalatal arch, **b.** Transpalatal bar.

Construction

- Bands are fitted on both the first permanent molars, impression is taken and a working cast is prepared with bands on molars.
- Archwire is constructed with heavy gauge stainless steel wire of thickness 0.9 mm or 0.036 inch which is adapted in close proximity of palatal contour but is 2-3 mm away from palatal mucosa.
- An omega loop is bent either mesially or distally in the middle of the palate and the wire is soldered to the bands on the palatal side. (Figs. **20a, b**)

Various advantages and disadvantages include (Fig. **21**) [6].

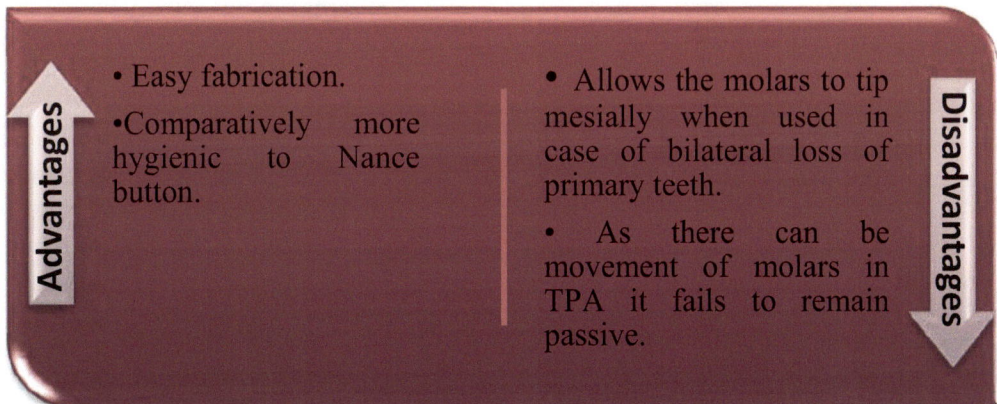

Advantages	Disadvantages
• Easy fabrication. •Comparatively more hygienic to Nance button.	• Allows the molars to tip mesially when used in case of bilateral loss of primary teeth. • As there can be movement of molars in TPA it fails to remain passive.

Fig. (21). Advantages and disadvantages of transpalatal arch space maintainer.

FIBRE-REINFORCED COMPOSITE RESIN SPACE MAINTAINER

With the advent of acid etching and the introduction of bondable composite materials in dentistry, esthetics have gained importance in dentistry over the years. One such bondable composite material, Glass Fibre-reinforced composite resin (GFRCR), is widely used in removable prosthodontics, orthodontics and periodontal splints. Even though conventional band and loop space maintainers are widely used and have a high success rate, it has a few disadvantages like the disintegration of cement, caries at the level of the band on abutment tooth and plaque accumulation. Hence in quest of need for an alternative material, GFRCR emerged, which is now used as a space maintainer, which overcomes many disadvantages of the regular band and loop space maintainer [1].

Fibre-reinforced composite resin (FRCR) is translucent in colour consisting of resin matrix and fillers. Resin matrix acts as a carrier, load splicing medium and protector, which is light curable. Mechanical properties are improved by adding specifically oriented fillers like glass fibres, carbon/ graphite fillers, ultra-high molecular weight polyethylene (UHMWPE) fibres, and aramid fibres which acts as a skeleton for the composite resin.

Various available bondable reinforced fibres include

- Vivadent, StickTech, Pentron (Fibers impregnated with resin)
- GlasSpan, Polydentia (Glass fiber)
- Ribbond (Ultrahigh molecular weight polyethylene fibre)

Method of Construction

Distance from mesiobuccal line angle of primary canine to distobuccal line angle of deciduous second molar is measured and FRCR material is cut to that required length. Abutment teeth are cleaned, polished, acid etched and a bonding agent is applied, cured for 20 secs. Flowable composite is applied to the buccal surface of the abutment tooth and ends of FRCR material are placed on it and cured for 40 secs, a similar procedure is repeated on the lingual surface. Uncovered surface of the fibres is coated with flowable composite and cured. Gingival clearance or any occlusal interference are checked and corrected accordingly, finishing is done with composite finishing burs. Fibre framework is applied with the bonding agent and cured at multiple points which reactivate the fibres [1].

Another method includes forming a loop using wetted FRCR material simulating a loop of the conventional band and loop space maintainer. A thin layer of composite is applied to the loop formed and cured for 40 secs to its entire length for initial handling, adaptability and rigidity. Loop is detached from the tooth and the composite is applied on its entire length, cured for 40 secs, finished and polished. Loop is then bonded to the etched buccal and lingual surface of the distal abutment tooth (Figs. **22 and 23**) [8].

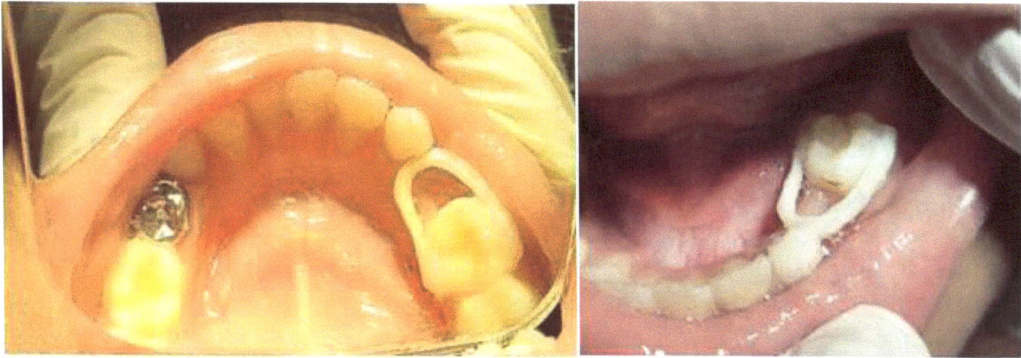

Fig. (22). GFRCR space maintainer.

Advantages	Disadvantages
•Aesthetic and Hygienic •Provides cost and time savings as it does not require lab procedure and needs less appointments. •Can be used in children with metal allergy. •Demineralisation of enamel, caries formation by metal bands, tissue irritation can be overcome with use of GFRCR system. •Adhesion is long lasting which overcomes the problem of solder failure, disintegration of cement . •Annual removal of conventional space maintainers to inspect, clean and fluoride application to tooth is avoided.	•Debonding might occur at enamel-composite interface, fiber composite interface or fracture of fiber frame work. •Failure might occur if proper isolation is not done during placement.

Fig. (23). Advantages and disadvantages of GFRCR.

REMOVABLE SPACE MAINTAINERS

They include removable partial dentures and Hawley's type of appliance.

Indications

• Unilateral or bilateral early loss of both the deciduous molars.
• Early loss of anterior teeth.
• When a space maintainer is required for a short time interval.
• Cleft palate cases where palatal defect needs closure.
• Permanent molar is not fully erupted to place the band for a fixed maintainer.

Contraindications

- When patient compliance is difficult to achieve.
- Epileptic children with uncontrolled seizures.
- Patients who are allergic to acrylic resins.

Appliance Design

An acrylic extension is shorter on the buccal or labial side and wider on the lingual side; this design does not hamper lateral jaw growth. If a tooth is present distal to the appliance, distolingual acrylic extension should be till the centre of that tooth for better retention of the appliance. An anterior lingual aspect of the acrylic should be away by 1-2 mm to prevent untoward movement of erupting teeth. Clasps and cribs should be avoided if a tooth is present distal to the edentulous space, if required appliance is stabilised by a bow or simple clasp like Adams clasp [6]. (Figs. **24a, b**) Removable space maintainer can be non-functional with only acrylic base plate or functional with artificial teeth placed in the acrylic base plate to restore function and esthetics.

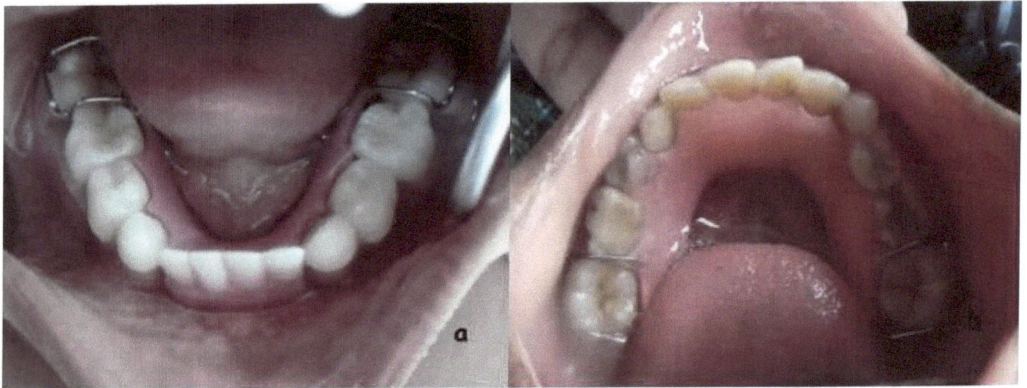

Fig. (24). a. Removable anterior space maintainer. **b.** Removable functional space maintainer.

Various advantages and disadvantages include (Fig. **25**) [6].

Advantages

• It restores phonetics, esthetics and masticatory function

• Appliance is easy to clean and can be used in conjunction with other preventive procedures.

• Band construction is not necessary.

• Vertical dimension of the jaw is maintained

• Follow up appointments for detection of dental caries or soft tissue health is easy.

• Restriction of abnormal tongue habits.

Disadvantages

• Poor retention of the appliance on continuously wearing and removing.

• Poor compliance by the child in using the appliance.

• High chances of misplacing or breakage of the appliance especially in preschool children.

• If clasp are incorporated, it might hamper lateral jaw growth.

• Irritation of underlying mucosa.

Fig. (25). Advantages and disadvantages of removable space maintainer.

SPACE REGAINING

Premature loss of primary teeth leads to space loss resulting in erupting permanent tooth may remain impacted, or it may erupt buccally or lingually if space maintenance is not planned (Fig. **26**).

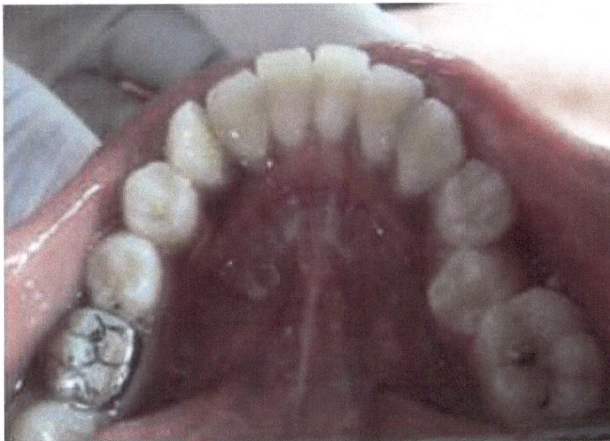

Fig. (26). Mandibular right premolar erupted lingually due to space loss during the mixed dentition stage.

Some of the most common causes of space loss within the arch are [2].

- Primary teeth with interproximal caries
- Alteration in the sequence of eruption
- Transposition of teeth
- Loss of primary molars without proper space management
- Dental impaction
- Ectopically erupting teeth
- Ankylosis of a primary molar
- Abnormal resorption of primary molar roots
- Premature and delayed eruption of permanent teeth
- Congenitally missing teeth
- Abnormal dental morphology

Evaluation of the loss of space in the dental arch, which interferes with the succedaneous tooth eruption, should be done.

Diagnosis: Diagnosis plays an important role before planning space management procedures.

RADIOGRAPHIC DIAGNOSIS

- To diagnose whether the tooth has tipped axially or moved bodily into the edentulous space
- Positions of the tooth present distal to the tooth to be moved; by severe distalization of the first molar, there is greater potential for the second permanent molar to get impacted.
  a. Study model analysis includes
- Mixed dentition analysis for determining the measurement of space loss against the estimation of space needed by the unerupted permanent tooth
- Visualization of vertical, transverse and sagittal dental relationships that might hinder the stability of Moyer's mixed dentition analysis
- Alignment or rotation of the tooth
- Improper contacts and transverse relation of teeth.

Indications

- Space loss in cases with Class I occlusion
- With adequate anchorage
- Second permanent molar is unerupted, having a favourable relationship with the first permanent molar.

Various removable and fixed appliances are used for space regaining in mixed dentition [9] (Fig. **27**). Until a subsequent comprehensive orthodontic treatment plan is initiated or adjacent permanent teeth have erupted completely, space regained should be maintained.

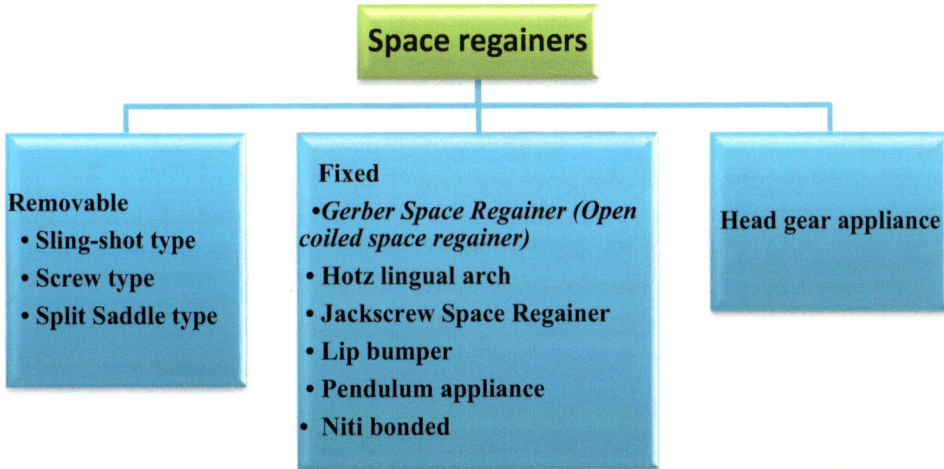

Fig. (27). Types of Space regainers.

GERBER SPACE REGAINER (OPEN COILED SPACE REGAINER)

Gerber space regainer is a chairside appliance that may be fabricated in a relatively short period, and it does not demand extensive laboratory procedures.

Nickel-titanium (Ni-Ti) open coil springs are the main component that produces a relatively more constant force on the tooth to be moved because of shape memory. Since it is a fixed appliance, patient acceptance has to be good and maintain good oral hygiene (Fig. **28**) [10].

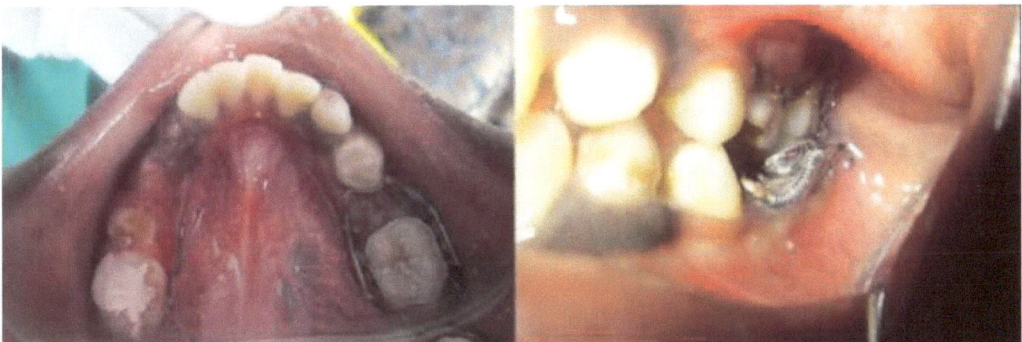

Fig. (28). Open Coiled Space Regainer.

Appliance: Band is selected on the abutment tooth, and molar tubes are welded or soldered on it. SS wire is placed through the buccal tube, extended anteriorly till reaching the distolabial surface of deciduous canine, then bent lingually around the deciduous canine and finally returned posteriorly, till reaching the lingual tube. Mating was done by assembling the mesial opening of the tube and the distal free end of the arm and then moving the SS arm into the distal end of the tube by dragging.

Open coil spring is inserted into the SS wire, and the length of open coil spring is measured by establishing the assembly in the desired position and the distance between mesial contact or solder point to the entry of wire in the tube and add the amount of space required or regained, along with 1-2 mm additional length to ensure activation of spring. Open coil spring is placed in a compressed state and the whole assembly is cemented onto abutment tooth.

HOTZ LINGUAL ARCH

Another method for moving molars distally is by using the looped Hotz lingual arch (Hitchcock 1974).

Indication

When the permanent tooth moves mesially rather than the distal movement of tooth mesial to edentulous space and also in cases where sufficient space is present for an eruption of the permanent second molar.

The lingual arch provides compound anchorage from all the other teeth that it touches. A horizontal spur can be soldered perpendicular to the archwire contacting the distal surface of the premolar or canine to reinforce the anchorage additionally. Periodically once a month, the loop on the active side is adjusted. After adjustment, the wire is forced forward and then slipped down into the appropriate space to contact the teeth (Fig. **29**).

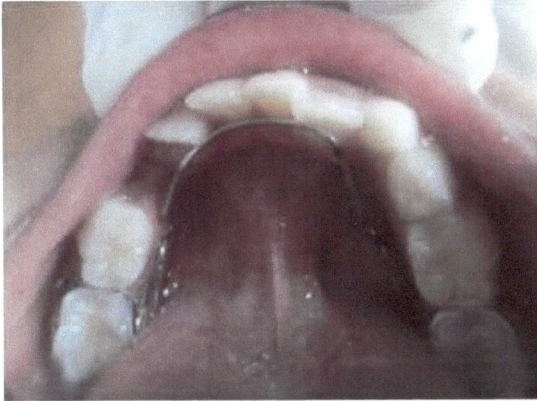

Fig. (29). Hotz lingual arch.

LIP BUMPER

It is given in the mandibular arch, and its counterpart in the maxillary arch is called Denholtz appliance. It is used to distalize and uprighting the mesially tipped permanent molars to regain space. Force is transferred from the muscles of the lips to the molar by lip bumper resulting in space regaining.

It can be fixed, semi-fixed or removable. In the case of fixed regainers, permanent molars are banded and labial archwire with a labial acrylic button is soldered to the buccal surface of molars. In semi-fixed regainers, molar bands are placed on permanent molar welded with buccal tubes and labial archwire with an acrylic button is inserted into the buccal tubes and stabilised with ligature wire or elastic module (Fig. **30a**).

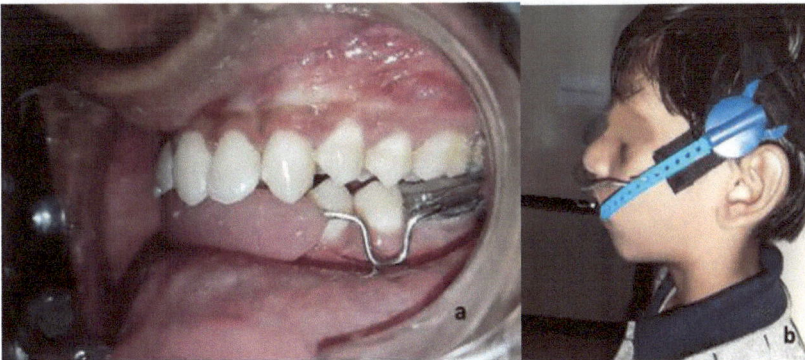

Fig. (30). **a.** Semi fixed lip bumper, **b.** High pull head gear.

Headgear: Both low pull and high pull headgear are used to distalize the molars and regain space (Fig. **30b**).

NITI BONDED SPACE REGAINER

It is a simple chairside method that uses the property of shape memory of Niti alloy aiding in distalizing the molar and regaining the space.

A composite dimple is bonded on the buccal surface of the permanent first molar. With the explorer or probe, a tunnel is created in the composite, which is open only on the mesial side and is cured. A small piece of 0.016 Niti of the required length is cut and is bonded to the buccal surface of tooth mesial to edentulous space. Free end of the Niti wire is placed in the tunnel in the composite on the permanent first molar with the help of a bird beak plier. A small amount of composite is placed at the opening of the tunnel and cured to stabilize the wire. Over time Niti wire becomes straight and regains the space, the same wire is left in its position to act as a space maintainer.

REMOVABLE SPACE REGAINERS

a) Slingshot: This appliance is named as it resembles a slingshot and has the advantage of offering light continuous force to the tooth in distalizing. The distal ends of the appliance consist of two hooks on the buccal and lingual sides extending on the permanent first molar. An elastic band is stretched between the hooks and the force produced by the elastic band results in distal movement of molars, thus gaining space (Fig. **31**). Force produced is light and physiological which distalizes molar up to 1-2 mm.

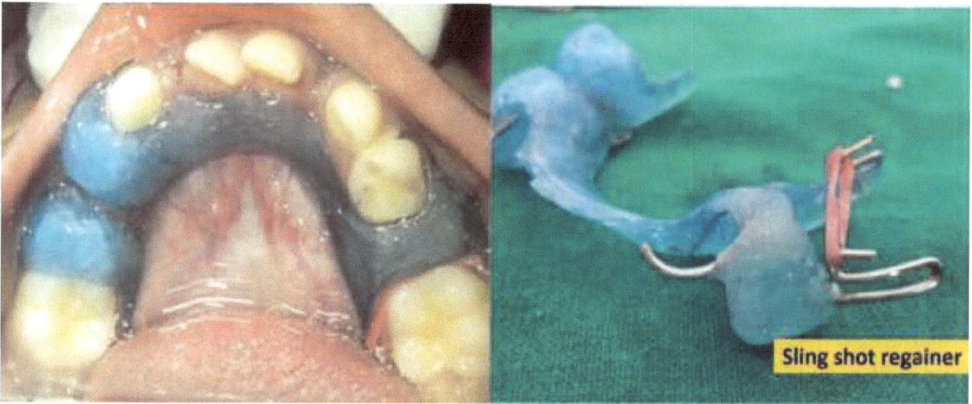

Sling shot regainer

Fig. (31). Sling shot removable space regainer.

b) Screw type: Jackscrew is incorporated in the acrylic plate to distalize molar and a maximum of 3mm space can be regained. Screw should be expanded once a week and is best suited when only distalization is required without rotation correction.

c) Spring type: A spring made of 0.7mm wire is used to distalize the molar and is incorporated into the split acrylic plate. Spring is activated twice a month, thus creating an increment of force for tooth movement.

d) Split saddle: Used in mandibular arch and regains up to 1-2 mm space. The bent portion of the wire which connects the split saddles of the acrylic plate is flattened to regain the space (Fig. **32**).

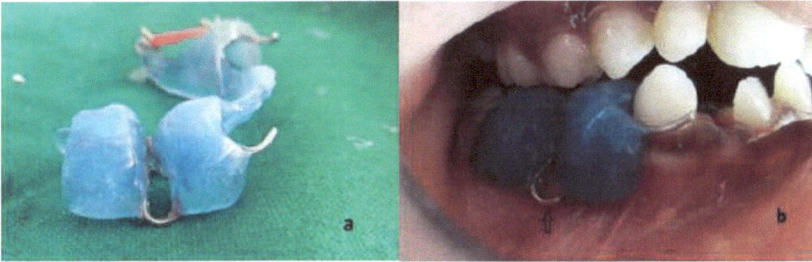

Fig. (**32**). a, b Split saddle space regainer. Arrow indicates activation point of the bent portion of wire.

SPACE SUPERVISION

It is carried out in doubtful situations over space availability after mixed dentition analysis. The prognosis of space supervision is doubtful, but it gives a better chance of getting through mixed dentition with certain clinical guidance rather than with no treatment measures. It involves an element of calculated risk and should be undertaken after parental understanding and patient cooperation.

Basic Principles of Supervision Include

• It is not begun until one-fourth or one-third of the root of the mandibular cuspid and first premolar is formed.
• Deciduous teeth are extracted serially to facilitate the eruption of succedaneous teeth
• An effort is made to keep mandible ahead of than maxilla in terms of eruption
• Care should be taken that late mesial shift in the mandible does not occur.

Gross discrepancy problems: In this significant difference is present between the sizes of erupting permanent teeth and the space available for it in the alveolar perimeter. It can be treated at different ages usually depending on the time at which it is first observed. These gross problems are termed as Serial extractions in most of the literature.

CONCLUSION

Every effort should be made to preserve the natural deciduous tooth as it is the best space maintainer for the erupting permanent tooth. But in case loss of the deciduous tooth is unavoidable, space created by it, is maintained by suitable space maintainers till a permanent successor erupts, if there is space loss, space regainers should be given and in case of a doubtful situation over space availability, space supervision is done and for gross discrepancies, serial extraction is considered. These measures help in the smooth and harmonious transfer of deciduous dentition to permanent dentition and maintain the integrity of the dental arches.

CONSENT FOR PUBLICATION

Not applicable.

CONFLICT OF INTEREST

The authors declare no conflict of interest, financial or otherwise.

ACKNOWLEDGEMENT

Declared none.

REFERENCES

[1] Setia V, Pandit IK, Srivastava N, Gugnani N, Sekhon HK. Space maintainers in dentistry: past to present. J Clin Diagn Res 2013; 7(10): 2402-5.
[http://dx.doi.org/10.7860/JCDR/2013/6604.3539] [PMID: 24298544]

[2] Management of the developing dentition and occlusion in pediatric dentistry The Reference Manual of Pediatric Dentistry. Chicago, Ill.: American Academy of Pediatric Dentistry 2020; pp. 393-409.

[3] Watt E, Ahmad A, Adamji R, Katsimbali A, Ashley P, Noar J. Space maintainers in the primary and mixed dentition – a clinical guide. Br Dent J 2018; 225(4): 293-8.
[http://dx.doi.org/10.1038/sj.bdj.2018.650] [PMID: 30141512]

[4] Achmad H. taya. The use of space maintainer in paediatric dentistry: a systemic review. Eur J Mol Clin Med 2021; 8(2): 1532-45.

[5] Gurunathan D, Ravinthar K. Applicability of different mixed dentition analysis among children aged 11-13 years in Chennai population. Int J Clin Pediatr Dent 2020; 13(2): 163-6.
[http://dx.doi.org/10.5005/jp-journals-10005-1736] [PMID: 32742095]

[6] Laing E, Ashley P, Naini FB, Gill DS. Space maintenance. Int J Paediatr Dent 2009; 19(3): 155-62.
[http://dx.doi.org/10.1111/j.1365-263X.2008.00951.x] [PMID: 19385999]

[7] Ramakrishnan M, Dhanalakshmi R, Subramanian EMG. Survival rate of different fixed posterior space maintainers used in Paediatric Dentistry – A systematic review. Saudi Dent J 2019; 31(2): 165-72.
[http://dx.doi.org/10.1016/j.sdentj.2019.02.037] [PMID: 30983825]

[8] Yeluri R, Munshi A. Fiber reinforced composite loop space maintainer: An alternative to the conventional band and loop. Contemp Clin Dent 2012; 3(5) (Suppl. 1): 26.
[http://dx.doi.org/10.4103/0976-237X.95099] [PMID: 22629061]

[9] Nakhjavani YB, Nakhjavani FB, Jafari A. Mesial stripping of mandibular deciduous canines for correction of permanent lateral incisors. Int J Clin Pediatr Dent 2017; 10(3): 229-33.
[http://dx.doi.org/10.5005/jp-journals-10005-1441] [PMID: 29104380]

[10] Kamatchi D, Kumar SS, Vasanthan P. Orthodontic challenges in mixed dentition. SRM Journal of Research in Dental Sciences 2015; 6(1): 22-8.
[http://dx.doi.org/10.4103/0976-433X.149585]

CHAPTER 8

Oral Habits and its Prevention in Children

Dhanashree Sakhare[1,*]**, H. Sharath Chandra**[2] **and M.H Raghunath Reddy**[3]

[1] *Founder, Lavanika Dental Academy, Melbourne, Australia*

[2] *Reader, Department of Paediatric and Preventive Dentistry, SJM Dental College and Hospital, Chitradurga, Karnataka, India*

[3] *Professor and Head, Department of Paediatric and Preventive Dentistry, SJM Dental College and Hospital, Chitradurga, Karnataka, India*

Abstract: A habit is a repetitive action that is being done automatically and is resistant to change. In the infantile period, certain repetitive behaviours are common, the majority of them begin and stop spontaneously. If oral habits persist beyond a particular developmental age, it results in unfavourable outcomes for the developing teeth, occlusion and surrounding orofacial tissues. Oral habits are considered one of the main causes of malocclusion, leading to unfavourable growth and development of dentoalveolar, which starts in the early childhood and mixed dentition stage. The severity of malocclusion depends on the frequency, duration, and intensity of the habit. Early detection and interception of the habit should be done by parent/child habit awareness and counselling, elimination, etiology, behaviour modifications and correction of malocclusion.

Keywords: Oral Habits, Malocclusion, Mixed Dentition.

INTRODUCTION

Oral habits in children are a prime concern for the dentist, which applies negative forces to the teeth and dentoalveolar structures. The alignment and shape of the teeth play an important role in function and esthetics, and dentists are expected to treat cases that involve a multidisciplinary approach. The American Academy of Pediatric Dentistry (AAPD) recognizes that an infant's, child's, or adolescent's well-being can be affected by oral habits and encourages clinicians to take an individualized approach to the management of these habits [1]. The extent of dentoalveolar or skeletal deformations such as increased overjet, reduced overbite, open bite, posterior crossbite, or increased facial height depends on the following factors (Fig. **1**).

[*] **Corresponding Author Dhanashri Sakhare:** Founder, Lavanika Dental Academy (Melbourne, Australia; E-mail: avanika.23@gmail.com

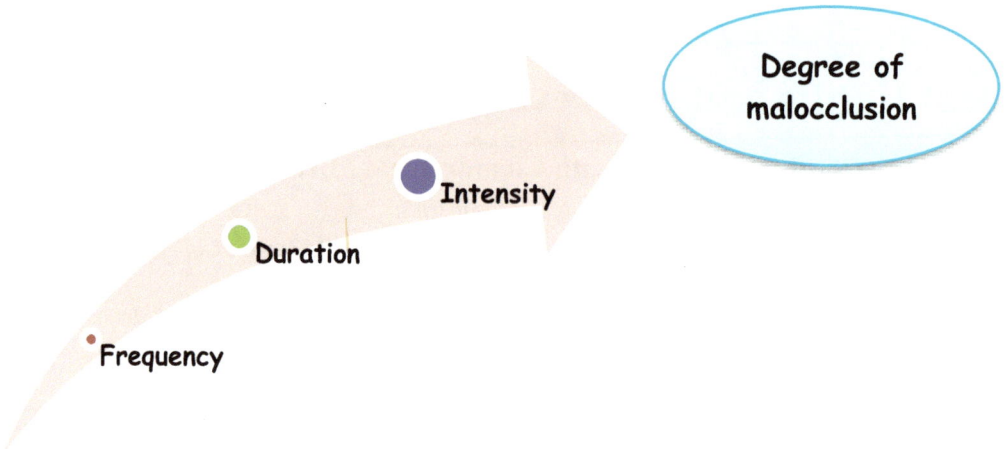

Fig. (1). Factors of oral habits influencing the degree of malocclusion.

- **Frequency:** Number of times the habit is practiced in a day
- **Duration:** Amount of time spent indulging in the habit
- **Intensity:** Force with which the habit is performed

Definition

According to ***Boucher O.C (1963),*** habit is defined as a tendency toward an act or an act that has become repeated performance, relatively fixed, consistent, easy to perform and almost automatic.

According to ***Mathewson (1982),*** oral habits are defined as learned patterns of muscular contractions.

Classification of Habits (Fig. 2a, 2b)

Acquired oral habits	• Learned and could be stopped easily and when the child grows up. • Child can give up that behaviour and start another one.
Compulsive oral habits	• Fixed in child and when emotional pressures are intolerable for the child • Child can feel safety with this habit, and preventing the child from these habits make him or her anxious and worried.

Fig. (2a). Classification of habits.

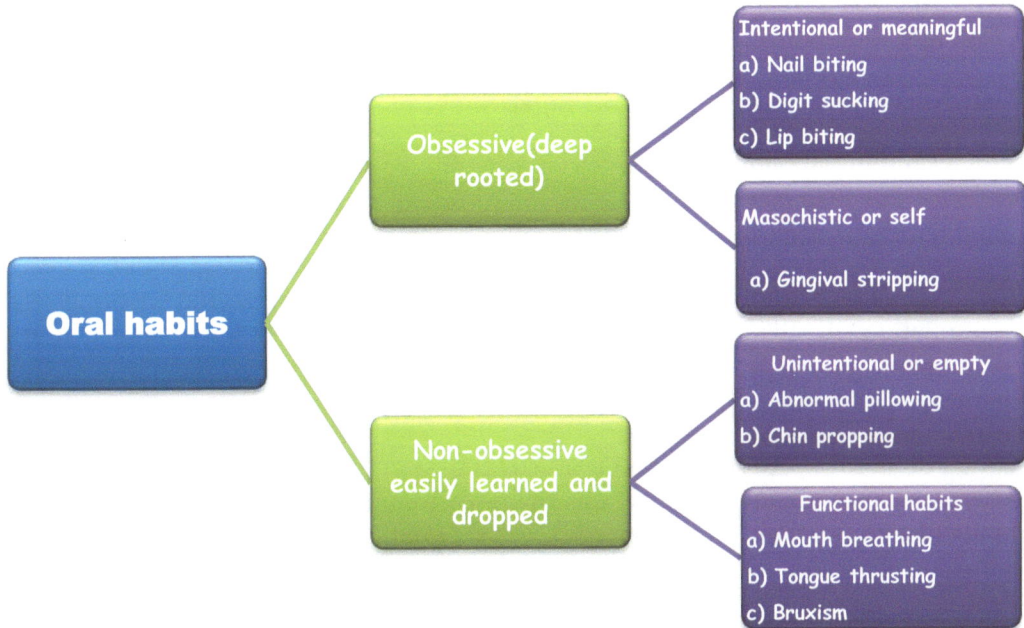

Fig. (2b). Classification of oral habits.

Treatment Objectives & Considerations

Treatment objectives are directed towards minimizing potential deleterious effects on the dentofacial complex by eliminating or decreasing the habit [1].

Habit interception should be done whenever the habit is associated with unfavourable dentofacial development of adverse effects on child health or when there is a reasonable indication that the oral habit will result in a developing permanent dentition in an unfavourable direction. This interception should be appropriate for the child's development, comprehension, and ability to cooperate.

Various treatment modalities include patient/parent counselling, behaviour modification techniques, myofunctional therapy, appliance therapy, or referral to other specialists like psychologists, myofunctional therapists, or otolaryngologists. The use of an appliance as a treatment modality will function as a reminder and would be beneficial only when the child wants to stop the habit.

Some of the habits which are of concern in growing dentition are

- Non-nutritive sucking (thumb/finger sucking, pacifier use)
- Tongue thrust swallow and abnormal tongue position
- Bruxism

- Obstructive sleep apnoea syndrome
- Self-injurious/self-mutilating behaviour

Non-Nutritive Sucking (Thumb/Finger Sucking, Pacifier use)

The term digit sucking is synonymous with finger sucking or thumb sucking and is defined as the placement of the thumb or one or more fingers at various depths into the mouth, according to *Foster.*

It is considered normal in infants and young children, but a long-term continuation of the habit is associated with various malocclusions. Early anticipatory guidance for cessation of the habit will prevent any deleterious effect on orofacial structures [2].

Based on clinical observation, thumb sucking is considered normal during 1st and 2nd year of life, then it disappears as the child matures and does not generate any malocclusion. When the habit persists beyond the preschool period, it is considered an abnormal habit and, if ignored, may cause deleterious effects on dentofacial structures. The prevalence of this habit is decreased as age increases, and it is stopped by 4 years of age [3].

Etiology

Insufficient Satisfaction of Sucking Needs During Childhood (As a Result of Insufficient Breastfeeding)

Breastfeeding helps in the development of breathing, swallowing, mastication and speech articulation, and any imbalance in these systems might lead to unsatisfied sucking needs. Maternal nipple deprivation leads to apparent emotional confusion and frustration, leading to an inappropriate replacement of the nipple by a digit or pacifier.

Learned Behaviour Theory

According to this theory, digit sucking is an innate behaviour that becomes a habit, and because it is soothing to the infant, the habit persists in some children when they are bored, anxious, or tired.

Emotional Theory

This theory is based on Sigmund Freud's psychosexual theory of child development and relates finger-sucking to the oral phase of child development in which the mouth is considered an Oro-erotic zone. The child hastened to place his fingers or any other object into the oral cavity. If this habit continues beyond the oral phase of child development, it becomes a fixation and at a later stage, it is usual, only considered a sign of regression. Fixation and regression are suggestive of emotional disturbance.

Phases of Development of Thumb Sucking (Moyers)

Phase I - Normal and Sub-clinically Significant Sucking

It is seen in the first three years of age, often seen in the ring weaning and teething period. It is often considered normal during this phase see, which is usually self-limiting.

Phase II - Clinically Significant Sucking

It extends between 3–6 years of age. The presence of sucking during this period is an indication that the child is under great anxiety, and treatment should be initiated by a definitive and firm program.

Phase III - Intractable Sucking

Any thumb sucking persisting beyond the 4th year, the child should alert the pediatric dentist as the psychological aspect of habit also should be considered along with associated malocclusion.

Classification

Substelny and Substelny have graded thumb sucking into four types:

Type A

- The Whole thumb is inside the mouth with the pad of the thumb pressing over the palate (Fig. **3**).
- Maxillary and mandibular contact is present.
- Seen in 50% of the children.

Type B

- Thumb is placed into the oral cavity without touching the vault of the palate (Fig. **3**).
- Maxillary and mandibular anterior contact is maintained.
- Seen in 24% of the children.

Type C

- Thumb is placed into the mouth just beyond the first joint and contacts the hard palate and only the maxillary incisors, but mandibular incisors are not in contact with the thumb (Fig. **3**).

• Seen in18% of the children.

Type D

• Thumb is not fully inserted into the mouth. The lower incisor makes contact at the approximate level of the thumbnail (Fig. **3**).
• Seen in 6% of the children.

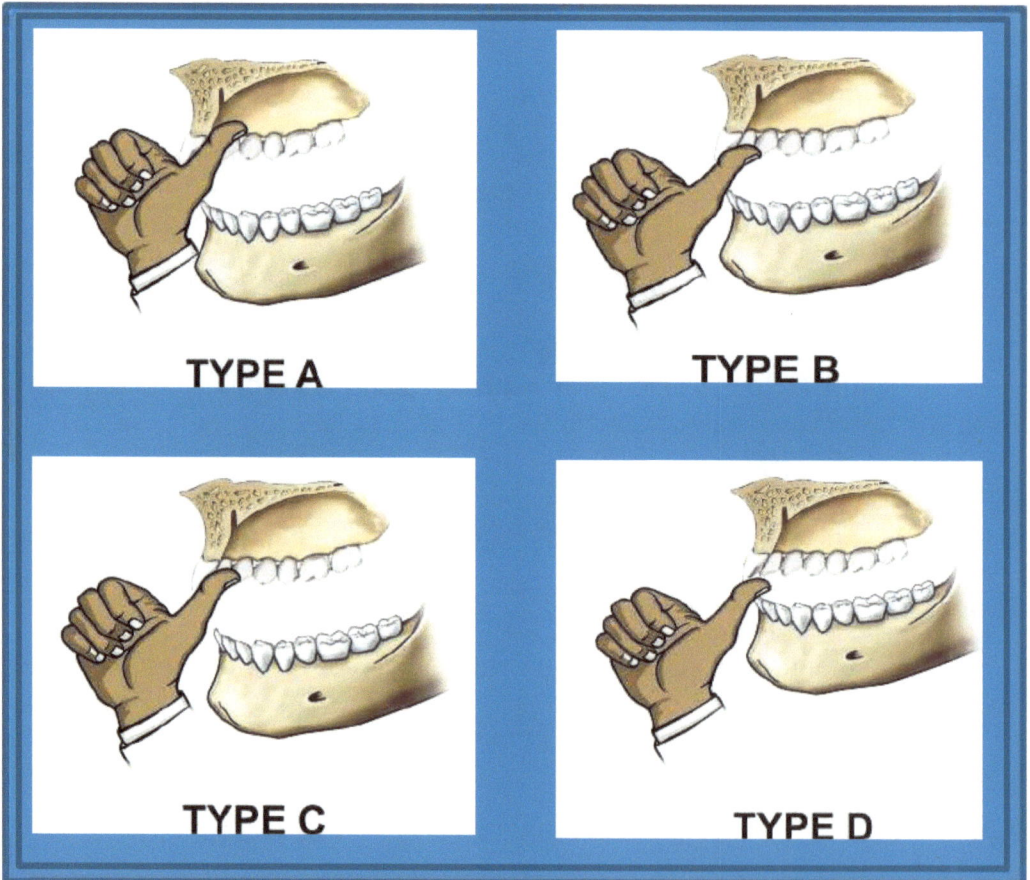

Fig. (3). Substelny and Substelny classification.

Clinical Features

Extraoral examination

• Digits, lips, and facial form are examined (Fig.**4**)

Intraoral Examination

- Labial inclination of the maxillary incisors with increased overjet. Intraoral frontal and lateral view. Increased overjet, decreased overbite, narrow palate.
- Anterior open bite.
- Spacing of the maxillary incisors.
- Increase in arch depth resulting in high palatal vault.
- Narrowing of the inter-canine and inter-molar arch widths.
- Class II canine and molar relationships and posterior crossbites have been observed in thumb-sucking individuals.
- In the mandible, increases in inter-canine arch widths have been detected, and the incisors may be labially or lingually inclined.

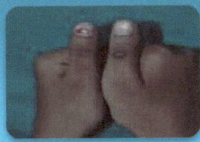

The digits:
- Digits that are involved in the habit will appear reddened, exceptionally clean, chapped and with a short fingernail, i.e., clean dishpans thumb.
- Fibrous roughened callus may be present on the superior aspect of the finger.
- The habit is also known to cause deformation of the finger.

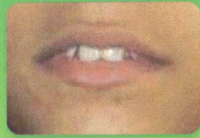

Lips:
- Upper lip may be short and hypotonic.
- Chronic thumb suckers are frequently characterized by a short, hypotonic upper lip.

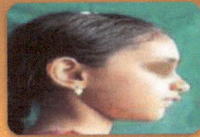

Facial form analysis:
- Mandibular retrusion, maxillary protrusion, high mandibular plane angle and profile.
- Facial profile is either straight or convex.

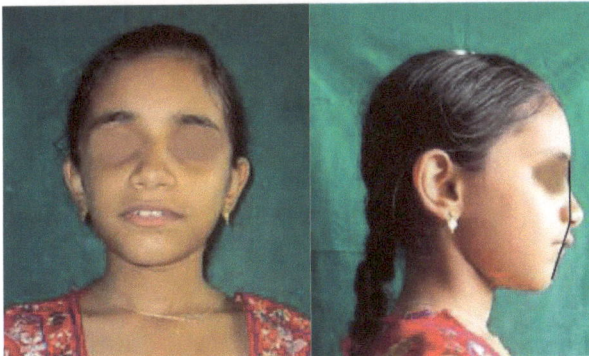

Fig. (4). Extraoral features. Short hypotonic upper lip, maxillary protrusion, mandibular retrusion, convex facial profile and high mandibular plane angle.

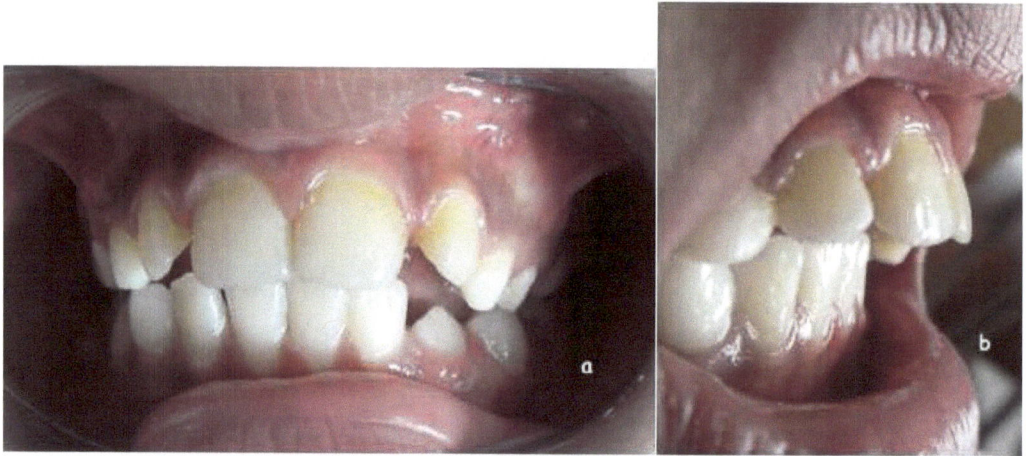

Fig. (5). Intraoral frontal and lateral view. Increased overjet, decreased overbite, narrow palate.

The digit is placed against the palate ventrally and also against the lingual surfaces of the upper incisors at an angle, forming a fulcrum that consists of the digit, the wrist, and the forearm. The force produced by this lever may be subdivided into horizontal and vertical vectors [4].

The vertical vector delays the vertical growth of the anterior maxillary base, which hinders the eruption of the anterior teeth while simultaneously allowing over eruption of posterior teeth. Hence open bite is created as the incisors cannot occlude.

The horizontal vector generates pressure anterior displacement of the anterior maxillary base, proclination of the maxillary incisors and spacing and splaying of the upper incisors, all increasing overjet. Overjet may be exacerbated by retroclined lingual incisors (Fig. **6**).

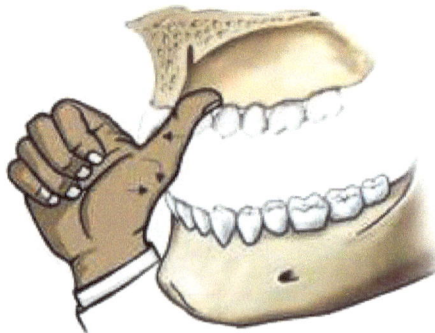

Fig. (6). Forces acting on the oral tissues during digit sucking.

Treatment Plan

The treatment plan can be broadly divided into the following:

- Preventive treatment
- Psychological therapy
- Reward system
- Reminder therapy
- Adjunctive therapy

Preventive Treatment [4]

- Babies' hunger should be satisfied whenever hungry in a natural way.
- Parents should give proper care, affection, and equal attention to all siblings and always make the child feel secure and well cared.
- Engaging the child in various recreational activities, which they can assume as hobbies like painting, crafts, and other outdoor activities, as a habit practiced when alone or bored (Fig. **7**).

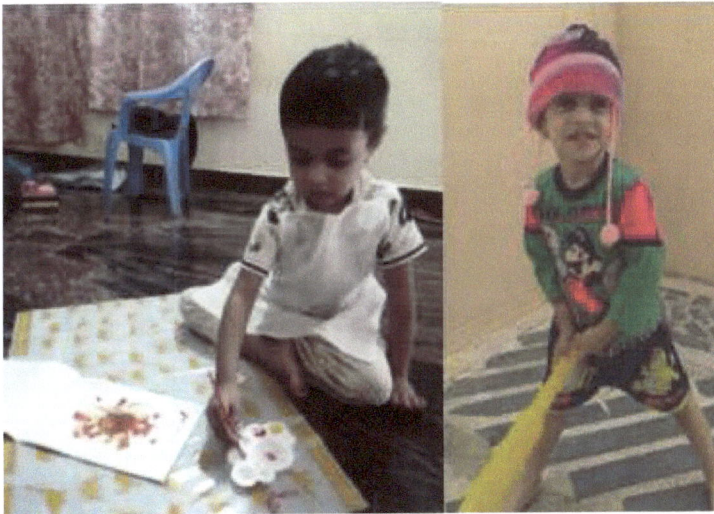

Fig. (7). Engaging child in recreational or outdoor activities.

Psychological Therapy

- ***Dunlop's beta hypothesis***: A child is asked to sit in front of a mirror and forced purposeful repetition of a habit which makes the s child experience unpleasant reactions, and the habit is abandoned.
- ***Six steps in cessation of habit (Larson & Johnson)***
  1. Screening for the psychological component.

2. Habit awareness.
3. Habit reversal with a competing response.
4. Response attention.
5. Escalated DRO (differential reinforcement of other behaviours)
6. Escalated DRO with reprimands. (Consists of holding the child, firmly admonishing the child to stop the habit by establishing eye contact)

- **Competing response therapy**: Squeezing an object whenever the child feels the impulse to thumb sucking.
- **Thumb - Home concept:** A small bag is tied around his wrist during sleep and explained that just as a child sleep in his home, the thumb will also sleep in its house and the o child is restrained from digit sucking furthering night.
- Elimination of chronic thumb sucking by preventing a Covarying response: "The behaviour is believed to lose its appeal by being reframed as a duty. Thus, make the child suck all ten fingers by forceful repetition for the same length of time so that it produces an unpleasant reaction and gradually it quits the habit."

Reward System

- Children should be encouraged and rewarded for not practising the habit.(Maguire, 2000)
- A contract made between the child and dentist or child and parent, called "Contingency Contracting", which states that the child should not suck their thumb for a specific period and in return will receive a reward, which is positive reinforcement.
- The reward does not need to be extravagant but must be special enough to motivate the child.
- Verbal praise from the parents and the dentist has a large role in placing reward stickers on a special personalized calendar given to the child by the dentist.
- Stick on stars are applied to the calendar on days when the child has avoided the habit and is evaluated at the end of a month or a specified period, verbal praise or a reward should be given for discontinuing the habit (Fig. **8a**).

Time-Out

- Removal of the reinforcer whenever thumb-sucking occurs. For example, a mother should stop reading a story whenever thumb-sucking occurred.
- When the child removed his/her thumb from their mouth, the mother immediately should resume reading the story.

Reminder therapy

- It is advisable for children who desire to stop the habit but need some assistance.
- These reminders make the habit unpleasant and difficult to practice.

- **Finn:** Habit reminders can be divided into extra-oral reminders and intraoral reminders.

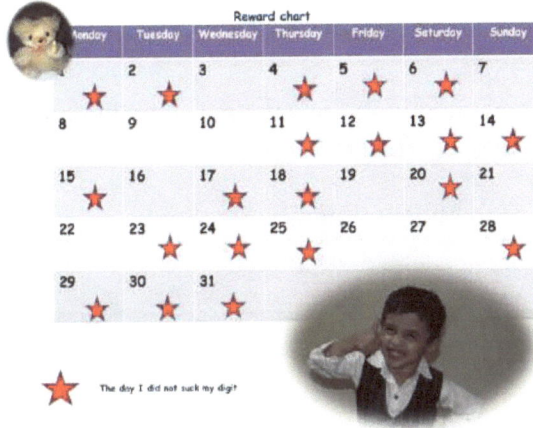

Fig. (8a). Reward chart.

Extra Oral Reminders

Chemical Method

- This is a negative or aversive therapy.
- Bitter and sour Chemicals like Quinine, Asafoetida, Pepper, and Castor oil are applied to the digit, which will have an unpleasant taste on sucking the finger.
- Anti-thumb sucking solutions like Femite, Thumb-up, and Anti-thumb are commercially available, but they have also had very moderate success.

Three Alarm System: (Norton & Gellin) (Fig. 8b)

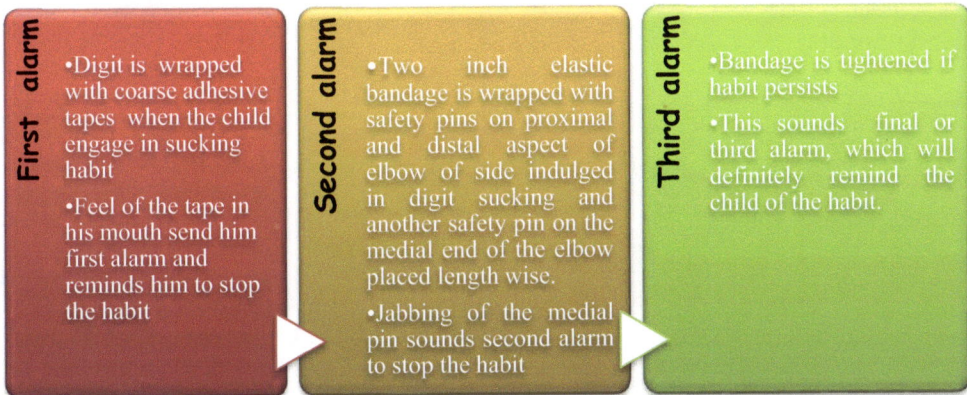

First alarm
- Digit is wrapped with coarse adhesive tapes when the child engage in sucking habit
- Feel of the tape in his mouth send him first alarm and reminds him to stop the habit

Second alarm
- Two inch elastic bandage is wrapped with safety pins on proximal and distal aspect of elbow of side indulged in digit sucking and another safety pin on the medial end of the elbow placed length wise.
- Jabbing of the medial pin sounds second alarm to stop the habit

Third alarm
- Bandage is tightened if habit persists
- This sounds final or third alarm, which will definitely remind the child of the habit.

Fig. (8b). Three alarm system.

Ace Bandage Approach (Figs 9a, b, c)

- Bandage should be wrapped around the finger and stars should be entered into the special personalised calendar on the days when the child does not suck the thumb.
- For every twenty stars entered in the calendar, the child should be rewarded.
- Thermoplastic thumb cap devised by Allen (1991) can also be used on the offending digit.
- A total of 6 weeks of treatment time was required for the elimination of habit.

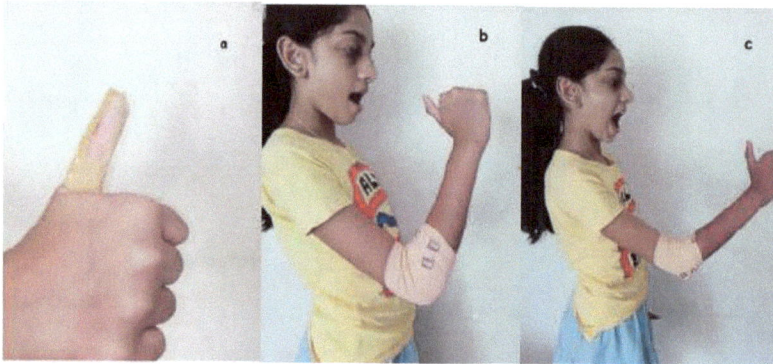

Fig. (9). **a** First alarm, **b-** Second alarm, **c-** Third alarm.

Current Strategies

- Thumb guard (T guard) (Fig. **10**)
- Use of long-sleeve nightgown **(Fig. 11a)**
- Thumb-sucking books **(Fig. 11b)**
- My special shirt
- Hand puppets

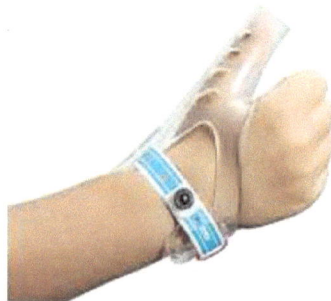

Fig. (10). Thumb guard (T guard).

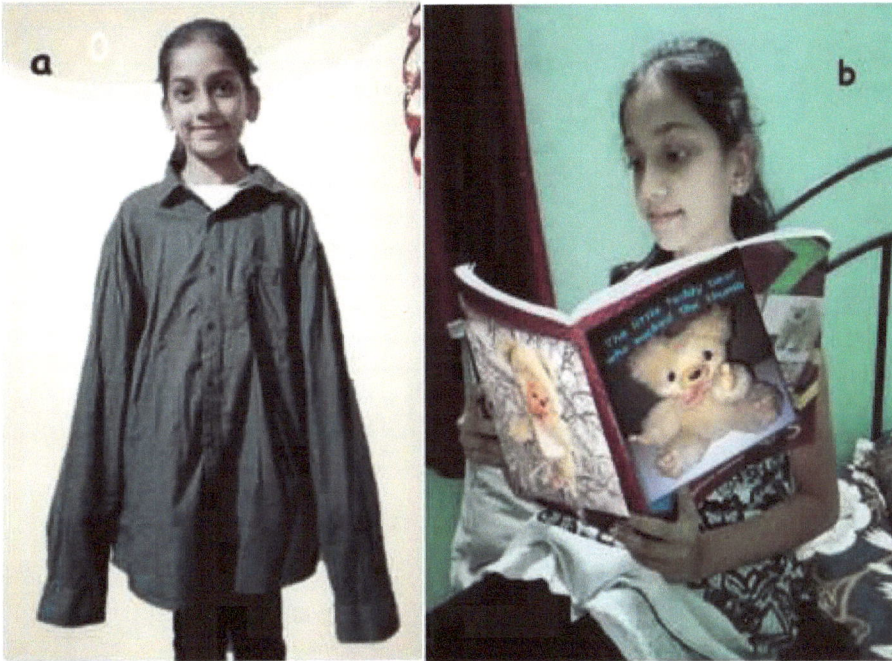

Fig. (11). a- Long-sleeve nightgown, b- Thumb sucking books.

Intraoral Reminders

• It is by removable or fixed intraoral appliances (Figs. **12 - 16**)

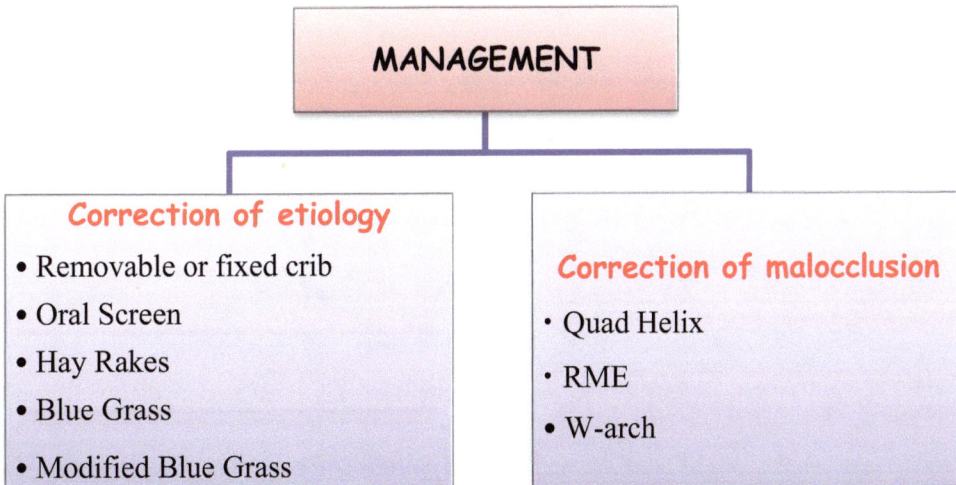

Fig. (12). Management of thumb-sucking habit.

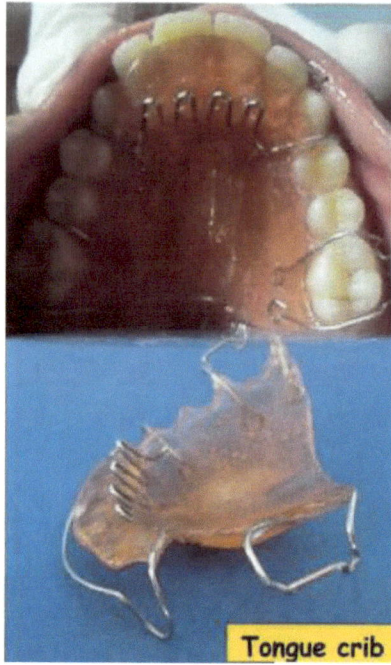

Fig. (13). Removable tongue crib.

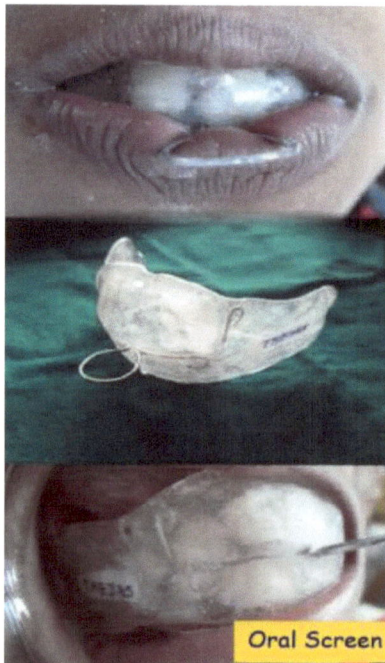

Fig. (14). Oral screen.

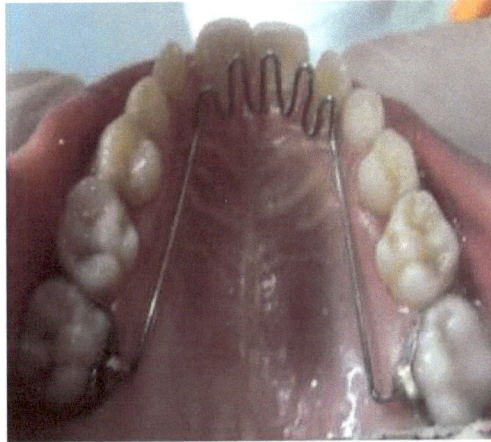

Fig. (15). Fixed tongue crib.

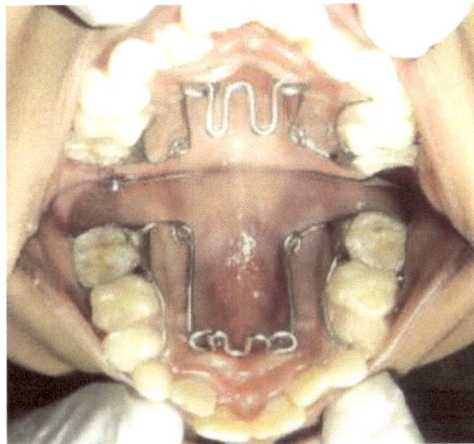

Fig. (16). Quad helix with the tongue crib.

TONGUE THRUSTING

Tongue thrusting is defined as a condition in which the tongue contacts any teeth anterior to the molars during swallowing.

Etiology

Factors which result in tongue-thrusting according to Fletcher:

a. Genetic or heredity factor: Certain anatomic or neuromuscular variations in the orofacial region can precipitate tongue thrust. *e.g.*, Hypertonic orbicularis oris activity.

b. Learned behaviour (habit): Tongue thrust can be acquired as a habit.

Predisposing factors that can lead to tongue thrusting:

1. Improper bottle-feeding
2. Prolonged thumb sucking
3. Prolonged tonsillar and upper respiratory tract infections.

Types of Tongue Thrust

1. *Physiologic:* Normal tongue thrust swallow of infancy.
2. *Habitual:* Tongue thrust swallow is present as a habit even after the correction of the malocclusion.
3. *Functional*: When the tongue is thrust, the mechanism is an adaptive behaviour developed to achieve an oral seal, it can be grouped as functional.
4. *Anatomic*: Persons having an enlarged tongue can have an anterior tongue posture.

Classification of Tongue Thrust by James S. Braner and Holt

Type I: Non-deforming tongue thrust
Type II: Deforming anterior tongue thrust
  ○ Subgroup 1: Anterior open bite
  ○ Subgroup 2: Anterior proclination
  ○ Subgroup 3: Posterior crossbite
Type III: Deforming lateral tongue thrust
  ○ Subgroup 1: Posterior open bite
  ○ Subgroup 2: Posterior crossbite
  ○ Subgroup 3: Deep overbite
Type IV: Deforming anterior and lateral tongue thrust
  ○ Subgroup 1: Anterior and posterior open bite
  ○ Subgroup 2: Proclination of anterior teeth
  ○ Subgroup 3: Posterior crossbite

Simple Tongue Thrust (Anterior Tongue Thrusting)

It is defined as a tongue thrust with teeth together swallow usually associated with the history of digit sucking. The features observed depend upon the duration, intensity, and frequency of the habit.

Complex Tongue Thrust (Anterior and Posterior Ongue Thrust)

It is defined as a tongue thrust with teeth apart swallow usually associated with chronic nasal respiratory distress, mouth breathing, tonsillitis, and pharyngitis (Table **1**).

Lateral Tongue Thrust (Posterior Tongue Thrust)

It is usually developed into a habit by laterally thrusting the tongue. A clinically lateral open bite can be seen. Depending upon the type of tongue thrust, it can be unilateral or bilateral.

Table 1. Differences between simple and complex tongue thrusting.

S.no	Simple	Complex
1.	Facial muscle contraction during swallowing is not seen	Facial muscle contraction can be seen during swallowing
2.	The mandible is stabilized by muscles of mastication	The mandible is stabilized by the muscles of lips and cheeks (facial muscles)
3.	Open bite is well defined with a definite beginning and ending	Open bite is diffuse, ill-defined
4.	Usually, will have a previous history of thumb sucking	Usually, will have a history of tonsillitis or airway obstruction
5.	Proper, secure, posterior occlusal fit	No proper posterior occlusal fit
6.	**Intraoral features** 1. Increased overjet. 2. Anterior open bite. 3. Retroclined or proclined lower anterior. 4. Posterior crossbites. 5. Tongue is thrust forward during swallowing to help establish an anterior lip seal.	**Intraoral features** 1. Bimaxillary protrusion 2. characterized by a teeth-apart swallow 3. Posterior open bite in case of lateral tongue thrust 4. Posterior crossbite
7.	Treatment is simple with less relapse tendency	Treatment is difficult with, more relapse tendency
8.	Occlusal equilibration may be needed	Occlusal equilibration is mandatory

An abnormal tongue position and deviation from the normal swallowing pattern result in abnormal speech, anterior open bite, and anterior protrusion of the maxillary incisors (Fig. **17**).

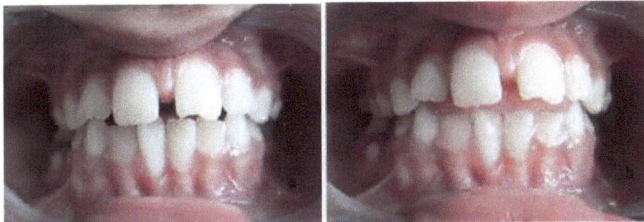

Fig. (17). Intraoral frontal view. Increased overjet, anterior open bite, tongue thrusting forward during swallowing.

Factors Influencing Treatment Planning

Interception of tongue thrusting habit depends on the following factors **[5] (Fig. 18a)**

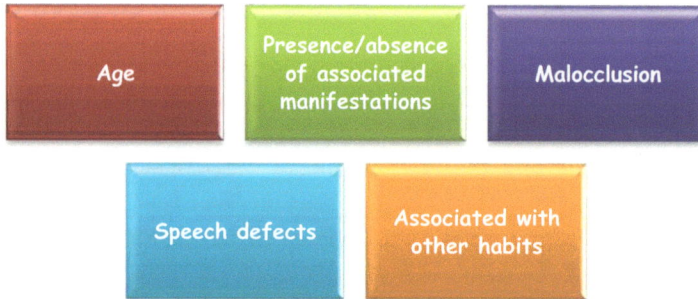

Fig. (18a). Factors influencing treatment planning.

Treatment options

- Training for correct swallowing and posture of the tongue
- Speech therapy
- Mechanotherapy
- Correction of malocclusion
- Surgical treatment

Training of Correct Swallow and Posture of the Tongue

Myofunctional Exercises

Educate the patient about normal swallowing by asking the patient to keep the tongue tip against the junction of the soft and hard palate. Various muscle exercises of the tongue can help in training it to adapt to the new swallowing pattern (Fig. **18b**).

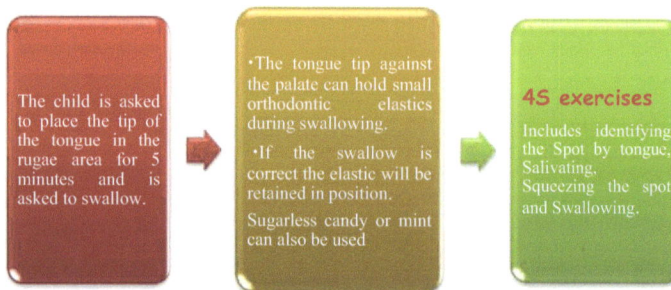

Fig. (18b). Myofunctional exercises.

The patient should practice the new swallowing pattern at least 40 times a day in 2/3 sessions. After learning the new swallowing pattern at a conscious level, it is necessary to reinforce it subconsciously for transforming the control of the reflex from the conscious to a subconscious level.

Guiding the Correct Positioning of the Tongue using Appliances

- **Myofunctional trainer appliance**: It is a prefabricated appliance which aids in the correct positioning of the tongue with the help of tongue tags. The tongue guards prevent the tongue from thrusting the teeth when the appliance is worn (Fig. **19**).
- **Nance palatal arch appliance**: Acrylic button of the appliance acts as a spot for training the correct position of the tongue.
- Mechanotherapy (Table **2**) (Figs. **20, 21a, b, c**).
- If the maxillary arch is constricted, cribs can be fabricated along with expansion devices like a quad-helix and expansion screw.

Table 2. Mechanotherapy for tongue thrusting habit.

Removable	Fixed
• Double oral screen • Hawley appliance with tongue crib/rakes/spikes (Fig. **22**)	Fixed tongue crib/rakes/spikes

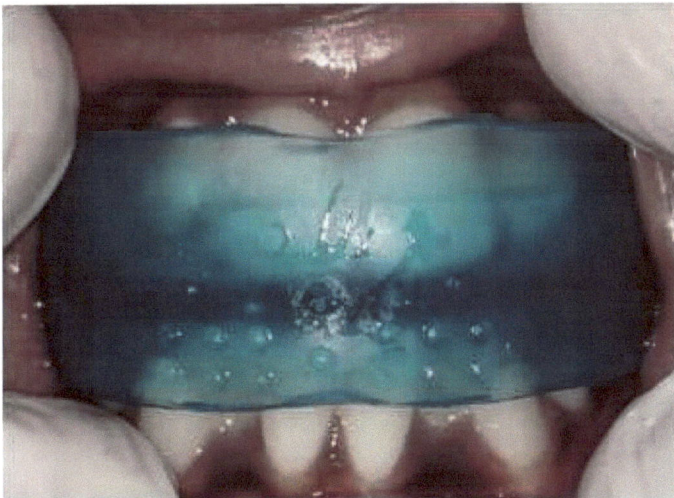

Fig. (19). Myofunctional trainer appliance.

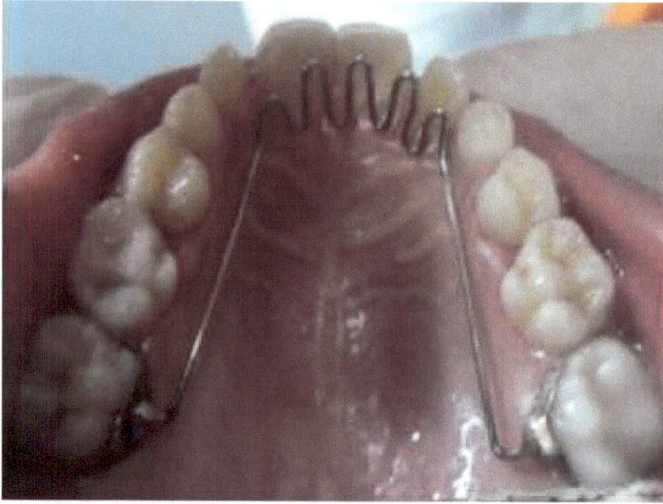

Fig. (20). Fixed tongue crib appliance.

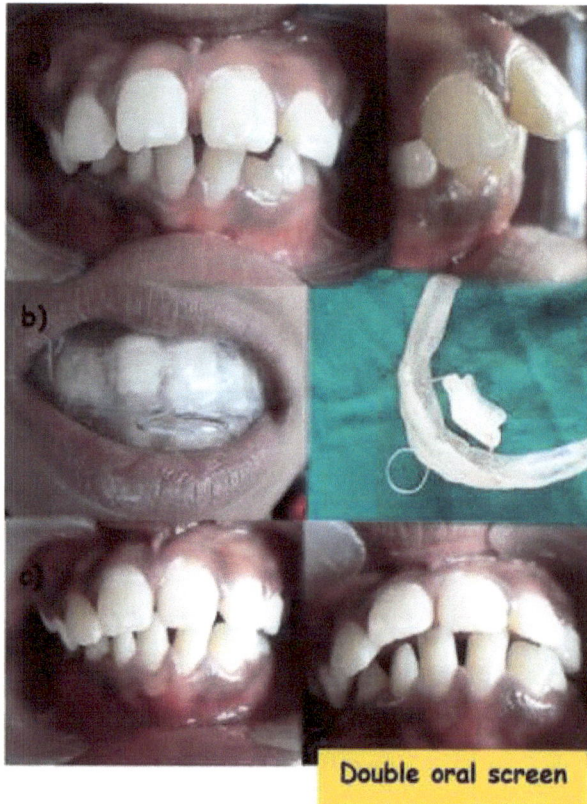

Fig. (21). a) Intraoral frontal view with proclined upper and lower anterior teeth, increased overjet and spacing, **b)** Double oral screen, **c)** Decreased spacing and overjet due to habit interception by the double oral screen.

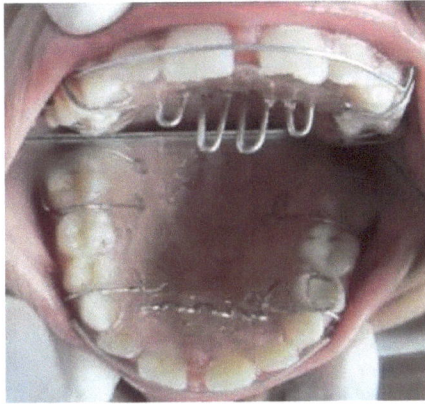

Fig. (22). Hawley appliance the tongue crib.

Mouth Breathing

Mouth breathing is defined as habitual respiration through the mouth instead of the nose.

Classification

Finn has Classified Mouth Breathing into:

a. *Anatomic:* Anatomic short upper lip does not permit complete closure of the lips.
b. *Obstructive:* Complete or partial obstruction of the nasal passage can result in mouth breathing. The following are some of the causes of nasal obstruction: Deviated nasal septum, Nasal polyps, chronic inflammation of nasal mucosa and Obstructive adenoids.
c. *Habitual:* The child continually breathes through his mouth by force of habit, although the abnormal obstruction has been removed.

Mouth breathing produces jaw deformities, inadequate position or shape of the alveolar process and malocclusion and results in the development of adenoid faces or long face syndrome.

Clinical Features of Mouth Breathing

- Long and narrow face which is often blank or expressionless.
- Narrow nose and nasal passage.
- Short and flaccid upper lip.
- Anterior marginal gingivitis can occur due to drying of the gingiva.
- Contracted upper arch with the possibility of posterior crossbite.

- Increased overjet because of flaring of the incisors.
- Anterior open bite can occur (Fig. **23**).

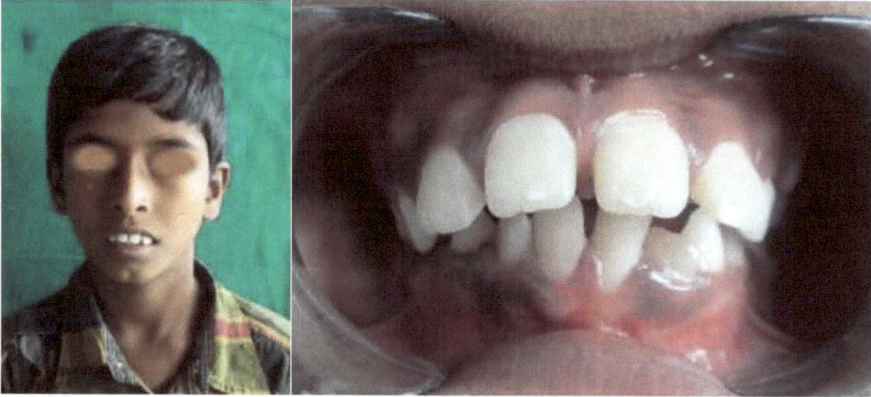

Fig. (23). Clinical features of mouth breathing habit. Long narrow face and nose with short flaccid upper lip, flaring of incisors with increased overjet, decreased overbite.

Diagnosis

History

Detailed history regarding the habit is recorded and also as nasal stiffness, nasal discharge, repeated attacks of cold and sore throat, restlessness at night, feeling thirst and hoarseness of voice [6].

Examination

• Lips are apart (incompetent) in mouth breathers whereas lips are competent in nasal breathers.

External nares do not change in size or shape during the respiratory cycle in mouth breathers [6].

Clinical tests

- *Mirror test*: Double side mirror is held between nose and mouth. Fogging on the oral side of the mirror indicates mouth breathing and on the nasal side, indicates nasal breathing. This is also called as fog test.

- *Massler and Zwemer Butterfly test/ cotton test*: Butterfly-shaped cotton strand is paced on the upper lip below the nostrils. If the fibres of cotton flutter downwards during exhalation, then the child is a nasal breather and if it flutters upwards, he is a mouth breather.
- *Water holding test*: The child is asked to hold water in the mouth. If the child is

a mouth breather, he cannot hold the water >2min.

- *Inductive Plethysmography (Rhinometry)*: Quantification of airflow through the nose and mouth is done using inductive plethysmography which gives a percentage of nasal and oral respiration.
- **Cephalometrics**: This is used to calculate nasopharyngeal space, size of adenoids and to know skeletal patterns of the child.

Treatment Considerations

Age of the Child

- With age, nasal passages increase as the child grows, relieving the obstruction caused due to the enlarged adenoids. Hence, mouth breathing could be expected to decrease over time.
- Mouth breathing is in many instances self-correcting after puberty [7].

ENT Examination

- Presence of enlarged tonsils, adenoids or deviated nasal septum should be evaluated.
- If identified, a pathological condition causing mouth breathing should be treated first.
- In habitual mouth breathers, the habit may continue even after the correction of the pathologic conditions [7].

Interception of the Habit

Lip Exercises

- Holding pencil between lips during daytime.
- Hold a sheet of paper between the lips.
- Tape the lips with surgical tape during night-time.
- **Button pull exercise**: Button with thread is placed behind lips and thread is pulled, button is restricted to pull by lip pressure.
- Stretch the upper lip as far as possible to cover the vermilion border under and behind the maxillary incisors to maintain lip seal (Fig. **24**).

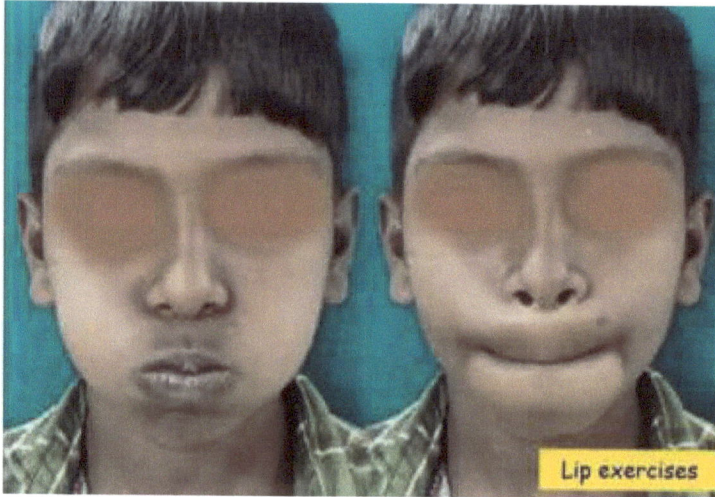

Fig. (24). Lip exercises to maintain lip seal.

Appliance Treatment

• Myofunctional trainer appliance (Fig. **25**) Oral screen (Fig. **26**).

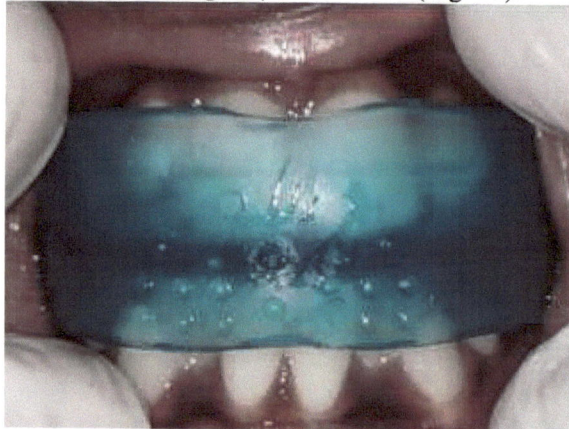

Fig. (25). Myofunctional trainer appliance.

Self-Injurious or Self-Mutilating Behaviour/ Sado Masochistic Habit

It is a rare and chronic condition which is a repetitive act that results in self-physical injury. It gives them a sense of pleasure. It is often associated with children with special health care needs, developmental delays or disabilities, traumatic brain injuries, and psychiatric disorders.

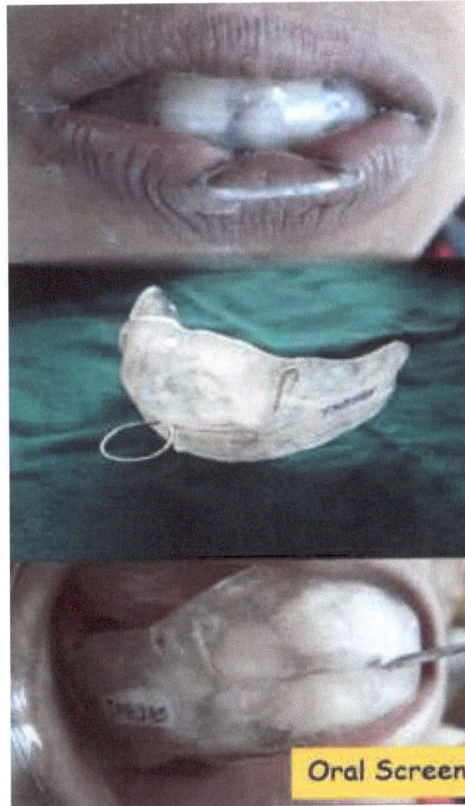

Fig. (26). Oral screen appliance.

Etiological Factors

1. **Organic factors**: It is seen in DeLange's Syndrome and Lesch Nyhan disease. Repetitive lip, tongue, finger, shoulder, and knee biting have been commonly observed.
2. **Functional: These are further** divided into:
   - *Type A*: Injuries which are layered on top of an established lesion.
   - *Type B:* Injuries occurring because of a previously developed habit. The self-destructive habit worsens the symptoms of the primary habit.
   - *Type C:* Injuries of unclear or complex etiology can occur. This type of habit is more psychogenic in nature. The child engages in a variety of self-destructive behaviors as a stress reliever.

Treatment options include

- Pharmacologic management
- Behaviour modification

- Physical restraint.
- Dental treatment modalities include lip-bumper and occlusal bite appliances, protective
- Padding and extractions.

BRUXISM

Bruxism is the habitual grinding of teeth when the individual is not chewing or swallowing (Ramfjord, 1966).

It is habitual non-functional and forceful contact between occlusal surfaces and can occur while awake or asleep.

Complications of bruxism include

- Dental attrition, headaches.
- Grinding or impacting sounds of teeth
- Temporomandibular dysfunction
- Soreness and hypertrophy of masticatory muscles (Fig. **27**)
- Hypersensitivity of teeth to cold air [8].

Juvenile bruxism does not endure in adults as it is self-limiting [1].

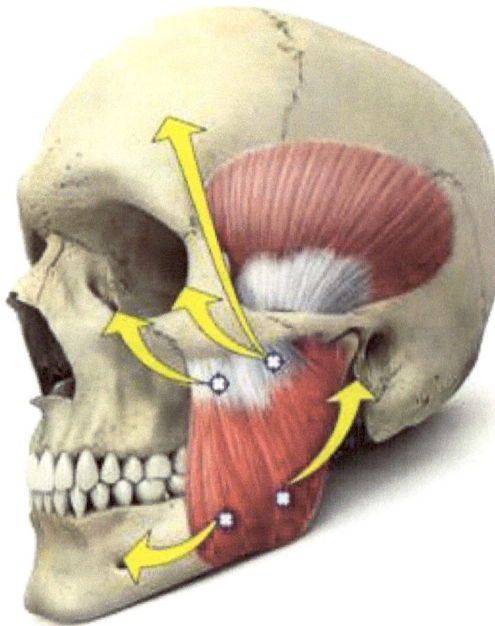

Fig. (27). Effects of Bruxism.

The Spectrum of Bruxism Management Ranges from

1. *Occlusal adjustments:* Prematurities or occlusal interferences in restorations should be corrected.
2. *Occlusal splints:* Occlusal surfaces of all the teeth are covered by vulcanite splints which prevents enamel loss during the habit. It can be prevented by the patented aero foil-shaped base and a double mouth guard design (Fig. **28**).

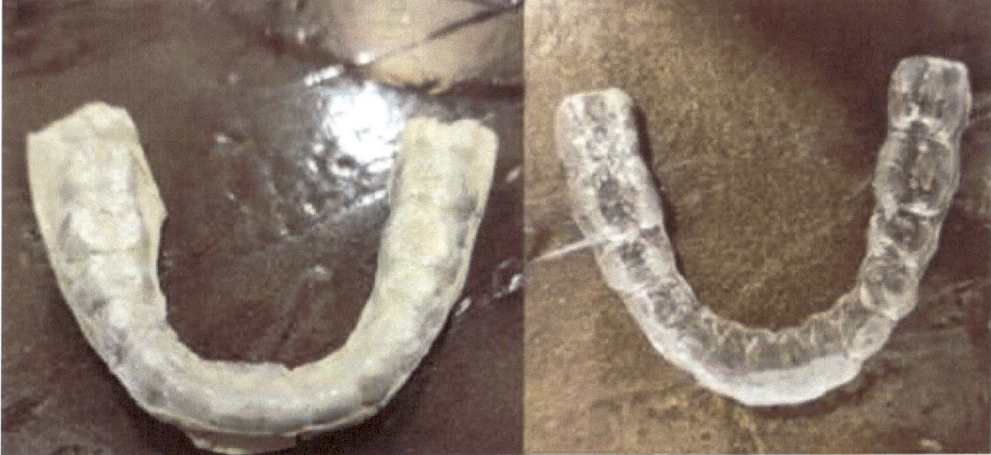

Fig. (28). Occlusal splints.

3. *Restorative Treatment*: Pulpal therapy with full coverage crowns is indicated if the attrition is so severe that penetration into the pulp chamber is seen.
4. *Psychotherapy*: Patient habit awareness is created and by counselling, voluntary control of the habit can be achieved which reduces bruxism.
5. *Relaxation training*: Training the patient to relax the tense muscle group voluntarily by relaxing. Hypnosis, conditioning, *etc.*, are also indicated for subjects in whom bruxism is due to a central cause.
6. *Biofeedback*: It utilizes positive feedback to able the patient to learn tension reduction. It is accomplished by allowing the patient to view an EMG monitor, while the mandible is postured with minimum activity.
7. *Electrical method:* Electro galvanic stimulation for muscle relaxation can be used.
8. *Orthodontic correction:* Certain malocclusions like Class II and Class III relation, frontal open bite and cross bites when associated with functional malocclusion may predispose to bruxism.
9. *Psychological techniques for medications:* Drugs like diazepam and clonazepam are effective [2, 8].

OBSTRUCTIVE SLEEP APNOEA SYNDROME

Obstructive sleep apnoea (OSA) is becoming a global problem with detrimental effects on general health and quality of life and is often seen in patients with a neurologic disease like stroke or medication-refractory epilepsy [9].

Associated with the following conditions

- Snoring
- Observed apnoea
- Restless sleep
- Daytime neurobehavioral abnormalities or sleepiness
- Bedwetting
- Signs of nasal obstruction, adenoidal facies, and enlarged tonsils
- Growth abnormalities
- Dental features include the constricted maxilla, crossbite, low tongue position, vertical growth, increased overjet, and open bite

Treatment Options for Obstructive Sleep Apnoea

a. Continuous Positive airway pressure (CPAP)
b. Oral appliances
   - Tongue-retaining devices
   - Mandibular advancement devices
c. Surgical
   - Phase I (nasal, palatal, tongue)
   - Phase II (maxillomandibular advancement)
   - Hypoglossal nerve stimulation
d. Adjunct
   - Weight loss
   - Positional therapy
   - Nasal expiratory PAP
   - Non-invasive oral pressure therapy
      The use of continuous positive airway pressure (CPAP) can improve sleep-related symptoms and quality of life and is considered the gold standard treatment for sleep apnoea [9].
      CPAP acts as a pneumatic splint that stabilizes the upper airway with constant positive pressure *via* a mask interface.

NOTE ON MYOBRACE

Myofunctional Orthodontic System has progressed over the past 20 years in which the Myobrace system by Myofunctional Research Co. (MRC) is advanced.

Modalities like habit correction, arch expansion and dental alignment are integrated into one system, Myofunctional Orthodontic System. It allows children to develop to their genetic potential along with being a less invasive way to straighten teeth without braces, it satisfies the demand from the parents.

THE MYOBRACE SYSTEM

Myofunctional pre-orthodontic treatment is less mechanical and more biologically based, offering a wide range of modalities that address the underlying causes of malocclusion and airway dysfunction. These appliances offer patients a more natural orthodontic solution which is ideally suited to treat children aged 3-15yrs by focusing on the correction of poor myofunctional habits affecting the teeth, jaws, and facial development [10].

The fundamental keys to this treatment are

- Obtaining correct nasal breathing
- Correcting tongue resting position
- Retraining the oral muscles to function correctly

Along with habit correction, these appliances apply light forces to the teeth to assist them to align into their natural position, usually with no need for braces or extractions in the future.

Appliance Usage

- The patient must wear the appliance for 1 to 2 hours during the daytime and overnight while sleeping.
- Good patient compliance is mandatory, and the appliance should be worn every day for successful results.
- At least one myofunctional exercise must be completed every day.
- The patient must learn how to swallow correctly and position the tongue in the correct place in the mouth.
- Mouth should be closed when not speaking or eating.

There are 3-4 stages of appliances that are designed for each dentition, which are specific to that age group. These appliances effectively train the tongue to its correct position in the maxilla, retrain oral musculature, expand the jaws, and align the teeth by exerting light forces. The effect of the correct tongue position and patented DynamiCore™ develops the arch form, allowing the better arch length and improving dental alignment

Components of Myobrace

• **Guides for teeth/tooth slots:** They promote correct alignment which is narrower anteriorly and wider posteriorly corresponding to the sizes of the incisal edges and occlusal surfaces of the teeth. The upper and lower channels are separated by a thermoplastic material of 2 mm in thickness [10, 11].

• **Labial and buccal shields**: Prevent the interposition of lips and cheeks and imparts a slight force on the front misaligned teeth.

•**Tongue guard**: Prevents tongue thrusting anterior teeth, forcing it in its natural position, stimulating the nasal breathing and discouraging deleterious habits.

• **Tongue tag:** Positioned at the retro-incisive papilla, acting as a proprioceptive stimulus to the tip of the tongue, and as a myofunctional trainer to correct the tongue posture.

• **Lip bumper:** Discourages hyperactivity of the mentalis muscle, hence relaxing the muscle.

• **DynamiCore with Frankel Cage** - Assists in widening and developing the jaws. (Fig. **29**) [12]

Types of Myobrace

1. **Myobrace for juniors (Three stages J1, J2, J3):** Used for 3-6 yrs. of age
   ◦ Stage 1 - Correct nasal breathing (J1)
   ◦ Stage 2 - Establish correct tongue position (J2)
   ◦ Stage 3- Maintain correct lip posture and swallow (J3)
2. **Myobrace for kids (Three stages K1, K2, K3):** Used for 6 - 10 years age group
   ◦ Stage 1 (habit correction) - establish nasal breathing.
   ◦ Stage 2 (arch development) - establish correct tongue position.
   ◦ Stage 3 (final alignment and retention) - maintain correct lip posture and swallow.
3. **Myobrace for teens T1, T2, T3, T4:** Used for 10 – 15 years age group
   ◦ Stage 1 (habit correction) - establish nasal breathing.
   ◦ Stage 2 (arch development) - establish correct tongue position, lip posture and swallowing.
   ◦ Stage 3 (dental alignment) - tooth alignment, once habits and compliance are good.
   ◦ Stage 4 (retention) - retain dental alignment while maintaining correct habits.
4. **Speciality Appliances -** The Lip Trainer

It is an adjunct to other Myobrace appliances and can be used at any stage for improving lip seal, strengthening, and stretching the lip muscles to reduce overactivity when swallowing.

5. Myobrace for adults A1, A2, A3
6. Myobrace for interceptive Class III
7. **Myolay:** Combination of composite buildup technique and Myobrace
8. Combination of Farrel bent wire system and myobrace appliance [11, 12].

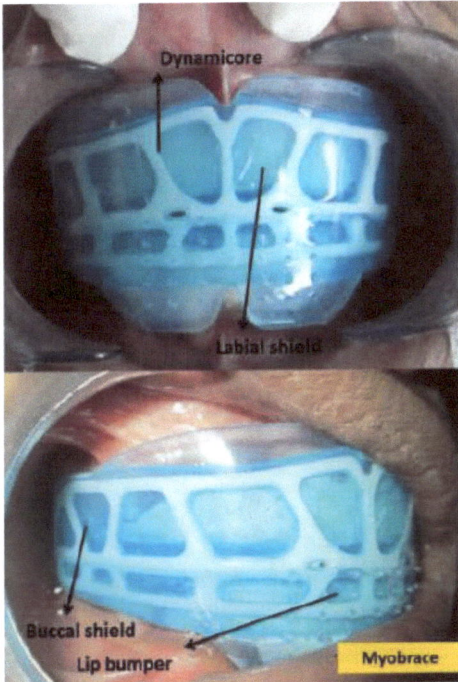

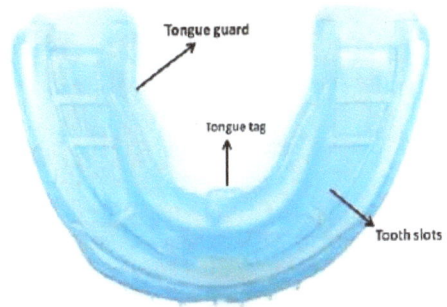

Fig. (29). Myobrace Myofunctional appliance.

CONCLUSION

Oral habits cause a deleterious effect on oral tissues leading to unfavourable dentofacial growth. A pediatric dentist plays a pivotal role in the early identification and interception of the habit so that potential unfavourable growth and development of dentofacial complex is minimised.

CONSENT FOR PUBLICATION

Not applicable.

CONFLICT OF INTEREST

The authors declare no conflict of interest, financial or otherwise.

ACKNOWLEDGEMENT

Declared none.

REFERENCES

[1]   Management of the developing dentition and occlusion in pediatric dentistry. The Reference Manual of Pediatric Dentistry. 2020; 393-409.

[2]   Shahraki N, Yassaei S, Moghadam MG. Abnormal oral habits: A review. J Dent Oral Hyg 2012; 4(2): 12-5.

[3]   Maguire JA. The evaluation and treatment of pediatric oral habits. Dent Clin North Am 2000; 44(3): 659-69.
        [http://dx.doi.org/10.1016/S0011-8532(22)01749-9] [PMID: 10925776]

[4]   Kamdar RJ, Al-Shahrani I. Damaging oral habits. J Int Oral Health 2015; 7(4): 85-7.
        [PMID: 25954079]

[5]   Singh S. Prerna, Kalia S. Habit breaking appliance for tongue thrusting – A modification. Indian Journal of Dental Sciences 2009; 1(1): 1-5.

[6]   Grippaudo C, Paolantonio eg, Antonini G, Saulle R, La Torre G, Deli R. Association between oral habits, mouth breathing and malocclusion. Acta Otorhinolaryngol Ital 2016; 36(5): 386-94.
        [http://dx.doi.org/10.14639/0392-100X-770] [PMID: 27958599]

[7]   Jain A, Bhaskar DJ, Gupta D, *et al.* Mouth breathing: A menace to developing dentition. Journal of Contemporary Dentistry 2014; 4(3): 145-51.
        [http://dx.doi.org/10.5005/jp-journals-10031-1085]

[8]   Maia LC, Soares-Silva L, Tavares-Silva C, Fonseca-Gonçalves A. Presence of oral habits and their association with the trait of anxiety in pediatric patients with possible sleep bruxism. J Indian Soc Pedod Prev Dent 2019; 37(3): 245-50.
        [http://dx.doi.org/10.4103/JISPPD.JISPPD_272_18] [PMID: 31584023]

[9]   Pavwoski P, Shelgikar AV. Treatment options for obstructive sleep apnea. Neurol Clin Pract 2017; 7(1): 77-85.
        [http://dx.doi.org/10.1212/CPJ.0000000000000320] [PMID: 29849228]

[10]   Farrell C. The Myobrace® System: Biologically focused treatment innovation. 2016; 74-8.

[11]   Aggarwal I, Wadhawan M, Dhir V. Myobraces: Say no to traditional braces. Int J Oral Care Res 2016; 4(1): 82-5.
        [http://dx.doi.org/10.5005/jp-journals-10051-0019]

[12]   Chrysopoulos KN. Interception of malocclusion in the mixed dentition with prefabricated appliances and orofacial myofunctional therapy. J Dent Health Oral Disord Ther 2017; 7(5): 343-5.
        [http://dx.doi.org/10.15406/jdhodt.2017.07.00255]

CHAPTER 9

Interceptive Orthodontics and Myofunctional Therapy in Pediatric Dentistry

H. Sharath Chandra[1,*], S.H. Krishnamoorthy[2] and Dhanashree Sakhare[3]

[1] *Department of Paediatric and Preventive Dentistry SJM Dental College and Hospital, Chitradurga, Karnataka, India*

[2] *Department of Paediatric and Preventive Dentistry, KVG Dental College and Hospital, Sullia, Karnataka, India*

[3] *Lavanika Dental Academy, Melbourne, Australia*

Abstract: Guidance of eruption and development of primary, mixed, and permanent dentition has a pivotal role in comprehensive oral healthcare in paediatric dentistry, which helps to achieve more stable, functionally, and aesthetically acceptable permanent dentition. Interceptive orthodontics includes procedures carried out in mixed dentition, and it takes advantage of the growth pattern and development during this phase. Early diagnosis and treatment of certain malocclusions will eliminate or reduce the severity of developing malocclusion, which would lessen the complexity of orthodontic treatment in the future, overall time, and cost. It also improves the child's self-esteem, confidence, and parental satisfaction. Overall clinical examination, radiographic evaluation, and study model analysis with thorough knowledge of growth and development help in diagnosing and carrying out appropriate interceptive treatments necessary.

Keywords: Early orthodontic treatment, Interceptive orthodontics, Mixed dentition.

INTRODUCTION

Early treatment means treatments undertaken during the most active stages of dentition and craniofacial skeletal growth to enhance dentoalveolar, skeletal and muscular development before the complete eruption of the permanent dentition. Historically, orthodontic treatment was provided for adolescents. But of late, the concept of early orthodontic treatment has gained approval, and many clinicians

---

* **Corresponding author H. Sharath Chandra:** Department of Paediatric and Preventive Dentistry SJM Dental College and Hospital, Chitradurga, Karnataka; E-mail: sharathchandrah2012@gmail.com

seek to modify skeletal, muscular and dentoalveolar abnormalities even before the eruption of full permanent dentition.

The early orthodontic intervention can be broadly classified as shown in Fig. (**1**).

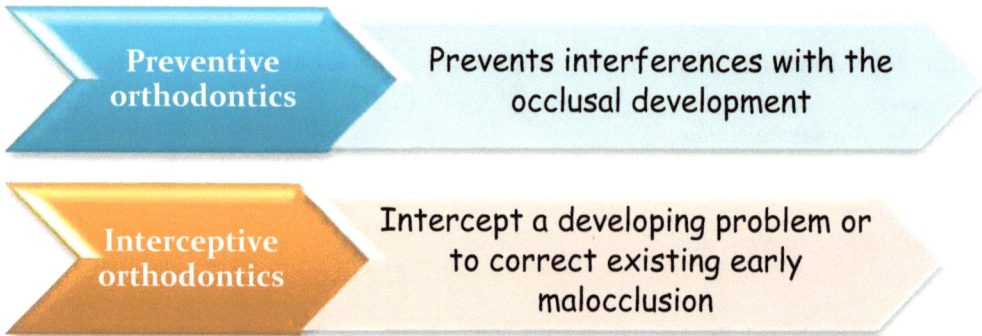

Fig. (1). Early orthodontic intervention.

BENEFITS OF EARLY TREATMENT

1. Certain malocclusions can be prevented or intercepted only at an early age.
2. More alternative treatment options are available at a young age.
3. Younger patients are often more cooperative and attentive.
4. Clinicians can utilize growth better at a younger age, and there is more growth remaining.
5. Psychological advantages in children by improving the esthetics of smile and the accompanying positive effects on self-image and improving the occlusion.
6. Compromise of quality of treatment is less as
   ○ It may remove etiologic factors and restore normal growth, and
   ○ It may reduce the severity of the skeletal pattern, making it possible, and easier and more precise tooth positioning in the adolescent.
7. Reduces the financial burden and is a much more affordable form of orthodontic treatment.
8. Possibility of achieving better results with modern precision bracketed appliances.
9. Early treatment of serious deleterious oral habits is easier than treating after years of ingrained habit reinforcement.

INTERCEPTIVE ORTHODONTICS

It is defined as "that phase of the science and art of orthodontics employed to recognize and eliminate potential irregularities and malposition's in the developing dentofacial complex"- *American Association of Orthodontists Glossary*.

In 1980, Ackerman and Proffit introduced Interceptive orthodontics as a means of correcting problems in the developing dentition and was considered efficient for improving oral hygiene, speech, masticatory efficiency, reduction of periodontal disease, the relief of temporomandibular disorder (TMD), resistance to trauma, and offer psychological benefits.

Interceptive orthodontics includes early diagnosis of certain features of malocclusion in the growing child and its early intervention by using removable appliances or simply fixed appliances by the dentist, will reduce the complexity of the malocclusion from developing as the child grows older. Thorough knowledge of craniofacial growth and development of the dentition must be used in diagnosing and reviewing possible interceptive treatment options before recommendations are made to parents.

Various Treatment Considerations are Addressed Based on Stages of Development of Occlusion [1].

Primary Dentition Stage

Oral deleterious habits and crossbites should be diagnosed and should be addressed as early as possible to facilitate normal occlusal relationships if they are not likely to be self-correcting.

Early-to-Mid mixed Dentition Stage

Treatments need to be addressed:

a. Crossbites
b. Arch length shortage
c. Intervention for crowded incisors
d. Intervention for ectopic teeth
e. Holding of leeway space
f. Oral deleterious habits
g. Soft tissue surgical needs
h. Adverse skeletal growth

Mid-to-Late Mixed Dentition Stage

Intervention for correction of skeletal disharmonies and crowding is initiated in this stage.

Adolescent Dentition Stage

Orthodontic diagnosis and treatment providing functional and esthetics occlusion.

Early Adult Dentition Stage

Evaluation of third molar position or space, extraction if indicated. Full orthodontic treatment should be recommended if needed.

Interceptive orthodontics includes crossbite corrections, Supernumerary teeth extractions, Oral habits interception, Managing crowding, Skeletal discrepancy correction, soft tissue surgical needs, Serial extraction, and Space loss.

CROSSBITE

According to Graber: Crossbite is defined as a condition where one or more teeth may be malposed abnormally buccally, lingually or labially concerning opposing tooth or teeth.

Causes

- Over-retention of deciduous teeth
- Irregular eruption pattern of permanent teeth
- Supernumerary teeth
- Cysts and tumours
- Malposition of permanent teeth
- Traumatic injuries
- Thumb sucking
- Swallowing in an abnormal way
- Mouth breathing habit

Classification: Crossbite can be classified in different ways as shown in Fig. (**2**).

Etiological factors: Dental, Skeletal and Functional

Number of teeth involved: Single and Segmental

Extent: Unilateral and Bilateral

ANTERIOR CROSSBITE

Anterior crossbite is defined as an abnormal reversed relationship of a tooth or teeth, to the opposing teeth in the buccolingual or labiolingual direction, and it is also known as reverse articulation - *American Association of Orthodontists glossary*

Anterior crossbite can lead to the following complication

- Dental and facial disharmony
- Gingival recession
- Mobility of the opposing mandibular tooth/teeth
- Enamel wears due to heavy contact between the opposing tooth/teeth at the incisal edge
- Thinning of the alveolar bone
- TMJ disorders

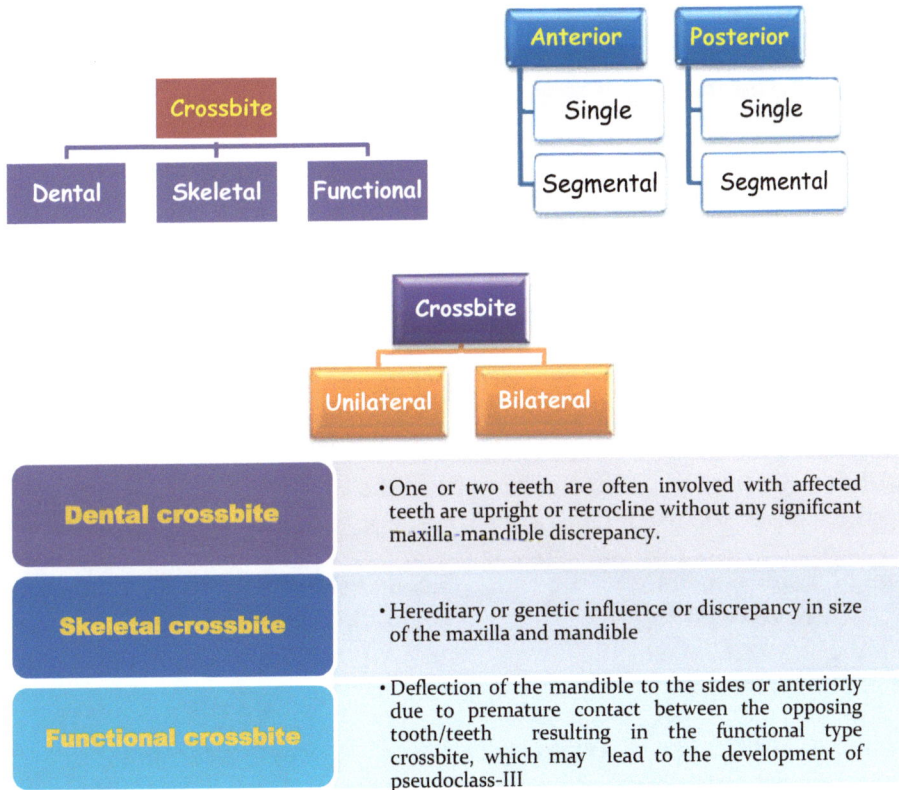

Fig. (2). Classification of Crossbite.

Hence anterior crossbite should be corrected in deciduous or early mixed dentition immediately once identified, to allow normal development of the occlusion and jaws. Any technique for correction of crossbite should be simple, non-invasive, require minimal patient co-operation, involve little chairside time, and gives rapid correction of the crossbite [2, 3].

A simple anterior crossbite of dental origin is the result of an abnormal axial inclination of maxillary anterior teeth with Class I molar occlusion. This condition should be differentiated from a Class III skeletal malocclusion where the crossbite is the result of the basal bone position.

Treatment Modalities

Correction of anterior dental crossbite requires first opening of enough space, then bringing the displaced tooth or teeth across the occlusion into the proper position. The appropriate method depends on the etiology of the crossbite, patient's age and compliance, space availability, eruption status of the teeth and treatment affordability [2].

Treatment modalities for correction of anterior dental crossbite are

- Tongue blades
- Catalan's appliance
- Removable acrylic appliances with Z springs
- Bonded resin-composite slopes
- Reverse stainless-steel crowns
- Bruckl appliance

Tongue Blade Therapy

Indications: The tongue blade can be used in the early stages of anterior crossbite development when the tooth/teeth are still erupting.

Method of use: The tongue blade is placed inside the mouth, contacting the palatal surface of maxillary teeth and on slight closure of the mouth, the opposite side of the blade contacts the labial aspect of the opposing mandibular tooth which acts as a fulcrum.

This results in the change of axial inclination of the erupting tooth, thus correcting crossbite. It is continued for 1-2 hrs a day for 2 weeks.

Catalan's Appliance

It is a lower inclined bite plane that works on newton's third law of motion and helps in reversing the bite.

Indications

- Catalan's appliance is used in the early mixed dentition stage (8-11yrs), where teeth are in the active stage of eruption.

- When there is enough space in the dental arch for labial movement of the upper incisors.
- Absence of crowding in mandibular anterior teeth.

Appliance

- Acrylic inclined bite plane with a slope of 45-degree angulations to the long axis of the tooth which facilitates tipping maxillary anterior teeth labially and mandibular teeth are tipped slightly in the lingual direction which is accentuated from the force of muscle while closing mouth, hence reversing the bite [3].
- The appliance is cemented onto the mandibular incisors and canines with zinc oxide eugenol cement, and the only contact point is present in the incisor region. The child is advised to maintain good oral hygiene and be on a soft diet for a few weeks. The child should be evaluated on a weekly basis for correction of bite, and the duration of the treatment should not exceed more than 6 weeks. Post correction, the appliance is removed, the enamel surface is polished and topical fluoride (APF) is applied.(Fig. **3a**, **3b,c**).

Advantages

- A safe, cost-effective, rapid, and easy alternative for the treatment of crossbite.
- As it is fixed to the tooth, the outcome does not depend on patient co-operation.
- Does not hamper the growth or cause any discomfort to the patient, and treatment is completed in a short period with a smaller number of visits.

Disadvantages

- Difficulty in speech and mastication.
- Risk of anterior open bite if the appliance is cemented for more than 6 weeks.

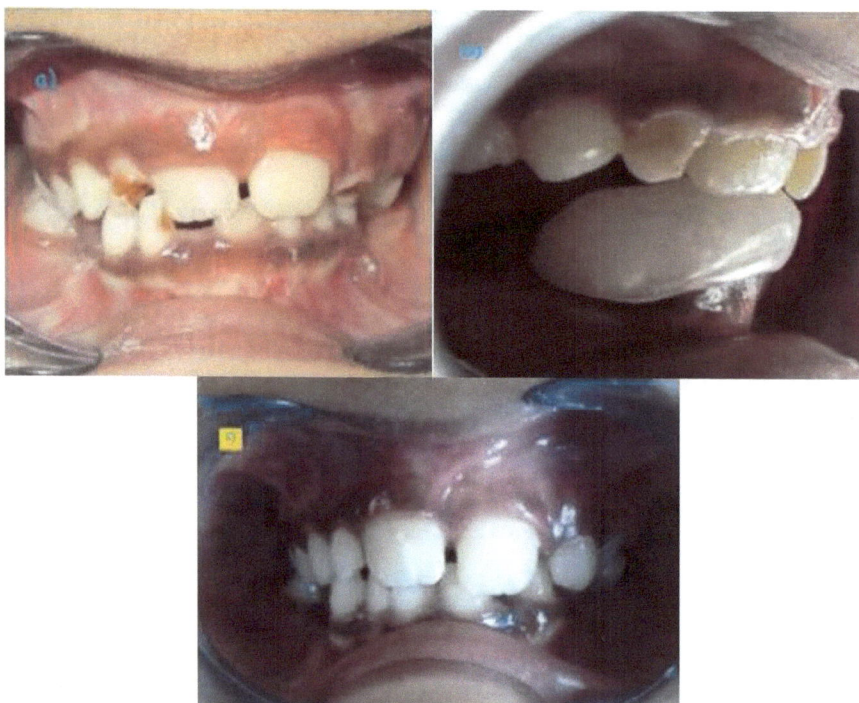

Fig. (3). a) Anterior crossbite of upper right central incisor **b)** Catalan's appliance for correction of crossbite cemented **c)** post-operative frontal view with correction of crossbite of the upper right central incisor.

Removable Appliance with Z Spring

Indications: Simple dental crossbite with no skeletal deformities and adequate space is present in the arch for labial movement of the tooth

Appliance: It is a removable Hawley's appliance with a Z spring incorporated for labial movement of the tooth. The posterior bite plane is incorporated to raise the bite by 2mm to facilitate labial movement of the tooth in crossbite without any hindrance by lower mandibular incisors.

Activation: The appliance delivers slow light continuous forces. The patient is followed every week, and the Z spring is activated by opening the helices by 2mm each time till correction s achieved. (Fig. **4a, b,c, d**) Relapse is prevented as normal overjet and overbite, which is achieved by correction by the appliance.

Advantages

- Helps in maintaining oral hygiene.
- Reduced chair side time.

Disadvantages

- Patient's compliance and supervision of parent are required.
- Chances of breakage or losing the appliance.

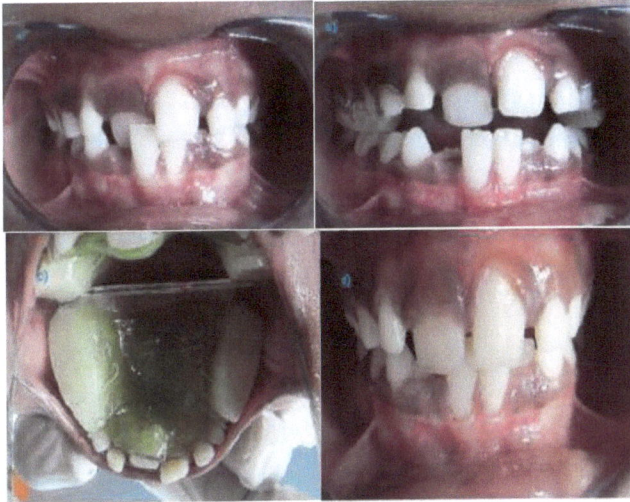

Fig. (4). a) Preoperative frontal view with anterior crossbite of tooth 11 **b)** Removable appliance with Z spring with posterior bite plane **c)** Occlusal view with the appliance **d)** postoperative view with correction of crossbite of tooth 11.

Bonded Resin-Composite Slopes

- Inclined slopes are formed on the labial surface of mandibular incisors using composite resins.
- The thickness of the resin is 3-4mm with resin slopes given at a 45° angle to the longitudinal axis of the tooth, which helps in labial movement of the teeth in crossbite, and the child is evaluated every week for treatment progress and periodontal health of the teeth [4].
- The children should be motivated to maintain good oral hygiene.

Reverse Stainless-Steel Crown

- Used for the correction of single tooth crossbite
- Oversized anterior preformed stainless-steel crown is trimmed and contoured to fit snugly to the tooth in crossbite and is cemented in the reverse direction. The slope of the labial side of the reverse crown helps in the correction of crossbite.
- Disadvantages include difficulty in the adaptation of the crown and the unesthetic appearance of the steel crown, which is often rejected by the child and parent.

Strip Crowns

It is another viable alternative for early anterior crossbite treatment in the primary dentition. Primary maxillary incisors are restored with esthetics paediatric strip crowns by slightly changing the longitudinal axis of the crowns. In this way, it will create interference when the teeth are occluded and guide the mandible to posturing backwards at the final occlusion of the teeth. It brings the child's occlusion into a normal relationship and permits dentofacial growth and development to continue into a more normal pattern (Figs. **5a, b**)

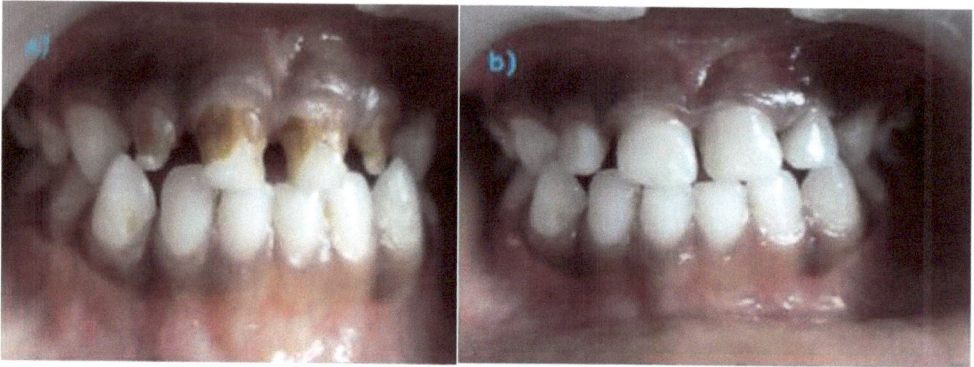

Fig. (5). a) Intraoral view with decayed maxillary anterior and lateral incisors in crossbite. b) Restoration of maxillary anterior teeth with strip crowns and correction of crossbite of 52, 62 by changing the axial inclination of strip crowns.

Bruckl Appliance

It is a removable functional appliance on the lower arch which has a simple design and works as an inclined plane [5].

Indications: It is used when there is an anterior crossbite involving several teeth (2-4) and vertical overbite 1/2-2/3 or more.

Appliance: Bruckl appliance is a mandibular Hawley type retainer with an inclined plane added to it. A labial bow incorporated into the appliance helps in the retraction of lower incisors. The inclined plane stimulates the forward or labial movement of maxillary incisors which are in crossbite and are accentuated by muscle force on closing the mouth (Figs. **6a, b, c** and **d**).

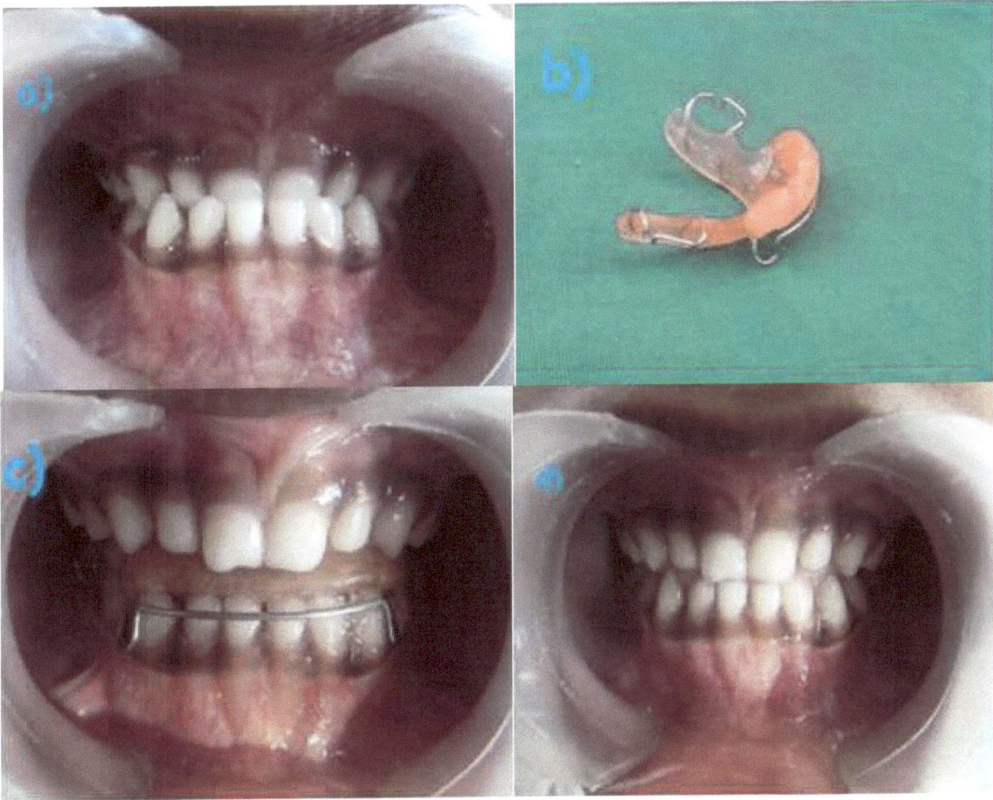

Fig. (6). a) Intraoral view with maxillary anterior in crossbite. **b), c)** Bruckl appliance. **d)** Change in axial inclinations of incisors resulting in correction of crossbite.

In closing, the upper incisors, which are in crossbite with lower incisors; bite on the inclined plane and the pressure of the bite (P) divides into two force vectors P1 and P2. Proclination of upper incisors is by pressure (P1) and intrusion of incisors is by pressure (P2). The steeper the plane, the greater the forward pressure on the maxillary incisors. (Fig. 7) The appliance should be worn full time, and the patient is instructed to adopt a soft diet until the incisor relationship is corrected and later appliance can be removed. The treatment duration is around 7-8 weeks.

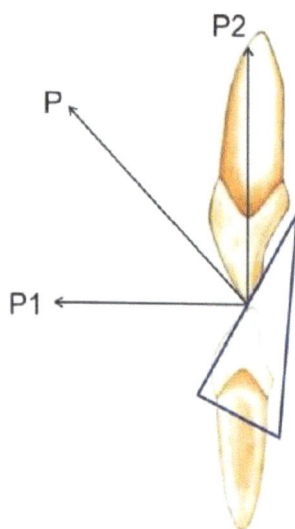

Fig. (7). Resulting force vector of the inclined plane.

Advantages

- It can be used as a retention appliance after active treatment
- It can be used as a removable space maintainer in the lower jaw in the case where there is a premature loss of the primary teeth incorporating acrylic teeth in the appliance.

TREATMENT MODALITIES FOR ANTERIOR CROSSBITE OF SKELETAL IN ORIGIN

Face Mask and Rapid Maxillary Expansion

Indications

- It is indicated when a skeletal-transverse deficiency occurs in the maxilla.
- Skeletal Class III malocclusion usually is a three-dimensional problem and patients have constricted maxilla with anterior and/or posterior crossbite.

Since maxillary growth is retarded, which is coupled with unimpeded growth of the mandible, hence sagittal discrepancy may worsen with age. Early interception with orthopaedic appliances would advance the maxilla and, at the same time, restrict the mandibular growth. This enables a morphologic and functional condition that favours normal facial growth, in addition to establishing more acceptable esthetics in the early stage.

Appliance

Use of rapid maxillary expansion (RME) has been recommended along with a face mask for protraction of the maxilla. RME will disarticulate the maxilla and initiate a cellular response in the circummaxillary sutures, bringing about a more positive reaction to protraction.

RME appliance can be bonded or banded to the maxillary arch. The patient activates the expander once or twice a day until the desired transverse relationship is achieved. Another protocol is the use of alternate rapid maxillary expansions and constrictions (Alt-RAMEC). Activation of expansion/constriction is 0.5mm daily to disarticulate the suture without overexpansion (Fig. **8a, b**) [6].

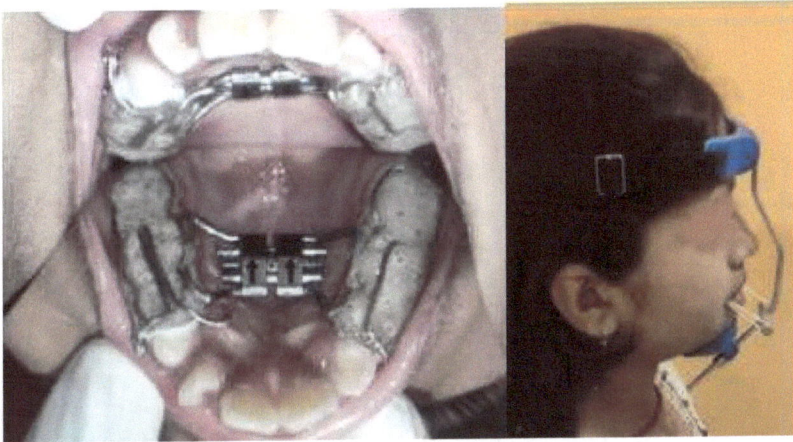

Fig. (8). a) Bonded hyrax Rapid Maxillary Expansion (RME) appliance with J hook b) Reverse pull head gear or Petit face mask.

Face mask/reverse headgear is an orthopaedic appliance that, when worn 10-14 hours a day for 9-12 months, can skeletally advance the maxilla in the range of 2-4 mm to correct the Class III malocclusion. Hence both anterior and posterior crossbites are corrected.

Frankel III Functional Appliance

Frankel III functional appliance is made while the mandible is positioned posteriorly. It has pads to stretch the upper lip and periosteum forward that stimulate forward growth of the maxilla, hence correcting anterior crossbite.

Chin Cap

In growing children with short lower facial height and mandibular prognathism, a chin cap is very effective which redirecting mandibular growth. Chin cup rotates the mandible backward, retards mandibular growth, and remodels the mandible, thereby, anterior skeletal crossbite is corrected. It also increases the anterior facial height.

Posterior Crossbite

Posterior crossbite may be the result of the bilateral or unilateral lingual position of the maxillary teeth relative to the mandibular posterior teeth due to tipping or alveolar discrepancy, or a combination.

Most often, bilateral crossbites with a functional mandibular shift will result in unilateral posterior crossbites. Dental crossbites may be the result of tipping or rotation of a tooth or teeth and are localized and do not involve the basal bone, whereas disharmony of the craniofacial skeleton results in skeletal crossbites.

This disharmony of the craniofacial skeleton occurs in two ways:

- Disharmony in transverse growth of the maxilla and mandible.
- Disharmonious growth in the anteroposterior or sagittal length of maxilla and mandibles.

Such growth aberrations can be due to inherited growth patterns, trauma, or functional disturbances that alter normal growth.

If space is needed, an expansion appliance also is an option. Posterior crossbite correction can accomplish the same objectives and can improve the eruptive position of the succedaneous teeth. Early correction of unilateral posterior crossbites has been shown to improve functional conditions significantly and eliminate morphological and positional asymmetries of the mandible. Functional shifts should be eliminated as soon as possible with the early correction to avoid asymmetric growth.

Important Considerations in Treating Posterior Crossbite

- All transverse alterations should be treated as soon as possible, ideally during mixed dentition
- If the transverse alteration is skeletal, the treatment should be even earlier, as soon as the first upper permanent molars erupt. Early treatment is essential for a stable result
- Treatment can be delayed until permanent dentition if the transverse problem is dentoalveolar, but only while patients are actively growing.
- Dentoalveolar transverse problems are corrected with a Hawley appliance with an expansion screw or with Quad-Helix.

- For skeletal transverse problems, the appliance of choice is a Rapid Maxillary Expander
- If there is transverse alteration along with vertical or anterior-posterior malocclusion, treating transverse alteration should be initiated first.
- After correcting the transverse malocclusion at an early age, the results must be stabilised with retainers until all the permanent teeth have replaced the deciduous teeth [7].

Treatment Options for Management of Transverse Maxillary Deficiency

- Hawley's appliance with jackscrew
- Coffin's spring
- Quad Helix
- Rapid maxillary expansion (RME)
- Fixed appliances (*e.g.*, archwires, auxiliary archwires and cross elastics)

Hawley's Appliance with Jackscrew

- Indicated for Dentoalveolar transverse expansion of maxillary arch.
- Expansion occurs by tipping of posterior teeth buccally with a small degree of skeletal expansion, by separation of the mid-palatal suture.

Appliance

It consists of Hawley's appliance with a jackscrew in the palatal region. The base plate of the appliance is separated in the middle so that an equal number of anchor molars on either side of the midline results in symmetrical expansion.

To produce asymmetric expansion, sectioning of the baseplate is done so that more teeth are in contact with it on the non-expansion side. Typically, the patients should be instructed to turn the expansion screw a quarter-turn (0.2 mm expansion) once a week. The rate of expansion may be monitored by measuring the intermolar distance with the calipers. Following expansion, the appliance is used as a retaining appliance for a minimum of three months. (Fig. **9**) [6]

Advantages

- It promotes greater post-expansion stability if an adequate retention period is given.
- Delivers constant physiological force.

Disadvantages

They are that removable appliance drawback.

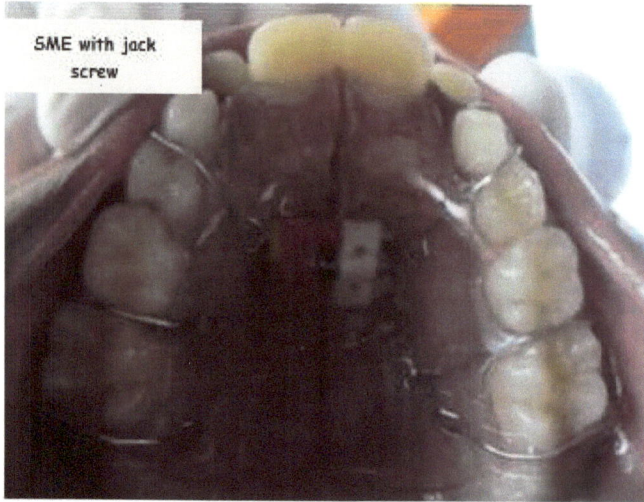

Fig. (9). Slow maxillary expansion with jack screw.

Coffin Spring

- It is indicated in young developing dentition for correction of posterior crossbite.
- It produces slow and bilaterally symmetric expansion, which is dentoalveolar.

Appliance

- Coffin spring is an omega-shaped wire appliance fabricated 1.25mm thickness wire placed in the midpalatal region with free ends of the wire embedded in acrylic covering slopes of the palate.
- Appliance is activated by using a three-pronged plier to flatten the omega-shaped wire to increase the space between the two halves of the base plate.

Quad Helix Appliance

It is a modification of Coffin's W-spring and was described by Ricketts as producing slow expansion, which is dentoalveolar in the ratio of 6:1 compared to skeletal expansion.

Appliance: It is laboratory constructed or prefabricated and is typically made from stainless steel or nickel-titanium. The latter delivers favourable force, which facilitates more physiological tooth movement with more rapid correction of crossbites due to the superelastic properties of the alloy. Four helices are incorporated into the W-spring to increase the flexibility and range of activation (Figs. **10a, b**).

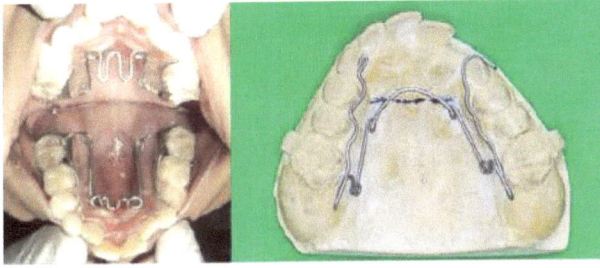

Fig. (10). a). Quad Helix for maxillary expansion with the incorporation of tongue crib for tongue thrusting habit **b)** Quad helix for maxillary expansion.

Depending upon teeth that are in a crossbite, the length of the palatal arms of the appliance can be altered. The appliance is soldered and retained by orthodontic bands cemented on the first permanent molars. Forces generated by the appliance can be controlled depending on the amount of activation. Reactivation is done using the three-prong pliers and is continued until the palatal cusps of the upper molars meet edge-to-edge with the buccal cusps of the mandibular molars. A degree of overcorrection is desirable to compensate for slight relapse.

Cross Elastics

- Used to treat localised posterior crossbite of dental origin.
- Cross elastics run from the palatal aspect of one or more maxillary teeth to the buccal aspect of one or more mandibular teeth (Fig. **11**).
- In addition to producing lateral forces, a vertical force vector is also produced, which tends to cause molar extrusion resulting in a reduced overbite or increased face height.
- Heavy rubber elastics are used at 0.25, *i.e.*, 3\16 6-ounce elastics are used.

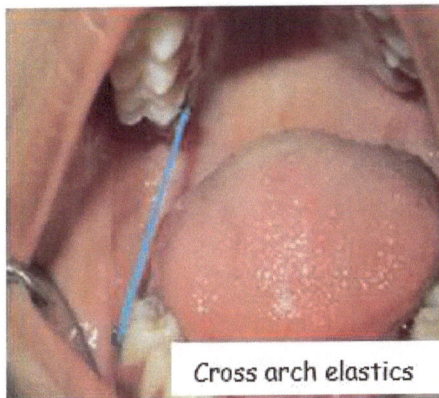

Cross arch elastics

Fig. (11). Cross arch elastics from the palatal aspect of maxillary molar to buccal aspect of mandibular molar.

Rapid Maxillary Expansion

The rapid maxillary expansion was first described by Emerson Angell and later re-popularized by Haas. The skeletal to dental movement ratio is improved, producing sutural expansion at the mid-palatal suture.

Indications

- Rapid maxillary expansion is indicated in cases with a transverse discrepancy equal to or greater than 4 mm, and where the maxillary molars are already buccally inclined to compensate for the transverse skeletal discrepancy.
- Used to facilitate maxillary protraction in Class III treatment by disrupting the system of sutures that connect the maxilla to the cranial base.
- Cleft lip and palate patients with the collapsed maxilla.

Contraindications

- Patients who have passed the growth spurt since there is a greater interlocking of the maxillary sutures, which may limit their separation
- Patients who have a recession on the buccal aspect of the molars
- Patients who show poor compliance

Appliance: Rapid maxillary expansion can be banded or banded and can be classified as Tooth & tissue borne and Tooth borne (Figs. **12a**, **b**).

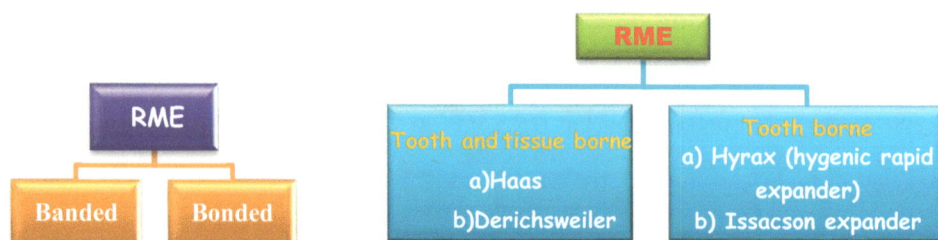

Fig. (12a, b). Classification of Rapid maxillary expansion appliance.

Clinical Management: Upper midline diastema will form during the expansion phase, which should be informed before to the patient and they should be reassured as it will close spontaneously. Patients should be instructed to turn the expansion screw one-quarter turn twice a day (am and pm). Force levels tend to accumulate following multiple turns and can be as high as 10 kg following many turns, which may cause minor discomfort. The activating key should be attached to a handle or tied to a piece of dental floss to prevent swallowing or aspiration should it be dropped in the mouth (Figs. **13a - e**).

Active treatment is usually required for 2–3 weeks, after which a retention period of three months is recommended to allow for bony infilling of the separated suture. During retention, ligature wire can be tied around the expansion screw or closed using resin to prevent it from turning inadvertently [6].

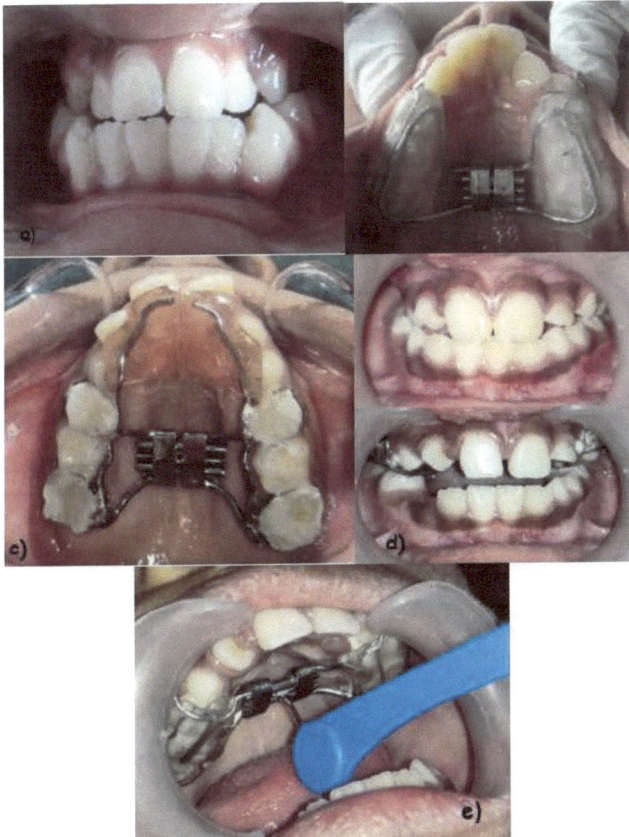

Fig. (13). a) Narrow constricted maxilla with a posterior crossbite, **b)** Bonded hyrax Rapid Maxillary Expansion appliance to expand maxilla and correct posterior crossbite. **c)** Banded hyrax rapid maxillary expansion appliance **d)** Upper midline diastema formed after activation **e)** Activation of the appliance by activation key.

Functional Crossbite

Functional crossbite occurs due to mandibular shifting into an abnormal position which is often a more comfortable position during the closure of the jaw.

Etiology

- Mandibular deviation during jaw closure occurs due to the presence of occlusal interferences.

- Other causes include decayed teeth, ectopically erupted teeth, and early loss of deciduous teeth.

This functional shift may be anterior, lateral, or posterior, which may lead to temporomandibular joint dysfunction, the pain of the masticatory muscles and undesirable growth modifications. Sometimes this functional shift leads to pseudo-class III malocclusion. Treatment includes the elimination of occlusal prematurities.

Soft Tissue Surgical Needs

Includes removal of soft tissue and bony barriers to facilitate permanent tooth eruption.

Causes for failure of succedaneous teeth eruption [1]

- Over retained primary teeth
- Supernumerary teeth
- Cysts and tumours
- Large frenum (Fig. **14 a, b, c**)
- Ankylosed primary teeth
- Fibrous or bony obstructions

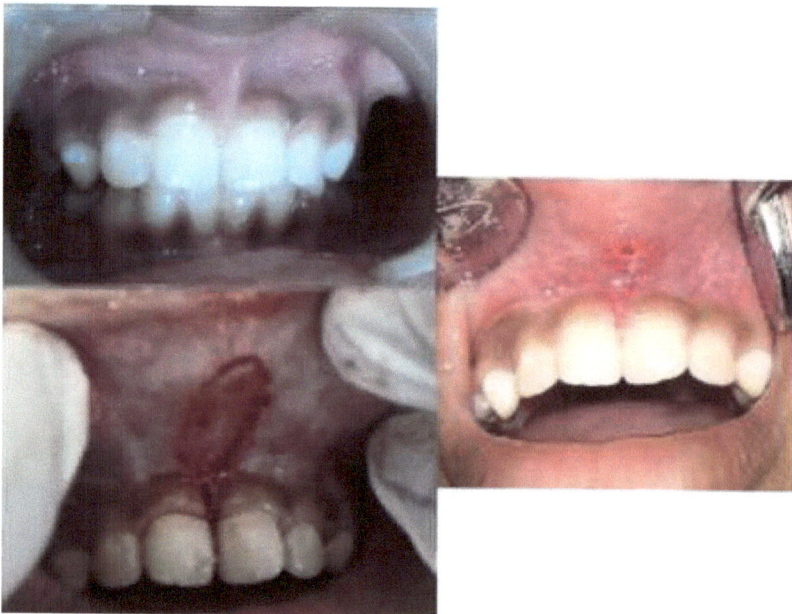

Fig. (14). Labial frenectomy.

The greater diameter of the crown should be exposed surgically to stimulate its eruption and surgical exposure should be greater than the dimension of the erupting permanent tooth. (Fig. **15 a - f,** & **16 a - e**).

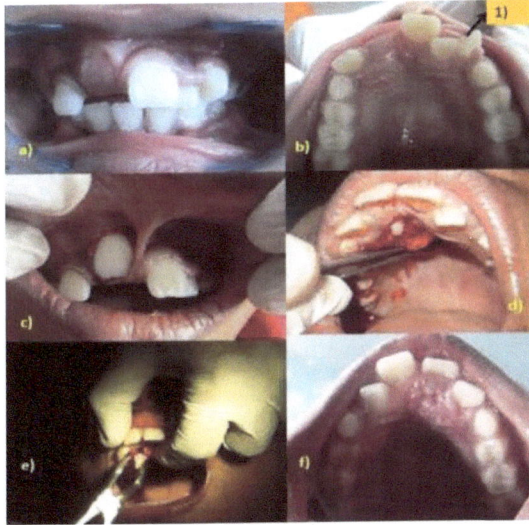

Fig. (15). a) Preoperative intraoral view with unerupted tooth 11, supplemental supernumerary tooth irt 22, **b)** 1. supplementary supernumerary tooth, **c)** Surgical exposure of clinical crown of 11 to stimulate eruption, **d), e)** Surgical removal of the supernumerary tooth, **f)** post-operative occlusal view.

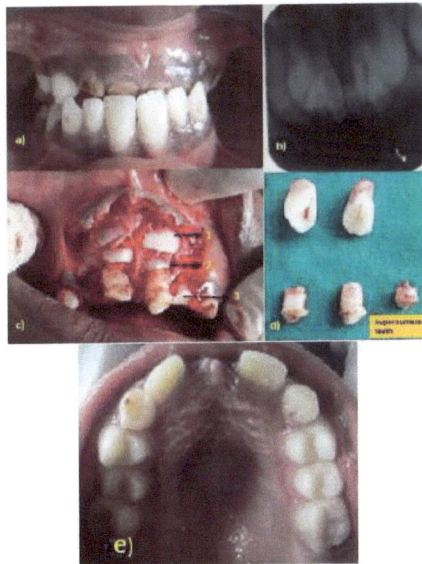

Fig. (16). a) Preoperative intraoral view with retained deciduous tooth **b)** Intraoral peri apical radiograph with supernumerary teeth irt 11, 21, **c)** Surgical removal of supernumerary teeth, **d)** Extracted supernumerary teeth and retained deciduous teeth. **e)** Central incisors eruption post-extraction. **1.** Permanent central incisors **2.** Supernumerary teeth, **3.** Retained deciduous tooth (51,6,62).

Tooth Size/Arch Length Discrepancy and Crowding

Arch length discrepancies represented in terms of a Bolton discrepancy include:

- Inadequate arch length and crowding of the dental arches
- Excess arch length and spacing
- Other etiological factors include missing teeth, supernumerary teeth, and fused or crowding may be found in conjunction with arch discrepancy, which will have a compounding influence, particularly in early mixed dentition [1].

Diagnosis: The patient should be evaluated comprehensively, which includes maxillary and mandibular skeletal relationships, direction and pattern of growth, facial profile, facial width, muscle balance, and dental and occlusal findings, including tooth positions, arch length analysis, and leeway space.

Treatment Objectives

Well-timed intervention can:

- Prevent crowded incisors.
- Increase long-term stability of incisor positions.
- Decrease ectopic eruption and impaction of permanent canines.
- Reduce orthodontic treatment time and sequelae.
- Improve gingival health and overall dental health.

Treatment Considerations

It may include, but are not limited to:

- Gaining space for permanent incisors to erupt and become straight naturally through primary canine extraction and space/arch length maintenance with holding arches. Extraction of primary or permanent teeth to alleviate crowding should not be undertaken without a comprehensive space analysis and a short- and long-term orthodontic treatment plan.
- Orthodontic alignment of permanent teeth as soon as erupted and feasible, expansion and correction of arch length as early as feasible.
- Utilizing holding arches in the mixed dentition until all permanent premolars and canines have erupted.
- Maintaining the patient's original arch form.
- Interproximal stripping of the enamel of mandibular primary canines to allow alignment of crowded lower permanent lateral incisors [1, 8].

Orthodontic Alignment of Permanent Teeth in Mixed Dentition

Minor orthodontic movements can be done by removable and fixed appliances using removable appliances with labial bows and springs to achieve tipping movements. Some commonly used removable appliances are listed in the text box (Figs. **17, 18a, b, d, e, f**).

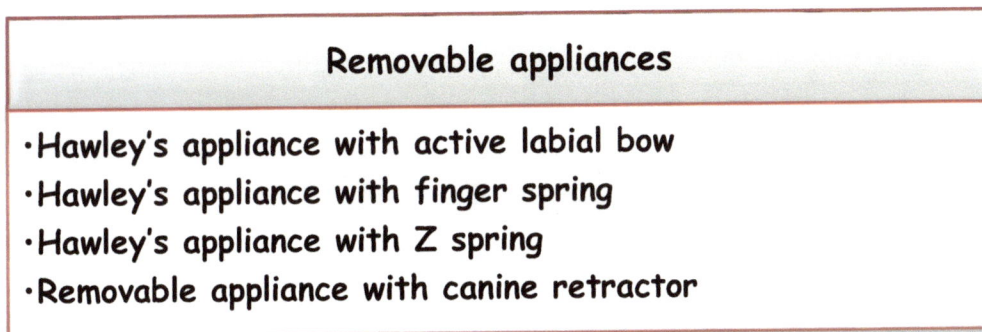

Removable appliances

- Hawley's appliance with active labial bow
- Hawley's appliance with finger spring
- Hawley's appliance with Z spring
- Removable appliance with canine retractor

Fig. (17). Removable appliances for minor orthodontic movements.

Disadvantages of Removable Appliances

- Appliance is rarely worn full time
  - Appliance damage/lost appliances
  - Difficulty in speech/eating
  - Gagging
  - Decalcification/caries
  - Gingivitis/palatal hyperplasia/fungal infections
  - Incorrect activation produces unhelpful changes
  - Allows only tipping of teeth

Advantages of Fixed Appliances

- Minimal discomfort
- Reduces need for patient co-operation
- Increase control of tooth movements
- Movement is possible in all three planes of space

Fixed Appliance Treatment in Mixed Dentition

A simply fixed appliance such as the 2 × 4 appliances can intercept some of the malocclusions in the mixed dentition stage. A desire to help patients with concerns and self-esteem considerations might fulfill using a partially fixed orthodontic appliance without waiting for the full permanent dentition for ideal results [9].

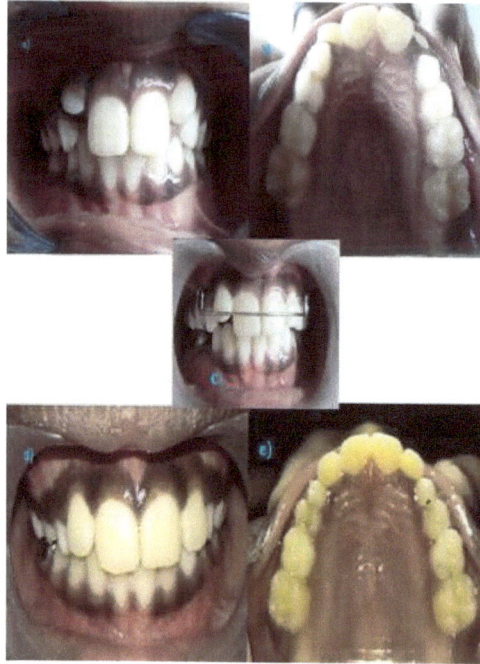

Fig. (18). a) & **b)** Intraoral preoperative view with tooth size arch length deficiency with crowding in the upper anterior region, **c)** Hawley's appliance with active labial bow and jack screw for slow maxillary expansion, **d)** & **e)** postoperative intraoral view with aligned tooth and dento alveolar expansion.

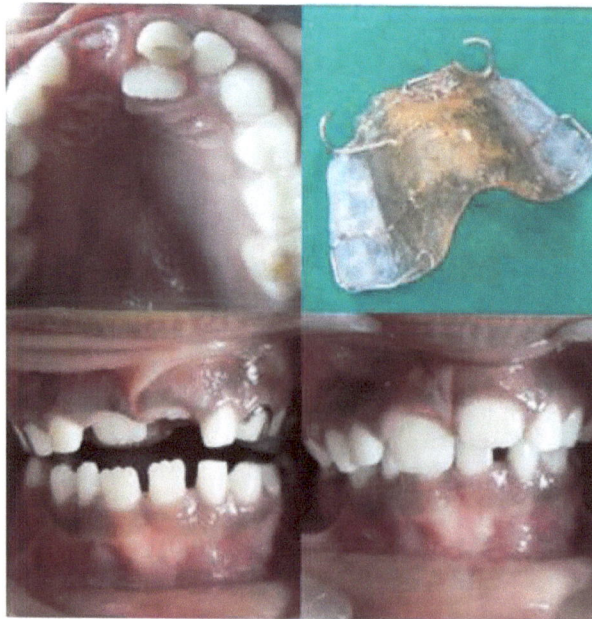

Fig. (18f). Removable appliance with Z spring for correction of anterior dental crossbite.

2 x 4 Appliances

- 2 bands cemented on both first permanent molars and 4 brackets bonded onto the erupted incisors.
- Continuous archwire provides complete control of the anterior dentition as well as a good arch form [10].
- Supporting steel tubing between the lateral incisors and first permanent molars. This tubing, if carefully shaped, maintains the correct arch form and strengthens the long unsupported span of wire, protecting it from occlusal forces and potential distortion during function.
- Utility arches placed along with the 2 × 4 appliances produce intrusion, protraction or retraction of incisors depending on the treatment needs.
- A quad helix can be soldered to molar bands or palatal sheaths welded for the provision of a removable quad helix if correction of a posterior crossbite is required simultaneously.

Various developing malocclusions treated by 2 by 4 appliances

- Crowding of anterior teeth (Fig. **19**)
- Proclination related to class II div 1
- Retroclination related to class II div 2
- Crossbites
- Single tooth anomalies.
- Severely rotated teeth (Fig. **19**).

Advantages

- Minimal patient discomfort and hence improved co-operation
- Increased control of force magnitude and that controlled tooth movement is possible in all three planes of space.
- The complexity and duration of this may be significantly reduced if definitive treatment is necessary for permanent dentition [9, 10].

Duration of fixed appliance treatment in mixed dentition

- Once the child is cooperative enough for placement of separators, cementation of bands, and bonding of brackets, treatment should be started.
- Treatment carried out in the mixed dentition stage may take as little as a couple of weeks, but in the more difficult cases can take longer.

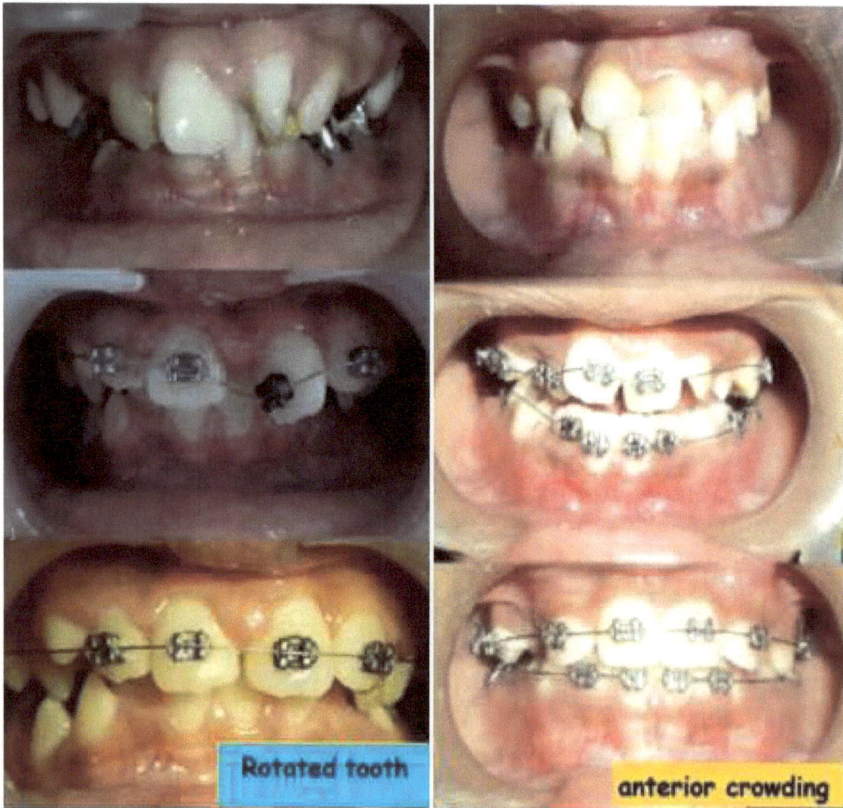

Fig. (19). 2 by 4 appliance for rotated tooth and anterior crowding treatment in mixed dentition.

Serial Extraction

Serial extraction is an interceptive orthodontic procedure usually initiated in the early mixed dentition to guide the erupting permanent teeth into a more favourable position, during the transition from the primary to the permanent dentition.

Definition

PROFFIT – Timed extraction of primary and permanent teeth to relieve severe crowding.

DEWEL –An orthodontic treatment procedure that involves the early removal of selected deciduous and permanent teeth in a predetermined sequence.

History

The concept of serial extraction was developed by Kjellgren of Sweden, Hotz of

Switzerland, Heath of Australia and Nance, Hoyd, Dowel and Mayne of the United States.

Nance has been called the father of serial extraction philosophy in the United States and presented clinics on his technique in 1940. Kjellgren, in 1940, termed this extraction procedure as a "Planned or progressive extraction procedure of teeth."

Hotz named the same procedure "Guidance of eruption," which is considered comprehensive and encompasses all measures available for influencing tooth eruption.

Principles of Serial Extraction

It is based on two principles (Fig. **20**)

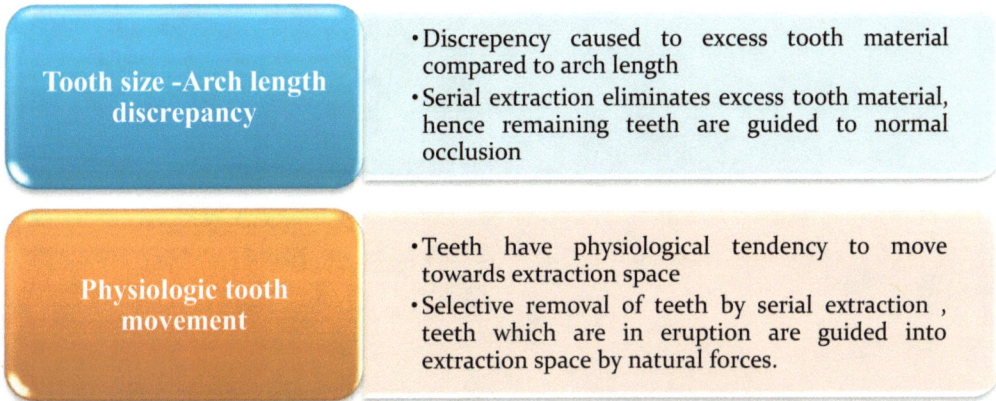

Tooth size -Arch length discrepancy	• Discrepency caused to excess tooth material compared to arch length • Serial extraction eliminates excess tooth material, hence remaining teeth are guided to normal occlusion
Physiologic tooth movement	• Teeth have physiological tendency to move towards extraction space • Selective removal of teeth by serial extraction , teeth which are in eruption are guided into extraction space by natural forces.

Fig. (20). Principles of Serial extraction.

According to Moyers

When a case satisfies the requirements of all following rules, it may be treated by the protocol that follows with a reasonable chance for success and a minimum chance of trouble.

Rule 1: There must be a Class I molar relationship bilaterally.
Rule 2: The facial skeleton must be balanced Antero posteriorly, vertically, and mediolaterally.
Rule 3: The discrepancy must be at least 5 mm in all four quadrants.
Rule 4: The dental midlines must coincide.
Rule 5: There must be neither an open bite nor a deep bite.

Indications for the Serial Extraction Procedure

- Class I malocclusion with tooth size- arch length deficiency of 5 mm or more per quadrant (10 mm or more for an arch) with no discrepancy in normal eruption sequence and skeletal growth pattern.
- Lingual eruption of the permanent lateral incisor
- Absence of physiologic spacing.
- Class I malocclusion cases with maxillary, mandibular dentoalveolar protrusion (bimaxillary dentoalveolar protrusion).
- In mesial step terminal plane in mixed dentition developed into class I permanent relationship with malocclusion.
- The patient should be in early mixed dentition, *i.e.*, between 8 to 9 years of age and the incisor crowded [11].
- Tooth size- jaw size discrepancy with severe arch length deficiency, which could be: (Fig. **21**)

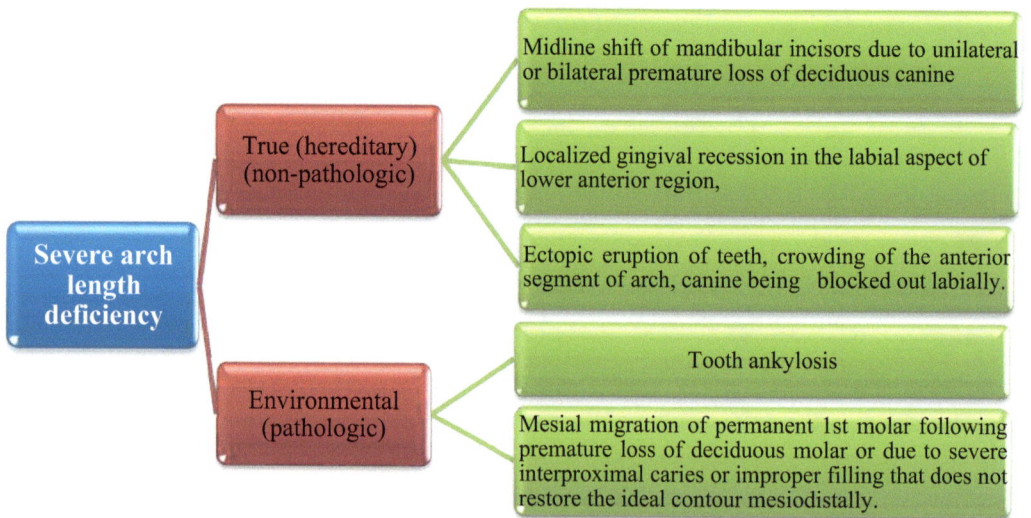

Fig. (21). Tooth size- jaw size discrepancy with severe arch length deficiency.

Contraindications

- Mild to moderate crowding, *i.e.*, tooth size arch length deficiency < 5 mm per quadrant, may lead to more residual space at the end of serial extraction.
- Congenital absence of teeth providing space
- Spaced dentition
- Midline diastema
- Cleft lip and palate
- Severe Class II, III of dental or skeletal origin because the closure of extraction spaces would be affected by how the skeletal problem was being treated.

- Open or Deep bites.
- Malformations in the unerupted teeth like dilacerations.
- Extensive caries or heavily filled first permanent molars, which cannot be preserved.

Advantages of the Serial Extraction Procedure

- Teeth are guided into normal positions by physiologic eruptive forces.
- Teeth erupt over the alveolus and through keratinized tissue avoiding ectopic eruption.
- Reduce the duration & cost of active orthodontic treatment at the later stage.
- More stable result.
- Less retention period is required.
- Oral hygiene can be maintained better.
- Iatrogenic orthodontic damage like root resorption and enamel decalcification since the health of investing tissues is preserved.
- Improved psychologic state and better patient compliance as a result of improved alignment.
- Cost is minimal [11].

Disadvantages of the Serial Extraction Procedure

- Prolonged treatment time with multiple visits (2-3 years), so patient follow-up is important.
- No single approach can be universally applied and thorough knowledge of growth, development, eruption sequence and calcification of permanent teeth.
- Tendency to develop tongue thrust.
- Subjecting the child to multiple progressive extraction visits.
- It is done as inter-canine growth is occurring, and hence it is difficult to assess accurately how crowded the dentition will be.
- Tendency to cause deep bite, especially in Class II div 2 cases.
- Residual spaces can remain between the canine and 2nd premolar.
- Should be followed by active orthodontic treatment (fixed appliance) to achieve ideal levelling & aligning, root parallelism, closure of residual spaces, and correction of deep bite.

Diagnosis and Treatment Planning

The decision to carry out serial extraction should always be based on the comprehensive assessment of dental, skeletal, and soft tissues. Extraction of any tooth is a critical step in orthodontic management.

Serial extraction is a time-lined process, and the decision is by multifactorial considerations like amount of crowding, arch length requirements, and whether or when to extract the next set of teeth or not should be evaluated at each visit of the patient. Thus, serial extraction is a decision-making process periodically rather than a single-time diagnosis. (Fig. **22**).

Orthodontic study models	Radiographs	Photographs
• To perform model analyses • Assessing the morphology of teeth • Evaluation of occlusion • Assessing the dental arch form	• To carry out radiographic mixed dentition analysis • To detect congenitally missing teeth and supernumerary teeth • To assess dental age • To assess the amount of root development and possible eruption pattern • To detect any bony pathologies	• Pre, mid and post-treatment intra- and extra-oral photographs • Helps to access before and after treatment improvement. • Educate and motivate the patient.

Fig. (22). Diagnostic aids for serial extraction.

Procedure

A number of extraction sequences are used, and no single extraction sequence applies to all patients, the method should be decided on the individual case. Some of the commonly used methods are:

- Dewel's method
- Nance method
- Tweed's method
- Grewe's method
- Moyers Method

Dewel's Method (Extraction of CD4)

Dewel proposed a three-step serial extraction procedure which is widely used even today and gives the most satisfactory results (Fig. **23**).

Step 1: Extraction of deciduous canines	Step 2: Extraction of deciduous first molars	Step 3: Extraction of first premolars
• Carried out at around 8-9 years to create space for the alignment of the incisors. • Main objective is to establish the integrity of upper and lower incisors. • Prevents the development of lingual crossbite of maxillary laterals and resultant mesial migration of maxillary canines	• Carried out when first premolars reach half of the root length as evidenced by radiographs. • Carried out at 12 months after the extraction of deciduous canines at around 9-10 years of age. • Objective is to accelerate the eruption of first premolars. • This ensures that the first premolars emerge into oral cavity, before the eruption of permanent canines.	• Carried out when they are emerging into oral cavity and when the permanent canines have developed beyond half of the root length. • Facilitates proper eruption and alignment of permanent canines • Orthodontic mechanotherapy of minimal duration may be necessary for establishment of proper intercuspation in some cases

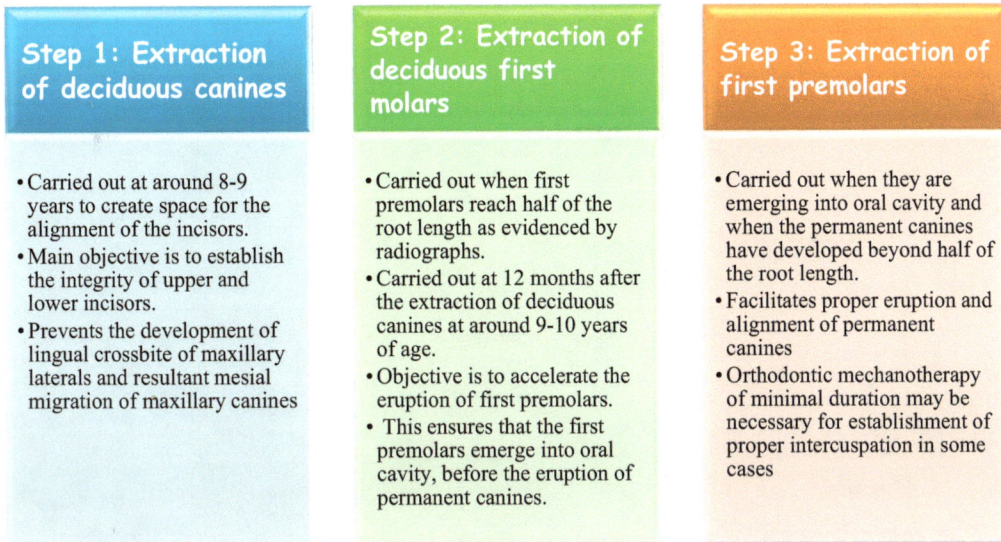

Fig. (23). Steps in Dewel's method.

Tweed's Method

This method involves extraction of deciduous first molar to facilitate first premolar eruption followed by extraction of erupted 1st premolar along with deciduous canine. This facilitates permanent canine eruption (Fig. **24**).

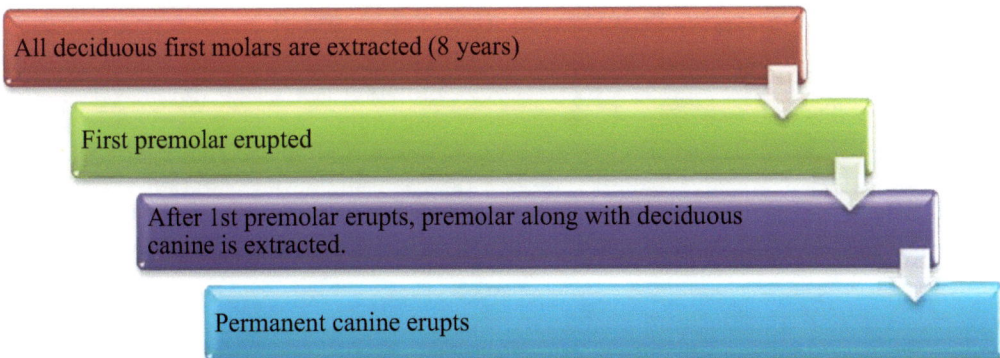

All deciduous first molars are extracted (8 years)

First premolar erupted

After 1st premolar erupts, premolar along with deciduous canine is extracted.

Permanent canine erupts

Fig. (24). Steps in TWEED's method.

Nance Method

This method is a modification of the tweed's method. It involves extraction of all deciduous first molars at the age of 8 years, extraction of the first premolar after eruption, followed by extraction of the deciduous canine (Fig. **25**).

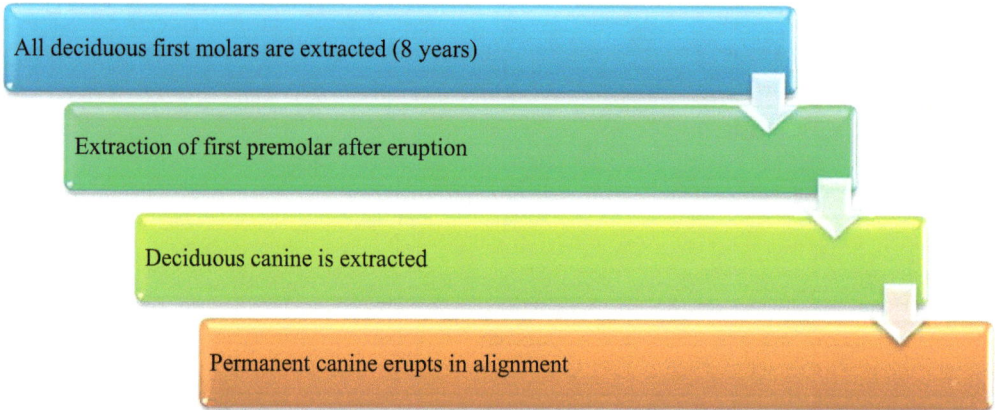

All deciduous first molars are extracted (8 years)

Extraction of first premolar after eruption

Deciduous canine is extracted

Permanent canine erupts in alignment

Fig. (25). Steps in the Nance method.

Moyers Method

This method involves treatment in 4 stages (Fig. **26**)

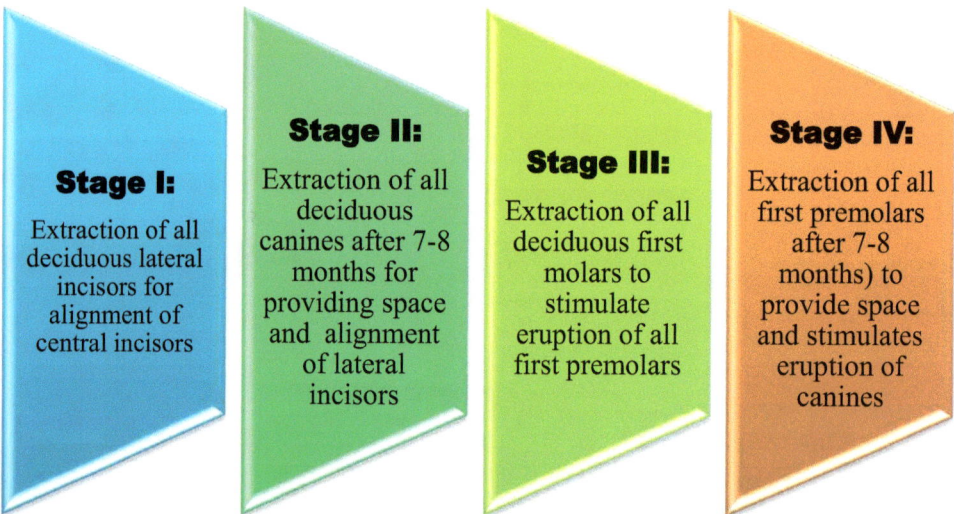

Stage I:
Extraction of all deciduous lateral incisors for alignment of central incisors

Stage II:
Extraction of all deciduous canines after 7-8 months for providing space and alignment of lateral incisors

Stage III:
Extraction of all deciduous first molars to stimulate eruption of all first premolars

Stage IV:
Extraction of all first premolars after 7-8 months) to provide space and stimulates eruption of canines

Fig. (26). Steps in Moyers method.

Interception of Skeletal Discrepancy

Skeletal discrepancies if diagnosed at early age should be intercepted to reduce the severity of malocclusion in the future. Interception of malocclusion helps to establish skeletal harmony and achieve a pleasing profile.

Class II malocclusion: Class II skeletal malocclusion usually occurs due to mandibular retrusion or maxillary protrusion or a combination of both. This may result in protruded upper incisors (increased overjet). Patients usually cannot close their lips and these protruded teeth are more prone to traumatic injuries. They may also have psychosocial problems from being teased by their peers and low self-esteem (Table **1**).

Table 1. Treatment options for various skeletal malocclusions.

S. No	Skeletal Malocclusion	Treatment Options
1.	Class II malocclusion due to mandibular retrognathism (Fig. **27b**)	Mandibular growth should be promoted by the myofunctional appliance • Twin block (Fig. **28**) • Herbst appliance • Functional regulator by Frankel 1 & 2 (Fig. **Fig. 29**) • Activator • Bionator
2.	Class II malocclusion due to maxillary prognathism. (Fig. **27c**)	Maxillary growth should be restricted • Headgear (high pull, cervical, occipital) (Fig. **30**)
3.	Class II malocclusion due to mandibular retrognathism and maxillary prognathism (Fig. **27d**)	Promoting mandibular growth and restricting maxillary growth • Twin block with high pull headgear
4.	Class III malocclusion due mandibular prognathism (Fig. **27e**)	Restrict mandibular growth • Chin cup, • Class III bionator
5.	Class III malocclusion due to maxillary retrognathism (Fig. **27f**)	Maxillary growth should be promoted • Face mask therapy (Fig. **31**) • Frankel 3
6.	Class III malocclusion due to maxillary retrognathism and mandibular prognathism (Fig. **27g**)	Promote maxillary growth and restrict mandibular growth. • Reverse pull headgear (Fig. **31**)

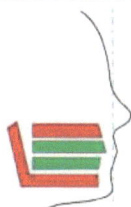

Maxilla and mandible are in harmonious relation with each other.

Skeletal Class I

Fig. (27a). Skeletal Class I.

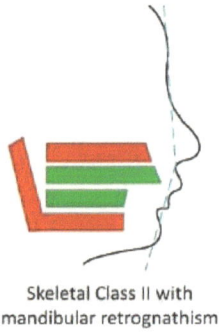

Mandibular growth should be promoted
Treatment options
- **Twin block (Fig. 28)**
- **Herbst appliance**
- **Functional regulator by Frankel 1 & 2 (Fig. 29)**
- **Activator**
- **Bionator**

Skeletal Class II with
mandibular retrognathism

Fig. (27b). Class II malocclusion due to mandibular retrognathism.

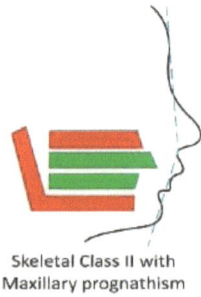

Maxillary growth should be restricted
Treatment options
- **Headgear (high pull, cervical, occipital) (Fig. 30)**

Skeletal Class II with
Maxillary prognathism

Fig. (27c). Class II malocclusion due to maxillary prognathism.

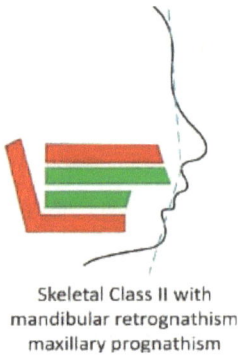

Promoting mandibular growth and restrict maxillary growth
Treatment options
- **Twin block with high pull headgear**

Skeletal Class II with
mandibular retrognathism
maxillary prognathism

Fig. (27d). Class II malocclusion due to mandibular retrognathism and maxillary prognathism.

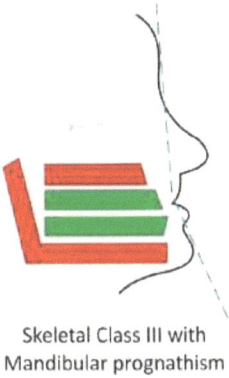

> **Restrict mandibular growth**
> **Treatment options**
> - Chin cup
> - Class III bionator

Skeletal Class III with
Mandibular prognathism

Fig. (27e). Class III malocclusion due mandibular prognathism.

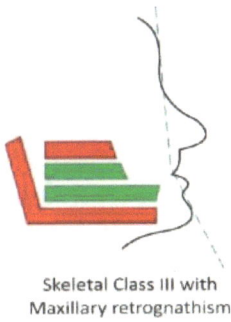

> **Maxillary growth should be promoted**
> **Treatment options**
> - Face mask therapy (Fig. 31)
> - Frankel 3

Skeletal Class III with
Maxillary retrognathism

Fig. (27f). Class III malocclusion due to maxillary retrognathism.

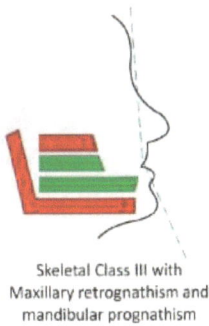

> **Promote maxillary growth and restrict mandibular growth**
> **Treatment options**
> - Reverse pull headgear (Fig. 31)

Skeletal Class III with
Maxillary retrognathism and
mandibular prognathism

Fig. (27g). Class III malocclusion due to maxillary retrognathism and mandibular prognathism.

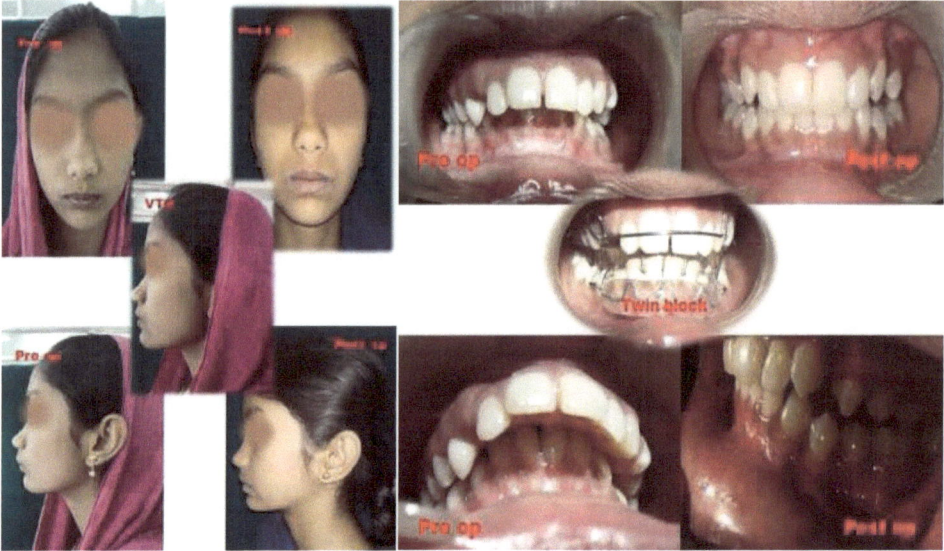

Fig. (28). Treatment of Skeletal Class II division 1 with retrognathic mandible by twin block with lip bumper.

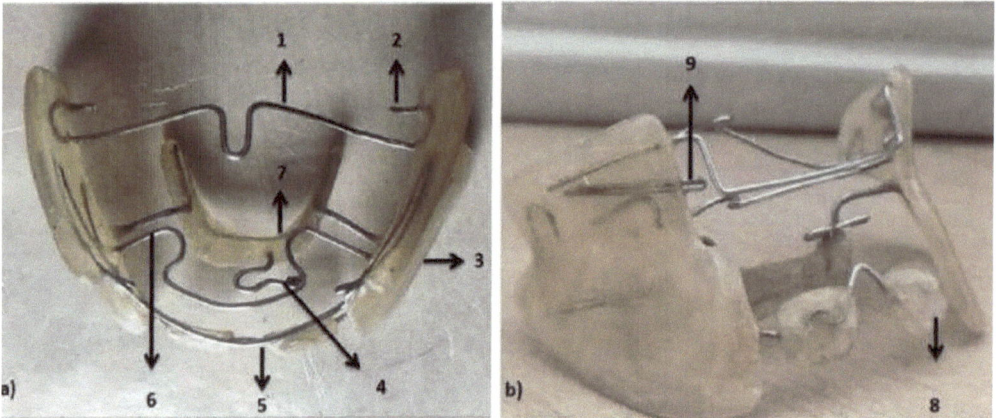

Fig. (29). a) Aerial view of Frankel 2 appliance b) Frontal view of Frankel 2 appliance 1. Stabilizing palatal bow, 2. Occlusal rest, 3. Buccal shield, 4. Lower lingual spring, 5. Passive maxillary bow, 6. Upper lingual wire, 7. Lingual shield, 8. Lip pad, 9. Canine clasp.

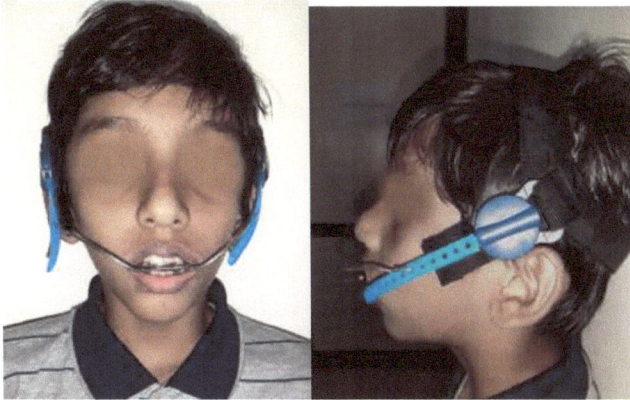

Fig. (30). High pull headgear.

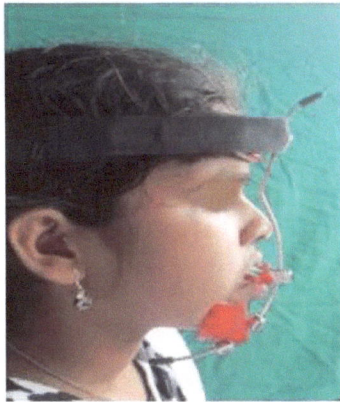

Fig. (31). Reverse pull headgear.

Treatment of a developing Class II malocclusion is aimed to improve an overbite, overjet, and intercuspation of posterior teeth and achieve an esthetic appearance and profile compatible with the patient's skeletal morphology.

Class III malocclusion: Class III skeletal malocclusion occurs due to asymmetry, mandibular prognathism, and/or maxillary retrognathism), the anterior functional shift of the mandible, or a combination of these factors.

Interception of skeletal Class III provides a more favourable environment for growth and may improve occlusion, function, and esthetics (Table **1**).

CONCLUSION

Interceptive orthodontics provides necessary, timely and more affordable treatment for orthodontic problems, reducing the burden of future orthodontic treatment. Children need not have to wait for permanent teeth to erupt for correction of certain malocclusions; interceptive orthodontic procedures can be carried out, which can make them more confident and increase self-esteem.

CONSENT FOR PUBLICATION

Not applicable.

CONFLICT OF INTEREST

The authors declare no conflict of interest, financial or otherwise.

ACKNOWLEDGEMENT

Declared none.

REFERENCES

[1]   Management of the developing dentition and occlusion in pediatric dentistry. The reference manual of pediatric dentistry. Chicago, Ill.: American Academy of Pediatric Dentistry 2020; 393-409.

[2]   Sockalingam SNMP, Khan KAM, Kuppuswamy E. Interceptive correction of anterior crossbite using short-span wire-fixed orthodontic appliance: a report of three cases 2018.
[http://dx.doi.org/10.1155/2018/4323945]

[3]   Prakash P, Durgesh BH. Anterior crossbite correction in early mixed dentition period using catlan's appliance: a case report. ISRN Dent 2011; 2011: 1-5.
[http://dx.doi.org/10.5402/2011/298931] [PMID: 21991464]

[4]   Bayrak S, Tunc ES. Treatment of anterior dental crossbite using bonded resin-composite slopes: case reports. Eur J Dent 2008; 2(4): 303-6.
[http://dx.doi.org/10.1055/s-0039-1697397] [PMID: 19212539]

[5]   Jirgensone I, Liepa A, Abeltins A. Anterior crossbite correction in primary and mixed dentition with removable inclined plane (Bruckl appliance). Stomatologija 2008; 10(4): 140-4.
[PMID: 19223714]

[6]   Agarwal A, Mathur R. Maxillary Expansion. Int J Clin Pediatr Dent 2010; 3(3): 139-46.
[http://dx.doi.org/10.5005/jp-journals-10005-1069] [PMID: 27616835]

[7]   Castañer-Peiro A. Interceptive orthodontics: the need for early diagnosis and treatment of posterior crossbites. Med Oral Patol Oral Cir Bucal 2006; 11(2): E210-4.
[PMID: 16505804]

[8]   Nakhjavani YB, Nakhjavani FB, Jafari A. Mesial stripping of mandibular deciduous canines for correction of permanent lateral incisors. Int J Clin Pediatr Dent 2017; 10(3): 229-33.
[http://dx.doi.org/10.5005/jp-journals-10005-1441] [PMID: 29104380]

[9]   Kamatchi D, Kumar SS, Vasanthan P. Orthodontic challenges in mixed dentition. SRM Journal of Research in Dental Sciences 2015; 6(1): 22-8.
[http://dx.doi.org/10.4103/0976-433X.149585]

[10]   Fiona McKeown H, Sandlerd J. The two by four appliance: a versatile appliance. Dent Update 2001; 28(10): 496-500.
[http://dx.doi.org/10.12968/denu.2001.28.10.496] [PMID: 11862851]

[11]   Naragond DA, Kenganal S. Serial Extractions – A Review. IOSR J Dent Med Sci 2012; 3(2): 40-7.
[http://dx.doi.org/10.9790/0853-0324047]

CHAPTER 10

Gingival and Periodontal Diseases in Children

Vinaya Kumar Kulkarni[1,*], Mala Dixit[2], Shruti Balasubramanian[3] and **Abdulkadeer Jetpurwala[4]**

[1] *Department of Pediatric Dentistry, SMBT Dental College and Hospital, Sangamner, India*

[2] *Department of Periodontics, Nair Hospital Dental College, Mumbai, India*

[3] *Government Dental College & Hospital, Nagpur, India*

[4] *Pediatric Dentistry, Nair Hospital Dental College, Mumbai, India*

Abstract: Pediatric population experiences a wide array of gingival and periodontal diseases. Studies have shown that gingivitis is almost universally prevalent among pediatric patients. However, lesser attention is given to periodontitis in children owing to the shorter life span of primary dentition. Periodontal assessment must be incorporated into the routine oral examination of the child since prompt diagnosis plays a crucial role in successfully managing periodontal conditions. Severe periodontal disease may also occur among children with concomitant systemic conditions. Therefore, the presence of a destructive periodontal condition may serve as an early indicator of an underlying systemic condition, and the dentist may be the first to notice such a condition. Hence, a thorough medical evaluation should be performed for children exhibiting severe periodontitis, especially for cases that appear resistant to therapy, to determine the systemic causes of the condition. Although at present, there is increased awareness regarding periodontal health and treatment modalities, it is restricted to adults with a negligible focus on children. Intraoral assessment of children is cecentredroundan examination of hard tissues with minimal focus on the health of soft tissue. Hence, this chapter enlightens various gingival and periodontal conditions and the importance of overall health during childhood.

Keywords: Children, gingiva, gingivitis, gingival disorders, periodontium, periodontitis.

INTRODUCTION

The soft tissue which surrounds the neck of the tooth, coronal to the alveolar bone crest and extends up to the mucogingival junction is known as the Gingiva. It is a component of the supporting structure of the, *i.e.* periodontium, along with cementum, periodontal ligament, and alveolar bone (Fig. **1**).

* **Corresponding author Vinaya Kumar Kulkarni:** Department of Pediatric Dentistry, SMBT Dental College and Hospital, Sangamner, India; E-mail: vinayakumar53@gmail.com

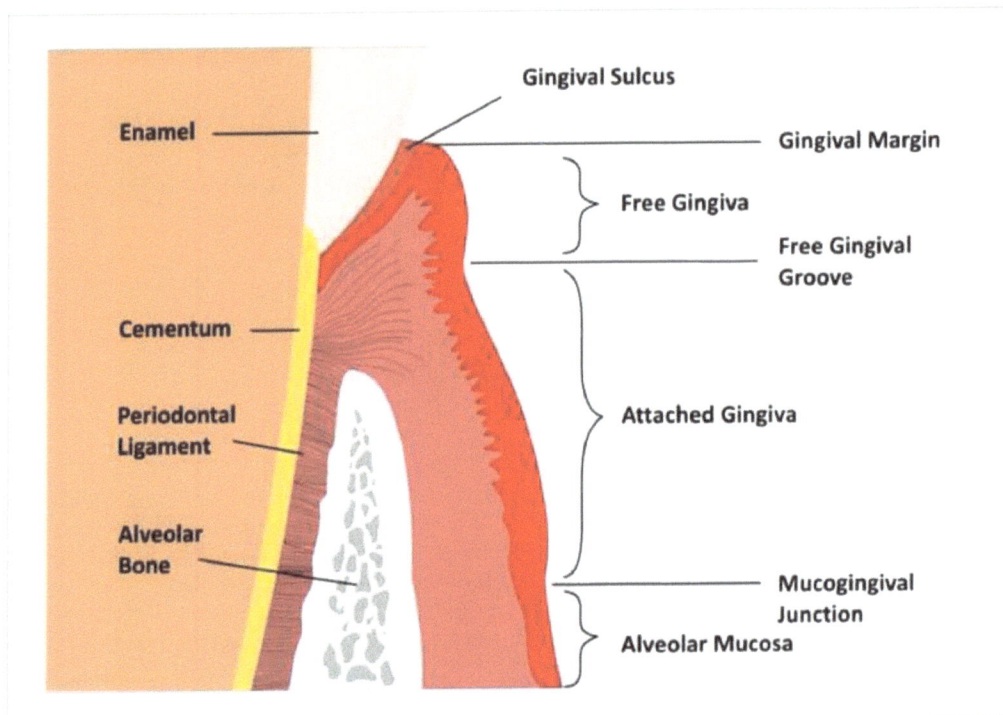

Fig. (1). Components of the periodontium.

Inflammation of periodontal tissues is common among children and adolescents. The inflammation is restricted to the gingival tissues in most cases. The presence of inflammation restricted to gingiva without associated loss of connective tissue or alveolar bone is the characteristic feature of gingivitis.

Children and adolescents present varying manifestations of periodontitis, just like adults. Presently, both aggressive (severe and rapidly progressing type) and chronic (slow progression of the disease) variants are observed and distinguished.

NORMAL PERIODONTIUM IN PRIMARY DENTITION

The marginal gingiva of primary teeth appears rounded and bulky. The characteristic stippling develops around the age of 2-3 years. The interdental tissues are comparable to saddle areas, *i.e.*, those areas of primary teeth with diastema (Fig. **2a**).

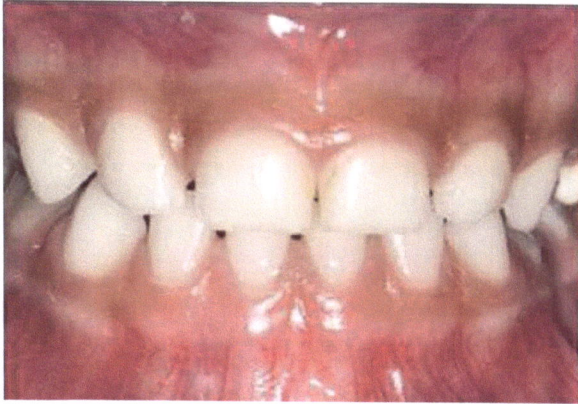

Fig. (2a). Clinical appearance of gingiva in children (Primary Dentition).

The interdental cleft and the retrocuspid papilla are the two unique anatomic features seen in the gingiva of children. The interdental cleft is present apical to the interdental area, whereas the retrocuspid papilla lies behind the mandibular canine below the marginal gingiva (Fig. **2b**). The retrocuspid papilla decreases with age and should not be confused with intraoral swelling.

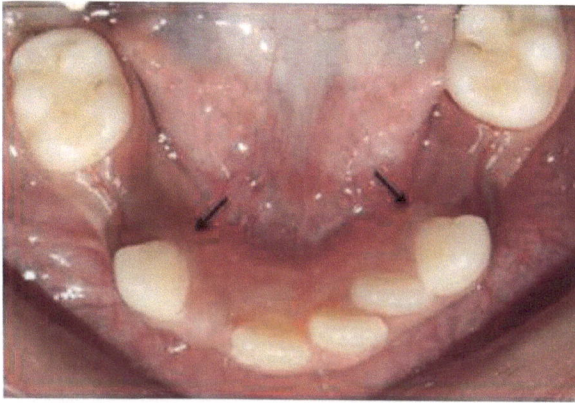

Fig. (2b). Retrocuspid papilla.

Once the molars establish proximal contact, the interdental region is filled with interdental papilla along with marginal concavity, *i.e.*, col, which corresponds to the shape of the contact area.

The composition of the connective tissue is similar to a young permanent tooth, but the primary teeth comprise a thicker junctional epithelium. It is more resistant to inflammation as it is less permeable. The alveolar bone comprises a relatively wider PDL membrane, and the lamina dura appears thin on radiographs. Also, larger marrow spaces and fewer trabeculae with rich blood supply are seen [1 - 4]. The root cementum is largely cellular and thin (Tables **1** and **2**).

Table 1. Clinical appearance and histological features of gingiva in primary dentition.

Clinical Appearance	Histological Features
Reddish in colour	The epithelium is thin with greater vascularity a and a lesser degree of cornification
Stippling not seen	Flatter and shorter papilla from lamina propria
Gingival margin is rolled and rounded	The eruption is accompanied by hyperemia oedema a.Thecervicall ridge on the crown of primary teeth is prominent
Greater sulcular depth: The mean sulcular depth is 2.1 mm ± 0.2 mm for primary dentition	The sulcus can be split by inserting a probe into the area of the crevicular margin which stimulates a pocket formation

Table 2. Differentiating features of the periodontium in children.

Gingiva	Connective tissue comprises lesser well-developed collagen fibres compared to adults. The surface of the col is covered with an ontogenically -derived epithelium which is atrophic with diminished proliferating capacity. Later, oral epithelium replacing the ontogenically -derived epithelium is necessary for periodontal health.
Periodontal Ligament	The periodontal ligament is wider and has less dense fibres, and has greater hydration along with increased vascular supply and lymphatic drainage as compared to adults. When the tooth is erupting, principal fibres align parallel to the long axis of the tooth and on encountering its functional antagonist, it arranges in the form of a bundle.
Cementum	It is less dense and thinner than that of adults. It has a tendency for hyperplasia of cementoid, which is present apically to the epithelial attachment.
Alveolar Bone	Lamina dura is thinner with larger marrow spaces and fewer trabeculae. It is less mineralized with higher vasculature and a flat alveolar crest.

NORMAL PERIODONTIUM IN PERMANENT DENTITION

Compared to the gingiva of primary teeth, the gingival margin of permanent teeth is relatively thinner and has a characteristic coral pink colour.

Healthy gingiva appears in 'coral pink' or 'salmon' colour (Fig. **3**). It may show pigmentation, which varies based on the ethnicity of the subject. The gingiva has a firm consistency and is firmly adherent to the alveolar bone. The surface is keratinized and may show a characteristic orange-peel appearance known as 'stippling ' (Fig. **4**). The marginal gingiva is present on the surface of enamel about 0.5 to 2 mm coronal to CEJ once the tooth is fully erupted [4].

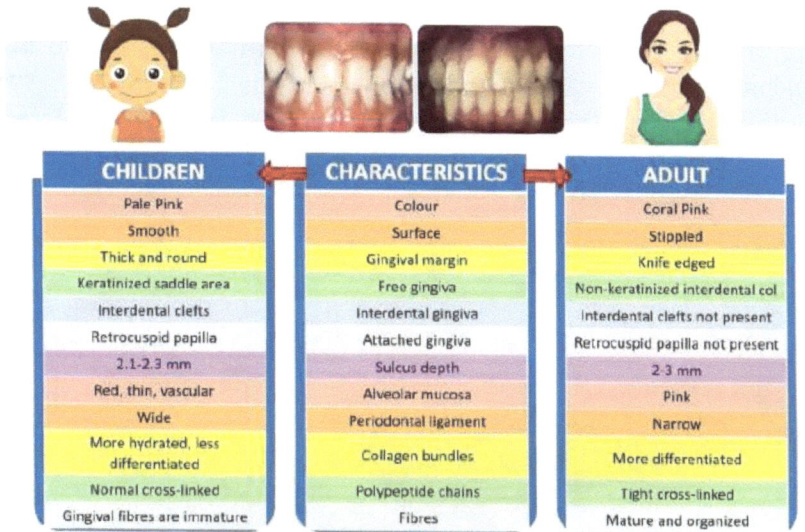

CHILDREN	CHARACTERISTICS	ADULT
Pale Pink	Colour	Coral Pink
Smooth	Surface	Stippled
Thick and round	Gingival margin	Knife edged
Keratinized saddle area	Free gingiva	Non-keratinized interdental col
Interdental clefts	Interdental gingiva	Interdental clefts not present
Retrocuspid papilla	Attached gingiva	Retrocuspid papilla not present
2.1-2.3 mm	Sulcus depth	2-3 mm
Red, thin, vascular	Alveolar mucosa	Pink
Wide	Periodontal ligament	Narrow
More hydrated, less differentiated	Collagen bundles	More differentiated
Normal cross-linked	Polypeptide chains	Tight cross-linked
Gingival fibres are immature	Fibres	Mature and organized

Fig. (3). Differences in periodontal characteristics of children and adult.

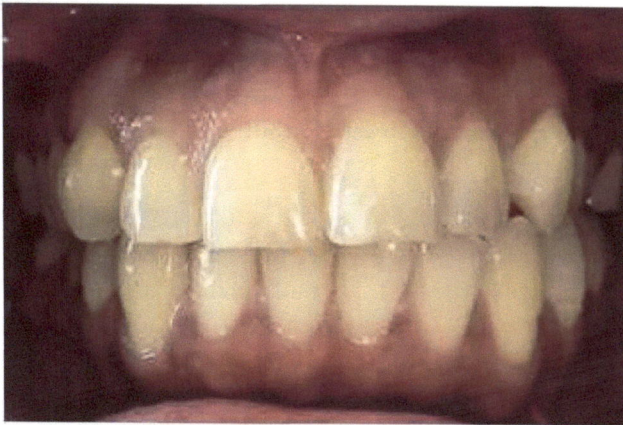

Fig. (4). Clinical appearance of gingiva in adults (Permanent Dentition).

Physiologic Gingival Changes Associated with Tooth Eruption

During the period of transition in the development of the dentition, changes are observed in the gingiva which is associated with the eruption of permanent teeth. It is important to recognize these physiologic changes and differentiate them from the gingival pathology [2].

Pre-eruption Bulge

The gingiva appears as a bulge which is firm, adheres to the contour of the underlying crown before the crown appears in the oral cavity and also shows slight blanching (Fig. **5**).

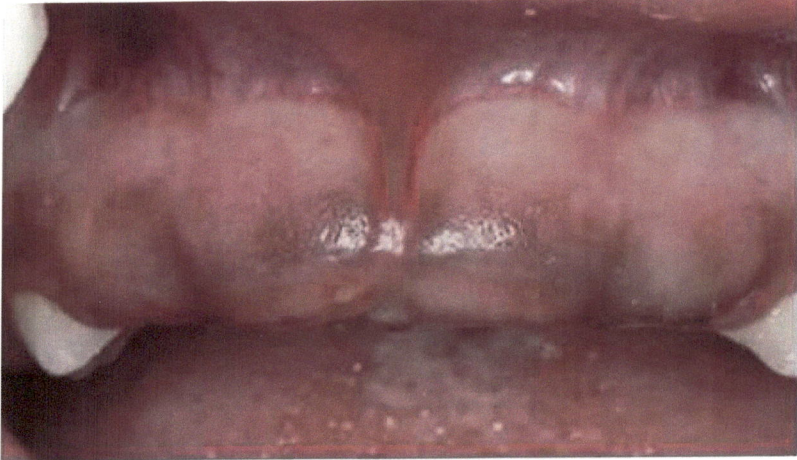

Fig. (5). Pre-eruption bulge.

Formation of the Gingival Margin

The gingival margin and sulcus develop as the crown penetrates the mucosa. The gingival margin is rounded, slightly reddened and edematous during the eruption.

Normal Prominence of Gingiva

In the mixed dentition phase, the marginal gingiva around the permanent tooth appears prominent, especially in the upper anterior portion. During this stage of the eruption, the gingiva is still adherent to the crown and is prominent when it superimposes on the underlying bulk of enamel.

Etiology

It is a fact that gingivitis is caused by dental plaque. The normal ecology of the oral cavity comprises a large number of bacteria. Studies assessing the microbial role in causing gingivitis have concluded that the number of bacteria is important for the pathogenesis of gingivitis. However, gingivitis should be considered a multifactorial disease since a multitude of extrinsic and intrinsic factors play a role in influencing its severity (Fig. **6**).

Factors influencing plaque formation
- Calculus
- Disturbances of the enamel mineralization
- Manifest carious lesions
- Restorations with defective margins
- Malocclusion and Fixed orthodontic appliances

Factors modifying the defence system
- Mouth breathing
- Hormonal changes
- Eruption of teeth

Systemic factors
- Haematological disturbances
- Malnutrition including vitamin and protein deficiencies
- Metabolic disorders like Diabetes Mellitus type I
- Hereditary and genetic factors
- Viral, bacterial and fungal infections

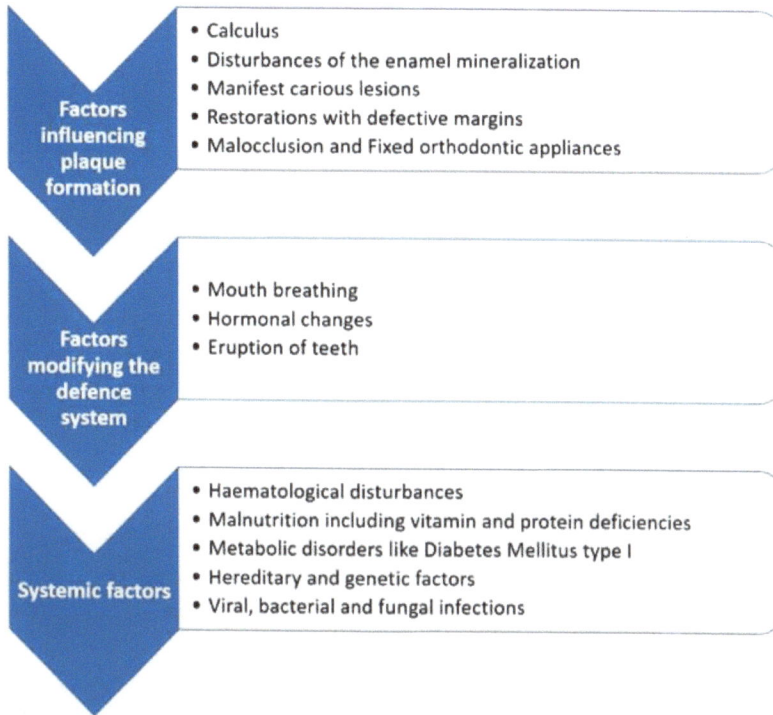

Fig. (6). Factors influencing gingival and periodontal diseases.

Classification of Gingival and Periodontal Diseases (Figs. 7 and 8) [5]

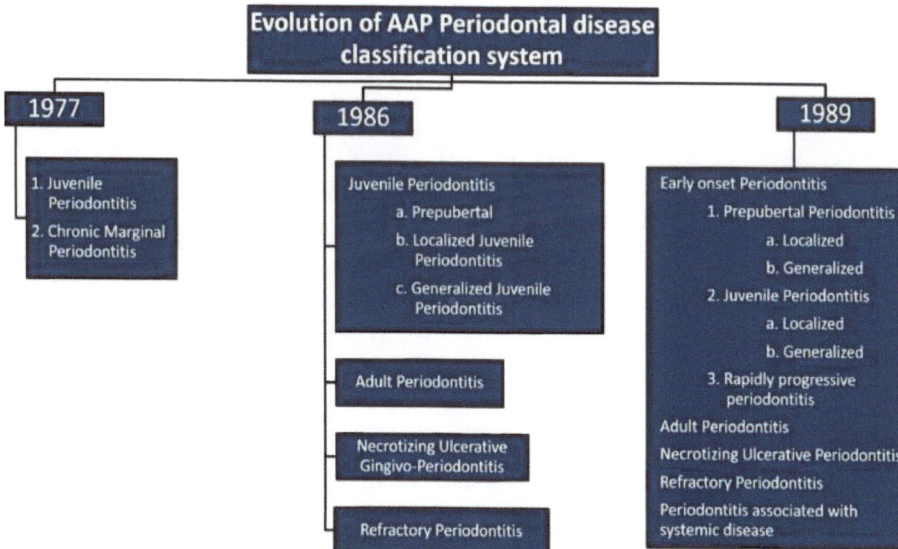

Evolution of AAP Periodontal disease classification system

1977
1. Juvenile Periodontitis
2. Chronic Marginal Periodontitis

1986
Juvenile Periodontitis
  a. Prepubertal
  b. Localized Juvenile Periodontitis
  c. Generalized Juvenile Periodontitis

Adult Periodontitis

Necrotizing Ulcerative Gingivo-Periodontitis

Refractory Periodontitis

1989
Early onset Periodontitis
1. Prepubertal Periodontitis
  a. Localized
  b. Generalized
2. Juvenile Periodontitis
  a. Localized
  b. Generalized
3. Rapidly progressive periodontitis
Adult Periodontitis
Necrotizing Ulcerative Periodontitis
Refractory Periodontitis
Periodontitis associated with systemic disease

Fig. (7). Classification of periodontal diseases by American Academy of Periodontology.

Periodontal diseases and conditions

Periodontal health, gingival diseases and conditions

Periodontal health and gingival health	Gingivitis: Dental biofilm induced	Gingival diseases: Non-Dental biofilm induced

Periodontitis

Necrotizing periodontal diseases	Periodontitis	Periodontitis as a manifestation of systemic disease

Other conditions affecting the periodontium

Systemic diseases or conditions affecting the periodontal supporting tissues	Periodontal abscesses and endodontic periodontal lesions	Mucogingival deformities and conditions	Traumatic occlusal forces	Tooth and prosthesis related factors

Peri-implant diseases and conditions

Peri-implant health	Peri-implant mucositis	Peri-implantitis	Peri-implant soft and hard tissue deficiencies

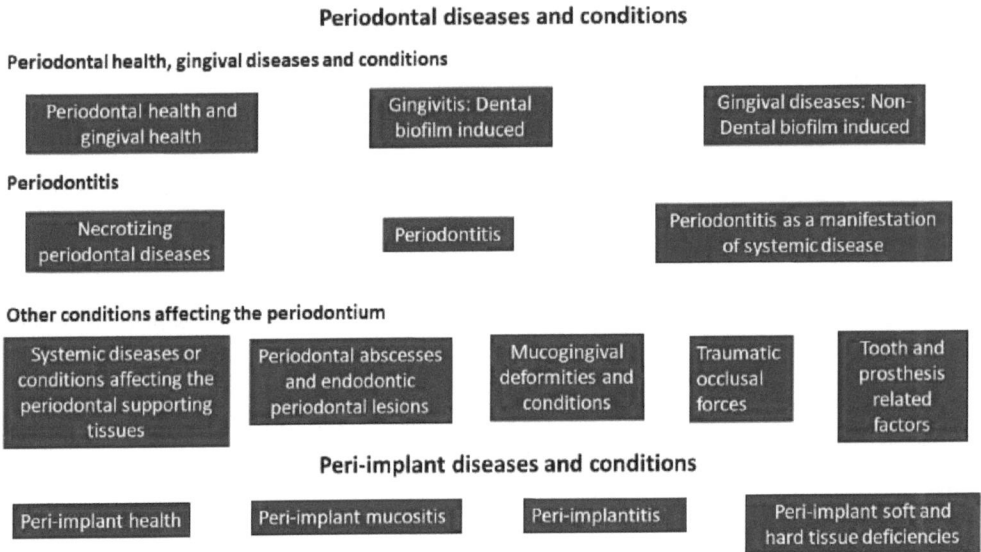

Fig. (8). Classification of periodontal and peri-implant diseases and conditions (2017 World Workshop).

GINGIVAL DISEASES IN CHILDREN

Gingivitis Associated with Dental Plaque

Without Local Contributing Factors

Dental Plaque is regarded as the primary cause of gingivitis in the absence of local contributing factors. Plaque formation seems to occur more rapidly among 8–12-year-old children in comparison to adults. Dental plaque-induced inflammation usually confines to the marginal gingiva (Fig. **9**). With time, the inflammation progresses to other parts of periodontal tissues. A fiery red appearance is seen on the surface, which superimposes the underlying chronic alterations. Changes in colour and swelling in the gingiva appear to be the more common clinical manifestations of gingivitis among children as compared to bleeding on probing and an increase in pocket depth [6]. The progranulocyte migration rate is lower among children in comparison to adults. The tendency for bleeding as well as production of GCF and leukocytes is lesser than in adults. The greatest degree of gingivitis is observed among 14-16-year-old [1, 2].

With Local Contributing Factors

Eruption Cyst & Hematoma

Erupting teeth may commonly be associated with eruption cyst, which is a type of dentigerous cyst. It usually presents as a translucent, fluctuant, and circumscribed swelling. Swelling appears fluctuant, circumscribed, and deep – blue/purple when the cystic cavity contains blood, termed eruption hematoma (Fig. **10**) These cysts usually rupture as the tooth erupts in the oral cavity, and no treatment is necessary. In case they bother, an incision can be made to expose the tooth to aid in its eruption.

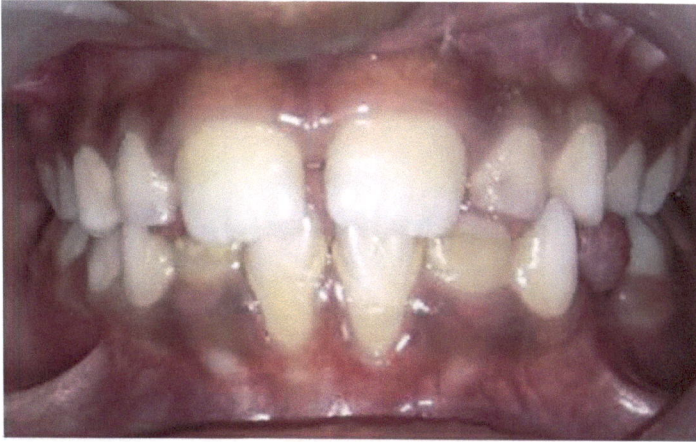

Fig. (9). Plaque-induced gingivitis.

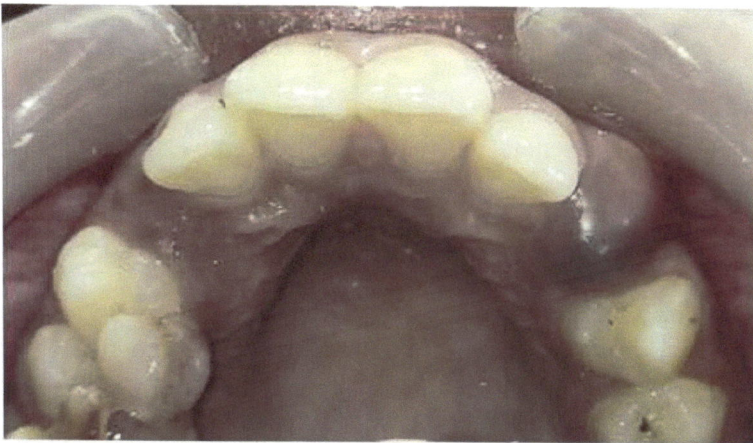

Fig. (10). Eruption hematoma.

Eruption Gingivitis

It is a transitory form of gingivitis which is frequently observed among young children at the time of eruption of primary teeth. It is localized and is associated with difficult eruption, which recedes after the emergence of a tooth into the oral cavity. Maximum incidence of gingivitis is seen in the n 6-7-year age group at the time of eruption of permanent teeth (Fig. **11**). Eruption gingivitis is prevalent in areas of shedding primary teeth and erupting permanent teeth due to difficulty in maintaining oral hygiene, which greatly predisposes the area to plaque accumulation. There is a lack of protection to the gingival margin from the coronal contour of the month during the initial stages of active eruption. Additionally, accumulation of material alba, food debris and plaque around the free gingival margin can cause exacerbation of inflammation. This inflammatory process is most often associated with the eruption of permanent first and second molars, which may develop into a painful condition, namely pericoronitis or peri coronal abscess [3].

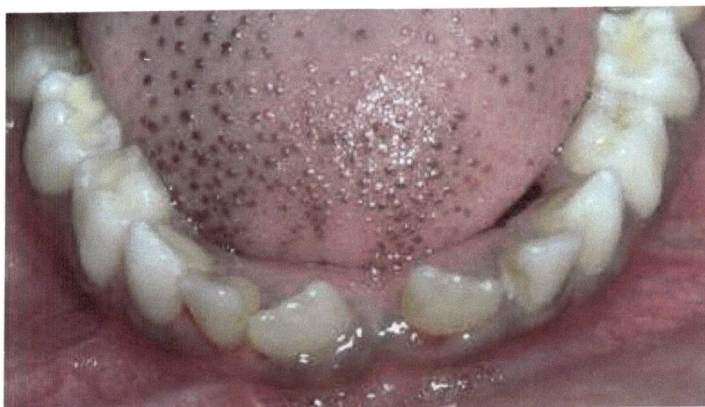

Fig. (11). Eruption of gingivitis.

Furthermore, sometimes an exaggerated response to the bacterial irritants may be observed owing to the degenerative changes exhibited by the epithelium at the site of fusion between oral and dental epithelium. This site presents a weak point of the epithelial barrier, and also, the increased permeability of the newly developed junctional epithelium makes it susceptible to microbial attack.

Another relevant factor is that once inflammation in gingiva is established, the internal enamel epithelium of erupting tooth may separate from enamel which creates a niche for pathogenic flora, thus risking the involvement of deeper tissue. Such an accumulation of subgingival plaque explains the reason for the difficulty in treating gingival inflammation in an erupting tooth as compared to a completely erupted tooth.

Mild cases of eruption gingivitis can be corrected by meagre improvement in oral hygiene. Painful pericoronitis may be relieved by local irrigation with counterirritants like Peroxyl. However, pericoronitis presenting with swelling as well as the involvement of lymph nodes is indicated for antibiotic therapy.

Gingivitis Associated with Orthodontic Appliances

Access for plaque control in the interproximal region is significantly reduced during fixed orthodontic treatment. This problem is aggravated when the tooth is banded instead of being bonded. Supragingival plaque shifts to the subgingival region as a result of tipping movements. Conversely, the bodily movement has a lesser chance of inducing such relocation of supragingival plaque. Hence, changes in gingiva may occur within 1-2 months of initiation of fixed therapy which are transient [1] (Fig. **12**).

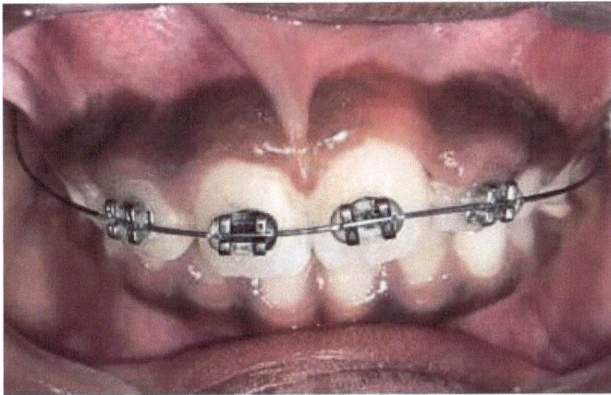

Fig. (12). Gingivitis associated with orthodontic appliances.

Mouth Breathing

Studies have associated mouth breathing and chronic gingivitis (Fig. **13**). Mouth breathing causes drying of the maxillary anterior gingiva, which in turn causes vasoconstriction and reduced host resistance [1].

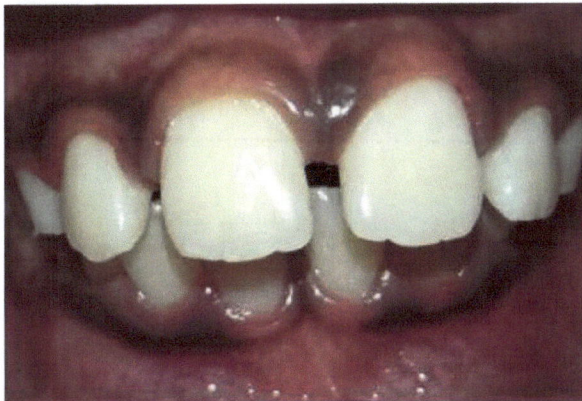

Fig. (13). Gingivitis associated with mouth breathing.

Other Factors

Other factors which frequently cause gingivitis are excessive overjet, overbite, partially exfoliated tooth, loose deciduous teeth, malposed teeth, and eroded margin of partially resorbed carious teeth.

Gingival Diseases Modified by Systemic Factors

Gingival Diseases Associated with the Endocrine System

Puberty Gingivitis

Exaggerated gingivitis without plaque accumulation occurs at the time of puberty (Fig. **14**). The cytoplasm of gingival cells contains specific receptors for both testosterone as well as estrogen. Receptors for estrogen are observed in the spinous as well as the basal layer of epithelium, in endothelial cells and fibroblasts of small blood vessels of connective tissue. Hence, the gingiva acts as a target for steroid hormones [7, 8].

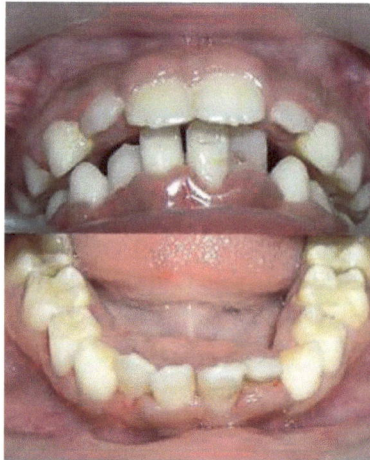

Fig. (14). Puberty gingivitis.

Gingivitis associated with puberty peaks among girls around 11-13 years and boys at around 13-14 years. Earlier peak observed among girls strengthens the association between the prevalence of gingivitis and increased levels of circulating sex hormones. Increased *P. intermedius* proportion *in vivo* correlates with plasma progesterone and estrogen levels, which shows that *P. intermedius* derives nutrients from these hormones. Puberty gingivitis clinically appears bluish-red, red discolouration with oedema as a result of exaggerated inflammatory response from local irritants [1, 3, 9].

Menstrual Cycle-associated with Gingivitis

Exaggerated inflammatory response occurs as a result t of an increase in circulating levels of sex hormones. Gingiva appears to be more edematous at the time of menses and appears erythematous before the commencement of menses. Increased hormonal gingival interaction is observed during the menstrual cycle. Increased gingival exudate is observed at the time of the menstrual period and is sometimes associated with a mild increase in tooth mobility. There is a higher incidence of post-extraction osteitis at the start of menses.

Increased estrogen and progesterone levels cause increased synthesis of prostaglandin E2 (PGE2), endothelial growth factors, angiogenetic factors, and tumour necrosis factor-alpha (TNF-α), which cause exaggerated gingival inflammatory response at the time of the menstrual cycle. At the time of mensan es, an increased level of progesterone is seen from the 2nd week and peaks at around 10 days and a dramatic drop in the levels is seen before menstruation. Progesterone causes an increase in microvasculature permeability, alters the rate of collagen formation, increases folate metabolism, and alters the immune response.

Progesterone stimulates PGE2 release, which mediates the inflammatory response of the body. PGE2 is majorly secreted by monocytes which increases during gingival inflammation.

Increased gingival bleeding and tenderness during menses require close monitoring. Hence, periodontal maintenance must be adapted to the individual patient's requirements Maintenance of oral hygiene must be emphasized, and the use of antimicrobial mouth rinse before cyclic inflammation may be suggested to the patients. It is recommended to schedule surgical visits after the menstruation cycle in patients with prior history of postoperative haemorrhage or excessive menstrual flow.

Diabetes Mellitus-associated Gingivitis

Insulin-dependent diabetes mellitus or Type 1 diabetes mellitus occurs more frequently among children and young adults, whereas non-insulin-dependent diabetes mellitus or Type 2 diabetes mellitus is observed among adults. Gingivitis and periodontitis are more prevalent among affected children than in unaffected individuals, similar to diabetic adults (Fig. **15**). Clinical consequences include premature loss of teeth and impaired immune response to microflora. The severity of the periodontal disease is worse among children with poorly controlled diabetes. Although destructive changes are rather rare in healthy children, periodontal destruction can be observed in diabetic children, usually appearing around the time of puberty and becoming progressively worse as children mature into adulthood. Disease prevention and fastidious oral hygiene measures should be highly promoted [10]. Diabetic children must be given instructions and adequately motivated regarding plaque control early on itself.

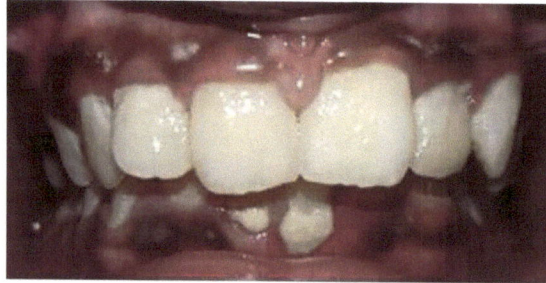

Fig. (15). Diabetes mellitus-associated gingivitis.

Gingival Diseases Associated with Blood Dyscrasias

Leukaemia

Leukemia is a malignancy caused by the abnormal proliferation of WBCs. It has acute and chronic types and has the potential to affect any WBC – lymphocytes, monocytes, or granulocytes. The acute form is common in young individuals lesser than 20 years. All is highly prevalent among children less than 10 years. Factors responsible for its etiology are chemical injury, radiation injury, immune deficiency, and viral infections. Signs and symptoms include fever, sore throat, malaise, lethargy, presence of petechiae and purpura, cervical lymphadenopathy, and hepatosplenomegaly [1, 9, 11]. Clinically, the gingiva is a red-deep purple and has a swollen and glazed appearance along with gingival bleeding. There is the diffused enlargement of gingiva along with discrete tumour-like mass seen interproximal. The gingiva has a firm consistency but tends towards being friable and prone to haemorrhage on slight provocation (Fig. **16**).

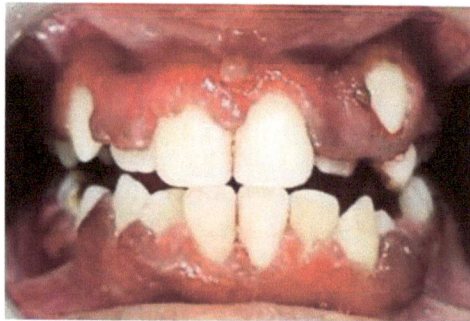

Fig. (16). Leukemic gingivitis.

Plaque control is necessary before medicinal and cytotoxic therapy. Maintenance of oral hygiene along with the use of chlorhexidine mouth rinse or topical antibiotics may regress the swelling but patients usually have a poor overall prognosis.

Gingival Diseases Modified by Medication

Drug-Induced Gingival Enlargement

Drug-induced gingival enlargement is a common entity, which occurs following the consumption of certain anticonvulsants, calcium channel blockers and immunosuppressants. This poses problems with speech, mastication, aesthetics as well as tooth eruption. A well-recognized unwarranted effect of certain drugs is an overgrowth of the gingiva. The most common causative drugs are phenytoin, nifedipine and cyclosporine. The interdental gingiva becomes nodular prior to enlarging diffusely, causing encroachment of labial tissues. The anterior portion of the oral cavity is frequently and most severely involved. The enlarged gingiva appears pink, and firm and shows stippling in patients with good oral hygiene. For patients with gingival enlargement refractory long-term term therapy, their physician can be requested modifications in the treatment regimen.

Drug-induced enlargement may be absent in patients showing an abundance of plaque accumulation and may occur in patients with little or no plaque [1, 2, 9]. Gingival overgrowth can be kept under check with rigorous maintenance of oral hygiene. However, in a few patients, gingivectomy may become essential and may be demanded by patients for esthetic concerns.

Anticonvulsants

First drug reported to cause gingival enlargement is phenytoin (Dilantin). Other hydantoins which cause gingival enlargement are mephenytoin (Mesantoin) and ethotoin (Peganone). Other anticonvulsants which cause drug-induced gingival enlargement are ethosuximide (Zarontin) and valproic acid (Depakene) (Fig. **17**). Studies have shown that phenytoin causes the proliferation of epithelium and fibroblast-like cells. Similar effects have been observed on fibroblast-like cells with 2 analogues of phenytoin (5-methyl 5- phenylhydatoinate and 1-allyl-5-phenyl hydantoinate). These fibroblasts have demonstrated an increase in the synthesis of glycosaminoglycans *in vitro*.

Phenytoin may reduce the degradation of collagen by producing inactive fibroblastic collagenase [9, 12, 13].

Immunosuppressants

Cyclosporine is a potent immunosuppressive agent which is used for treating autoimmune disorders and preventing organ transplant rejection. Its exact mechanism is unknown, but it may cause selective and reversible inhibition of helper T cells which play a key role in cellular and humoral immunity. Cyclosporin A, when administered more than 500 mg/day either orally or *i.v.*, is reported to cause gingival enlargement (Fig. **18**). The gingival enlargement induced by cyclosporine is more vascular compared to the enlargement induced by phenytoin. Its occurrence ranges from 25-to 70%, with children being affected more frequently. The severity of drug-induced gingival enlargement correlates more with the plasma concentration rather than the periodontal condition of the patient. Gingival enlargement is more among patients who are given both cyclosporines as well as calcium channel blockers. The microscopic picture of this condition shows the presence of plasma cells along with an abundance of amorphous extracellular substances, which suggests that the enlargement is a hypersensitive reaction to the drug [9].

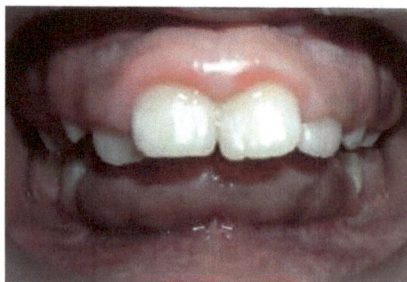

Fig. (17). Drug influenced gingival enlargement (Anticonvulsants).

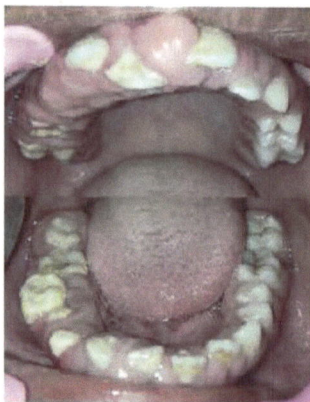

Fig. (18). Gingival enlargement associated with immunosuppressants.

Calcium Channel Blockers (CCBs)

This class of drugs are employed for treating cardiovascular conditions like hypertension, angina pectoris, cardiac arrhythmias, and coronary artery spasms. They act by inhibiting the influx of calcium ions across the cell membrane of heart cells and smooth muscle cells thus causing blockage of intracellular mobilization of calcium ions. This causes direct dilation of the coronary artery thereby causing improvement of oxygen supply to the heart and also causes dilation of peripheral vasculature thus reducing blood pressure. This class of antihypertensives comprise dihydropyridine derivatives (nifedipine [Adalat, Procardia], nicardipine [Cardene], amlodipine [Lotrel, Norvasc]), phenylethylamine derivatives (verapamil) and benzothiazine derivatives (diltiazem [Cardizem, Dilacor XR, Tiazac]). Few of these drugs tend to cause gingival enlargement (Fig. **19**). Nifedipine is the most commonly used CCBs, and it causes a gingival enlargement in 20% of patients. Other CCBs like felodipine, verapamil and diltiazem also lead to gingival enlargement. Dihydropyridine derivative such as isradipine does not cause gingival enlargement; hence can be used to replace nifedipine in certain cases. Nifedipine is used along with cyclosporine in patients who have undergone a renal transplant and combined usage of these drugs causes gingival overgrowth to a greater degree [9].

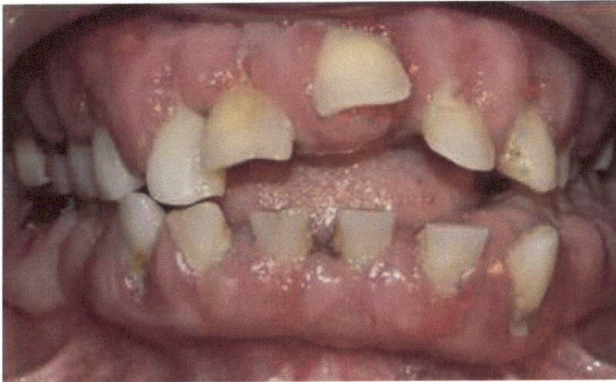

Fig. (19). Gingival enlargement associated with calcium channel blockers.

Gingival Diseases Associated with Nutritional Deficiency

Scorbutic Gingivitis

Scurvy is a nutritional deficiency disorder caused by inadequate consumption of Vitamin C. "Scorbutic gingivitis" occurs as a result of a combination of vitamin C deficiency and poor oral hygiene. Vitamin C deficiency leads to a predisposition to haemorrhage, degeneration of collagen and oedema of the connective tissue of the gingiva. Involvement of marginal gingiva and papillae is usually seen.

Gingiva has a soft, smooth, friable, and bluish appearance. Additionally, complaints of severe pain and spontaneous haemorrhage are common. The gingiva becomes boggy, ulcerates, and then bleeds (Fig. **20**). Surface necrosis along with pseudomembrane formation resulting from infarction in the capillaries supplying the gingiva is also observed. Apart from dietary deficiency, gingivitis associated with Vitamin C deficiency can be seen among both paediatric as well as adult cancer patients who are undergoing chemotherapy or radiotherapy. The mucosal lining of the intestinal wall is affected in these patients, which hampers the absorption of nutrients. Severe scorbutic gingivitis seems to be rare among children but may be observed among children exhibiting an allergy to fruit juice and concomitant supplementation of dietary vitamin C is neglected [1].

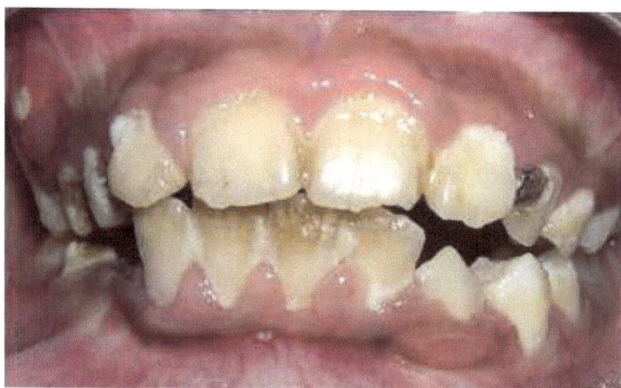

Fig. (20). Scorbutic gingivitis.

Scorbutic gingivitis shows a positive response to daily 250-500 mg of vitamin C in cases where blood studies have pointed towards vitamin C deficiency and excluded other possible systemic abnormalities. Inflammation of marginal gingiva and interdental papilla without the presence of local predisposing factors also may point towards scorbutic gingivitis. Enquiring the child and parents regarding the dietary habits along with the seven-day diet diary may frequently indicate inadequate consumption of vitamin C-containing foods. Complete dental care, along with improvement in oral hygiene and vitamin C supplementation, improves the gingival condition [12].

Non-plaque-induced Gingival Diseases

Bacterial Origin

The prevalence of gingival disease caused by specific bacteria is increasing. Lesions in the oral cavity may be caused by direct infection or may occur secondarily to systemic infections. Streptococcal gingivitis or gingivostomatitis occurs rarely and is an acute condition presenting with fever and malaise. Gingiva presents with acute inflammation and is the red, swollen, and painful way with a greater tendency to bleed and the occasional presence of a gingival abscess. Tonsilitis usually precedes the gingival infection and group A β- hemolytic streptococci are responsible for its causation.

Acute Necrotizing Ulcerative Gingivitis

Hyacinthe Jean Vincent, a French physician and Hugo Carl Plaut from Germany described the fusiform bacilli and spirochete-associated infection, which was later known as Vincent's angina. It is also known as trench mouth due to its classic presentation among military personnel during world war I. In developing countries, the prevalence of Necrotizing Ulcerative Gingivitis (NUG) is higher than in industrialized countries. In India, its prevalence ranges from 54-to 68% among children below 10 years of age. Prevotella intermedia, Fusobacterium and Treponemal species are predominantly implicated in NUG [2].

Necrotizing ulcerative gingivitis can most often be readily diagnosed due to its classical presentation. The gingiva exhibits a characteristic punched-out appearance due to ulceration and necrosis of marginal gingiva and interdental papilla. Ulcers are covered by greyish or yellowish-white slough known as pseudomembrane (Fig. **21**). Removal of this slough leads to bleeding and exposure of underlying tissues. This condition exhibits the varying intensity of fetor ex ore (halitosis). It is rarely associated with deep pockets due to extensive necrosis of gingiva and often also coincides with crestal alveolar bone loss. Systemic manifestations include fever (temperature as high as 40 °C), loss of appetite, generalized malaise along with fetid odour and enlarged lymph nodes. These patients usually present with poor oral hygiene [14].

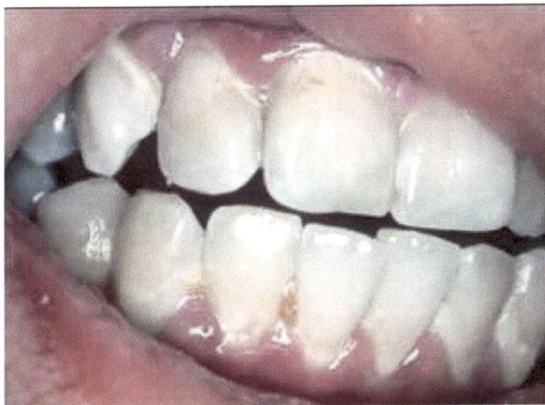

Fig. (21). Acute Necrotizing Ulcerative Gingivitis.

Treatment modality usually undertaken is subgingival curettage, debridement, and the use of oxidizing rinses like hydrogen peroxide. In cases presenting with acute and extensive inflammation of gingival tissues at the first visit, antibiotic therapy must be considered. Improvement in oral hygiene and the use of oxidizing solutions along with chlorhexidine mouthwash helps to overcome the infection. Usually, there may be no difficulty in differentiating NUG from acute herpetic gingivostomatitis, but sometimes confusion may be present in distinguishing the two clinical entities. Acute herpetic gingivostomatitis presents as round ulcers with red areolae on lips and cheek. Necrotizing ulcerative gingivitis responds favourably to subgingival curettage and debridement however, acute herpetic gingivostomatitis does not. The use of antibiotics causes a reduction in acute symptoms of NUG but has no impact on viral infections like acute herpetic gingivostomatitis. Acute herpetic gingivostomatitis is more prevalent among preschool children and has a rapid onset however NUG is rarely observed in this age group and tends to develop over a longer period. Necrotizing ulcerative gingivitis develops in the presence of several concomitant factors like poor oral hygiene, malnutrition, debilitating disease, and psychological stress. It has been observed that few acute oral conditions which were initially diagnosed to be NUG have been later understood to be an oral manifestation of xanthomatoses. Initial stages of certain conditions like Langerhans cell histiocytosis and Hand-Schülle--Christian disease overlap with several symptoms associated with NUG.

Viral Origin

Primary Herpetic Gingivostomatitis

Herpetic gingivostomatitis is caused by herpes simplex virus type 1 (HSV-1) which characteristically presents as high-grade fever along with painful oral lesions. It occurs most commonly among children of age 6 months-5 years but may also be seen in adults as well. This virus spreads through direct contact or also *via* oral secretions or lesions of symptomatic or even asymptomatic patients. After the primary infection with HSV, a recurrent infection can occur which is known as herpes labialis (cold sores) [1, 2, 15]. Clinically there is erythematous, diffuse involvement of the gingiva as well as of the adjacent mucosa associated with bleeding and oedema. There is the presence of discrete greyish vesicles that rupture, forming painful small ulcers with a halo li margin along with a depressed greyish-white or yellowish central part (Fig. **22**) [14].

Herpetic gingivostomatitis is generally a mild and self-limiting condition. Antiviral drug therapy significantly impacts the course of infection, provided the early diagnosis is made. Antibiotics aid in preventing secondary infections.

Topical anaesthetic gels and nonsteroidal anti-inflammatory drugs help in relieving associated discomfort.

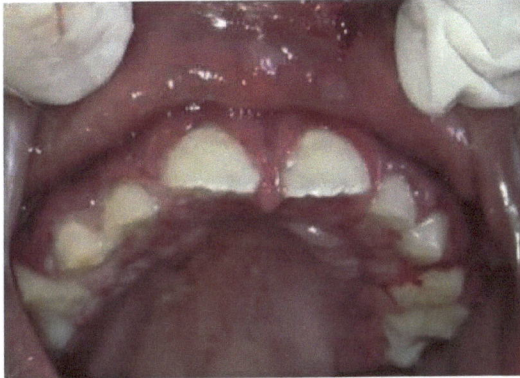

Fig. (22). Herpetic gingivostomatitis.

Recurrent Oral Herpes

Recurrent herpetic stomatitis is seen among adults and presents as an attenuated form of primary infection. Weathers and Griffin have stated that these recurrent herpetic lesions frequently involve the oral mucosa which is bound tightly to the periosteum, and rarely involve the mobile mucosa, which is in contrast to recurrent aphthous stomatitis, which invariably involves the mobile mucosa. Therefore, recurrent intraoral herpes most often involves the attached gingiva, hard palate, or alveolar ridge.

Up until recent times, only a little information was available regarding the actual treatment regimen for this condition except for providing symptomatic relief. However, over the years several drugs have been evaluated. Various antiviral drugs are available presently for certain HSV infections. Most popular among these are acyclovir (9– [2– hydroxyethoxymethyl] guanine), idoxuridine (5–iodo-2'-deoxyuridine) and vidarabine (adenine arabinoside). But their use must be based on specific indications only.

Varicella-zoster infections: Chickenpox is an acute, ubiquitous, extremely contagious disease usually occurring in children, and is characterized by an exanthematous vesicular rash. It is caused by the infection of Varicella zoster virus, which is a DNA virus. It causes two distinct lesions known as chickenpox, a primary lesion and a reactivated lesion known as herpes zoster. It is most common in the winter and spring months. The mode of transmission is by airborne droplets or direct contact with infected lesions. It presents clinically as small blister-like lesions involving mainly the buccal mucosa, gingiva, tongue, palate, and pharyngeal mucosa. The lesions present initially as slightly raised vesicles with erythema surrounding it, and they rupture to form small, eroded ulcers surrounded by a red margin, showing resemblance to aphthous ulcers [1].

Fungal Origin

Gingival infections caused by fungi are rare among immunocompetent individuals but are more common among immunocompromised patients and patients on broad-spectrum antibiotic therapy for a prolonged duration. Candidiasis is the most common fungal disease caused by *Candida albicans* seen in individuals on steroid therapy with reduced salivary flow, increased salivary glucose levels and patients with long-time denture wear. Candidal infections present clinically in the form of white patches involving the tongue, gingiva, or oral mucosa, which on removal with gauze leaves behind a red bleeding surface. In HIV patients, candidiasis presents as erythema involving the attached gingiva which has been termed *linear gingival erythema* [1, 14].

<u>*Acute Candidiasis (Thrush, Moniliasis, Candidosis)*</u>

Candida albicans is a fungus commonly inhabiting the mouth which may undergo rapid multiplication in cases of lowered host resistance leading to a pathogenic state.

Children develop a thrush post-antibiotic regimen which causes the proliferation of fungus. Candidiasis presents as white areas which can be removed, leaving behind a raw bleeding surface. Neonatal candidiasis is observed clinically in the first 2 weeks of life, contracted at the time of passage through the birth canal and is also a common occurrence in immunosuppressed patients.

This condition is treated with antifungal agents like nystatin suspension (1ml), and clotrimazole suspension (10mg/ml). These topical antifungals can be applied locally 4 times daily. Furthermore, systemic antifungals like fluconazole suspension (10 mg/ml) can be safely used in infants at a dose of up to 6 mg/kg/day.

<u>*Linear Gingival Erythema*</u>

In HIV-infected patients, candidiasis may present in the form of erythema involving the gingiva, which is termed *HIV-associated gingivitis* or *linear gingival erythema*. It is characterized by the presence of a 2-3mm band of intense erythema on the free gingival margin, which bleeds easily and extends to the attached gingiva as diffuse or focal erythema or extends beyond the mucogingival line involving the alveolar mucosa also. It may present as a localized or more commonly, as a generalized condition (Fig. **23**).

Histoplasmosis

Also called **Darling's disease**. The main causative organism implicated in this fungal disease is *Histoplasma capsulatum*. The infection is acquired *via* inhalation of dust comprising of fungal spores and contamination from bird excreta like pigeons and blackbirds. Levy and Stiff have reported that the oral lesions appear as nodular, vegetative, or ulcerated lesions involving the tongue, palate, gingiva, buccal mucosa, or lips. The ulcerated region is covered with a non-specific greyish membrane which shows induration and has rolled out and raised borders giving the appearance of carcinoma. It is advocated to preserve a portion of tissue during a biopsy to perform microbiological examination because the organism may be observed in certain tissue sections. This organism is isolated by inoculation in a blood agar medium comprising streptomycin and penicillin.

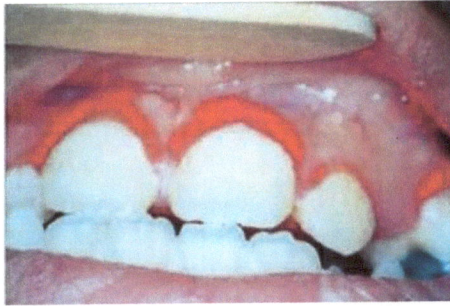

Fig. (23). Linear gingival erythema.

Congenital Anomalies

Hereditary Gingival Fibromatosis

Hereditary gingival fibromatosis is an idiopathic, benign condition affecting the maxillary as well as mandibular arch. It is an autosomal dominant condition affecting all genders equally. The gingiva is markedly enlarged, asymptomatic, non-hemorrhagic, and non-exudative. A relationship has been reported between this condition with deficiency of growth hormone. It presents clinically in a symmetric form or less commonly a nodular form. The onset of this abnormality coincides with the eruption of the permanent tooth. Hereditary gingival fibromatosis may predispose to functional and esthetic problems, malpositioning of teeth and retention of primary teeth. Treatment is usually a gingivectomy performed in one or several appointments. Recurrence is possible after some years [1, 9, 14].

Congenital Epulis

It is a rare tumour of newborns occurring along the alveolar ridge. It is also known as **Neumann's tumour**. It is usually not associated with other congenital malformations or developmental disturbances of the teeth. It is observed clinically as a well-defined smooth erythematous mass originating from the gum pad. It may sometimes have a size large enough to lift the upper lip. It does not usually affect the unerupted tooth. The treatment for the congenital epulis is surgical excision with little possibility of recurrence [2].

Gingival Manifestations of Systemic Conditions [14, 16]

Mucocutaneous Disorders

Lichen Planus

Oral lichen planus (OLP) is a common mucocutaneous disease which was described by Wilson for the first time. It has a worldwide prevalence of 0.5-1% and affects the skin or mucosa or both. Lichen planus in pediatric patients is a rare phenomenon. Clinically, there is the presence of white striations, plaque or papule bilaterally involving the buccal mucosa, gingiva, and tongue. Lesions of the oral cavity are different in appearance from skin lesions. They consist of velvety, radiating grey or white, thread-like papules arranged in a linear, retiform or annular pattern. Buccal mucosa shows the presence of reticular patches and streaks (Fig. **24**), but this presentation is less common on the palate, lips, and tongue. Wickham striae is a feature of lichen planus characterized by tiny elevated white dots present at the point where white lines intersect. Lichen planus of **atrophic** type presents as rendered-coloured smooth, poorly defined areas along with peripheral striae which may not be evident always. Chronic desquamative gingivitis is a condition wherein the gingiva is red, diffuse, and painful and is usually reported among postmenopausal women who are refractory to treatment. Lichen planus of **hypertrophic** variety resembles leukoplakia and appears as a white lesion which is elevated and well-circumscribed [14]. Oral lichen planus in pediatric patients can have a long-term psychological effect and impacts the overall quality of life of children. The presence of such lesions should be considered for a possible malignant transformation and hence, the patients must be encouraged to regular biannual evaluation. Sequential therapeutic modalities initial topical retinoids can be given in some cases.

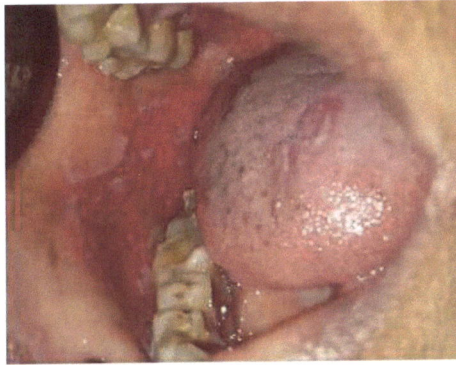

Fig. (24). Oral lichen planus.

Pemphigus Vulgaris

It is an autoimmune condition affecting the skin and mucous membrane. It is characterized as an intraepithelial, blistering disease which is mediated by circulating autoantibodies directed against the keratinocyte cell surface. This condition typically affects the mucous membrane first hence they precede the cutaneous lesion by months. The disease involves mucosa in 50–70% of patients. Intact bullae are rare in the mouth. Patients commonly present with irregular and ill-defined erosions on the gingiva, buccal mucosa or palate which are painful and heal slowly. These erosions are extensive and scattered involving any portion of the oral cavity. They may even cause involvement of the larynx leading to hoarseness subsequently. These lesions cause extreme discomfort to the patients posing difficulty in eating or drinking. Mucosal lesions may also be present on the oesophagus, conjunctiva, penis, urethra, cervix, vagina, and anus. The oral lesions are similar to the skin lesions [14]. Immunosuppression with corticosteroid therapy is the main treatment regimen. Oral pemphigusVulgariss occurring in childhood and adolescents is extremely rare.

Erythema Multiforme

It is an acute self-limiting condition characteristically showing eruptions present as iris or target lesion. Erythema multiforme is relatively common in children. Its severity ranges over a wide spectrum. The minor type of EM presents as a localized eruption on the skin with little or no mucosal involvement. The major type as well as the Steven-Johnson syndrome (SJS) presents with severe cutaneous and mucosal involvement and threatening. The major type of EM is present in 20-60% of patients with erythema multiforme along with mucosal involvement. Oral lesions are severe and extremely painful making mastication very difficult. Vesicles or bullae are seen which may rupture to leave behind a surface covered with whitish or yellowish exudate. Erosions are also present on the pharynx. Lips show painful ulceration with bloody crusting. Patients usually report the complcomplaintral lesions and are usually mistaken to be ANUG. Interestingly, it has been observed that the microorganisms responsible for ANUG are scarce among patients with EM. Steven Johnson syndrome shows more extensive and severe involvement of mucosa as compared to EM major [14].

Infectious Mononucleosis

Epstein – Barr virus is the main causative agent, and this disease occurs more commonly among children and young adults. Clinical presentation ranges from fever, sore throat, headache, enlarged tonsils, fatigue, and malaise to lymphadenopathy. The oral cavity shows gingival bleeding, ulceration of the gingiva, buccal mucosa and petechiae on the soft palate. Palatal petechiae are usually present even before the systemic symptoms become evident.

Herpangina

It is commonly seen in young children and is caused by the coxsackie group A virus. Clinical presentation includes multiple small vesicles which later on form ulcers on a grey base along with inflammation of the periphery. Ulcers are observed on the hard palate, soft palate, tongue, buccal mucosa, or posterior pharyngeal wall. These ulcers are generally not associated with pain and undergo a healing in a few days to a week [2].

Wegeners Granulomatosis

It is a systemic condition presenting as striking changes confined to the gingiva. There is a classical presentation of Strawberry gums wherein the gingiva exhibits erythema and enlargement bands [2, 12].

Kindlers Syndrome

It is a rare autosomal recessive condition characteristically presenting with acral blisters during infancy, which is followed by progressive poikiloderma, cutaneous atrophy and photosensitivity. It may also have oral manifestations with an appearance similar to desquamative gingivitis [2].

Periodontal Diseases in Children

Periodontitis is an inflammatory condition involving the gingiva as well as the concomitant tissues of the periodontium. It is characterized by clinical loss of attachment evident in the form of pockets along with alveolar bone destruction. Periodontal probing for detecting attachment loss and bitewing radiographs are the key diagnostic aids. Bitewing radiograph is used for detecting bone loss by comparing the height of the alveolar bone with the cementoenamel junction. Bone loss is usually evident in the region between primary first and second molars.

Chronic Periodontitis

This condition is most common among adults however it may also occur in young patients. It shows a minor loss of supporting periodontium and progresses slowly. These patients often exhibit considerable plaque deposition as well as subgingival calculus.

The loss of periodontal attachment usually manifests as a single lesion in primary molars in young children. The presence of deep periodontal pockets is limited around affected primary teeth. Scandinavian studies have reported that 2-4% of 7–9-year-olds have shown isolated areas of bone loss around deciduous dentition evident radiographically. Most of these areas may be considered to have incidental attachment loss which occurs in association with local trauma or factors relating to the development of the dentition. Such a defect may even represent a previous inflammatory process which had undergone healing. But such a defect may, more importantly, represent the early stage of progressive periodontal disease.

Epidemiological studies regarding loss of periodontal support conducted in developed countries report frequencies of lesser than 5%. The number of affected sites and the amount of loss of attachment show s increasing tendency with age. Permanent first molars are usually affected [3].

Chronic periodontitis is classified into localized (lesser than 30% sites are involved) and generalized (more than 30% sites are involved) types. It is also further categorized based on the amount of clinical attachment loss (CAL):

Slight – 1-2 mm CAL

Moderate – 3-4 mm CAL

Severe - >5 mm CAL.

Aggressive Periodontitis (Early-onset Periodontitis)

Aggressive periodontitis (Early-onset periodontitis, Juvenile periodontitis) is defined by Baer as a "disease of the periodontium occurring in an otherwise healthy adolescent, which is characterized by a rapid loss of alveolar bone around more than one tooth of the permanent dentition." It is divided into two types: localized and generalized aggressive periodontitis.

Case definition (According to 1999 American Academy of Periodontology workshop)

Primary features common to both localized and generalized variants are as follows:

- Patients are systemically healthy
- Familial tendency
- Presence of rapid clinical attachment loss and destruction of alveolar bone

Secondary features (not always but often associated with the condition) common to both localized and generalized variants are as follows:

- Disease severity is not consistent with the amount of plaque
- Elevated proportion of Aggregatibacter actinomycetemcomitans and Porphyromonas gingivalis
- Abnormalities in phagocytic function
- Elevated levels of PGE2 and IL-1β

Following specific features are used for defining the two types:

Localized Aggressive Periodontitis

- Circumpubertal onset
- Localized involvement of permanent first molars and incisor with attachment loss on at least two permanent teeth (one being permanent first molar) and involving no more than two teeth other than the first molar and incisor
- Robust serum antibody response to infectious agents

Generalized Aggressive Periodontitis

- Usually affects individuals <30 years but older patients may also be affected
- Generalized attachment loss affecting at least 3 permanent teeth other than first molars and incisors
- Episodic nature of periodontal destruction
- Poor serum antibody response to infectious agents

Aggressive periodontitis involving the primary dentition can occur in a localized form although a generalized form is frequently seen. Localized aggressive periodontitis (LAP) is a localized loss of attachment and alveolar bone in primary teeth around the age of 4 years in children who are otherwise systemically healthy. Radiographic examination reveals bone loss in the incisor and/or primary molar region. Abnormal probing depth, rapid alveolar bone loss with minimal gingival inflammation and varying plaque accumulation is seen at the affected site. Abnormal host defence mechanism, familial history of periodontitis and presence of proximal carious lesion which aid as a plaque retentive site is seen with LAP. With the progress of the disease, gingival inflammation with clefts in gingiva and ulceration of marginal gingiva is seen.

GENERALIZED AGGRESSIVE PERIODONTITIS

This condition begins soon after the eruption of deciduous teeth and causes severe inflammation of gingiva, generalized loss of attachment, rapid alveolar bone loss, increased mobility of teeth along with premature exfoliation. Gingiva initially exhibits minor inflammation along with minimal plaque deposits. There is a rapid progression of alveolar bone destruction leading to loss of deciduous teeth by 3 years of age. Affected teeth show the presence of a relatively higher number of non-motile, gram-negative facultative anaerobes (majorly Porphyromonas gingivalis) in GAP as compared to LAP. Predominant microorganisms include Aggregatibacter actinomycetemcomitans, Porphyromonas gingivalis, Prevotella intermedia, Capnocytophaga sputigena, Fusobacterium nucleatum and Bacteroides melaninogenicus. According to Asikainen *et al.*, several periodontal pathogens are transmitted across family members.

Neutrophils have suppressed chemotactic ability in patients with GAP. These patients show prominent periodontal inflammation along with heavy plaque accumulation. These individuals may also exhibit abnormalities in leucocyte adherence and impaired host defence mechanism.

LOCALIZED AGGRESSIVE PERIODONTITIS

This condition was previously known as localized juvenile periodontitis. It occurs in otherwise systemically healthy children and adolescents. It has a classical pattern demonstrating rapid alveolar bone loss which involves mostly permanent incisors and first molars (Fig. 25 **a,b**). It is a self-limiting condition, and it has been suggested that primary teeth exhibiting bone loss can serve as an early indicator of this condition. The estimated prevalence ranges from 0.1 to 1.5%. These patients exhibit less gingival inflammation along with less supragingival plaque accumulation. But they do have subgingival plaque deposits which are both teeth as well as tissue associated. Bone loss progresses at a rate 3-4 times greater than chronic periodontitis.

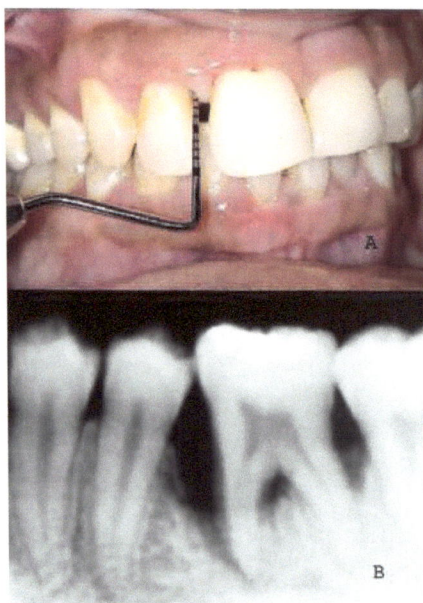

Fig. (25). Localized aggressive periodontitis; **(A)** - Loss of alveolar bone around incisors; **(B)** - Loss of alveolar bone around the first molar.

This condition does not represent a single disease entity. A wide array of defects in neutrophils have been observed among patients with LAP. As per Page and colleagues, LAP patients exhibit chemotactic abnormalities in leukocytes. Additionally, defects in phagocytosis, leukotriene B4 generation and other anomalies have been reported. Page and colleagues have suspected a hereditary basis of LAP wherein certain authors believe in an autosomal recessive mode of inheritance and others believe in X-linked dominant inheritance [3].

Treatment

In all periodontal treatment regimens, maintenance of oral hygiene is the mainstay for a successful outcome. Both chronic and aggressive periodontitis have shown that the progression of the disease correlates with the amount of plaque. The treatment regimen instituted comprises a preventive component to reduce plaque accumulation. Scaling and root planning are effective in removing subgingival deposits, causing a reduction in inflammation, and promoting healing. Cases of chronic periodontitis are managed by standard periodontal therapy, but cases of aggressive periodontitis respond lesser to conventional therapy thereby concomitant administration of antibiotics is required to improve the outcome. The patient should be kept under a rigid maintenance schedule post-treatment.

Periodontitis as a Manifestation of Systemic Diseases

Down's Syndrome

It is a congenital abnormality occurring as a result of chromosomal aberration *i.e.*, trisomy of chromosome 21. Affected individuals present with growth retardation and mental deficiency. Periodontal disease is highly prevalent in Down's syndrome patients, especially among those lesser than 30 years of age. Even though these patients have poor oral hygiene and show plaque deposits, the severity of periodontal destruction exceeds that explainable by the meagre presence of local factors. These patients show the presence of deep pockets, moderate gingivitis and substantial plaque deposition which are usually generalized but have a tendency to be more severe in the mandibular anterior region. Moderate gingival recession can also be appreciated in this region. Increased prevalence and severity of periodontitis among Down syndrome patients can be due to poor chemotactic and phagocytic abilities [17, 18].

Papillon-Lefevre Syndrome

It is an autosomal recessive condition that presents with both skin and oral manifestations. The characteristic skin lesions consist of palmar and plantar keratosis. The oral lesions are aggressive periodontitis causing severe alveolar bone destruction involving primary and permanent dentition. Due to rapid bone destruction, pathologic migration and mobility are observed which results in the loss of entire dentition at a very young age. The localized form shows vertical bone loss around the permanent incisors and first molar in systemically healthy individuals around puberty. Arc-shaped bone loss can be appreciated by extending from the distal surface of the second premototill methe sial surface of the second molar along with periodontal ligament space widening. This vertical bone loss may be more extensive on one tooth than the adjacent tooth and differs from the horizontal pattern of bone loss observed in cases of chronic periodontitis. In chronic periodontitis, several teeth are involved with the same level of severity hence the bone loss is horizontal. The treatment modality includes plaque control, removal of inflamed periodontal tissues along with administration of antibiotics. Periodontal surgical procedures must be done under antibiotic coverage along with post-operative use of chlorhexidine mouth rinse. Periodic maintenance visits are recommended due to the possibility of reinfection [18].

Chediak-Higashi Syndrome

This was described by Beguez Cesar (1943), Steinbrinck (1948), Chediak (1952) and Higashi (1954). It is an autosomal recessive condition characterized by abnormal intracellular protein transport. Ulcerations of the oral mucosa, severe gingivitis and glossitis are the commonly described oral lesions. Hamilton and Giansanti have observed that periodontal breakdown, probably related to defective leukocyte function, may also be a common oral feature.

Ehlers-Danlos Syndrome

It is comprised of more than 10 inherited disorders all involving a genetic defect in connective tissue, collagen synthesis and structure. This condition can affect the joints, skin as well as blood vessels. It is a clinically heterogeneous entity with each type exhibiting a different collagen abnormality. Barabas and Barabas have given a detailed description of the oral manifestations. In their series of cases, they observed that the oral mucosa had a normal colour but showed excessive fragility and a tendency to bruise easily. Even though the mucosa may not be able to hold sutures properly, there was only slight retardation in healing with no scar formation. They did not report any marked hyperextensibility of mucosa and patients had no difficulty wearing dentures. The gingival tissues appeared fragile and bled after toothbrushing; gingival hyperplasia and fibrous nodules were also noted. Tooth mobility was not increased.

Hypophosphatasia

It is a hereditary condition described by Rathbun transmitted as an autosomal recessive trait. Its earliest manifestation includes abnormal loosening and premature exfoliation of primary teeth, especially incisors. There are varying reports of gingivitis, but it is not a consistent feature of this condition [18].

Necrotizing Periodontal Diseases

Necrotizing Ulcerative Periodontitis

This term was adopted for the first time at the 1989 World Workshop in Clinical Periodontics. Earlier, it was termed "necrotizing ulcerative gingiva-periodontitis" in 1986. This term was used to represent recurrent NUG which progresses to chronic periodontitis with attachment as well as alveolar bone loss. The feature distinguishing NUP is the rapidly progressing disease showing marked destruction including clinical attachment as well as alveolar bone loss. They typically show the presence of deep osseous craters interdentally. In these cases, conventional deep pockets are not present due to the ulceration and necrosis of the gingiva which leads to the destruction of marginal epithelium and connective tissue and causes recession of the gingiva.

In usual cases of periodontitis, the reason for pocket formation is due to apical migration of junctional epithelium to cover the region where connective tissue is lost. This occurs because of the viable cells of the junctional epithelium. However, in cases of NUG and NUP, the junctional epithelium undergoes necrosis thereby preventing its apical migration and subsequent pocket formation. Advanced cases of NUP show the presence of severe alveolar bone loss, increased mobility and ultimately loss of a tooth. The general manifestations include fever, malaise, oral malodor, and lymphadenopathy.

This condition occurs with greater frequency in HIV-positive patients. This may occur as an extension of NUG wherein clinical attachment and alveolar bone loss is present. Necrotizing ulcerative periodontitis is characterized by rapid destruction of periodontium, soft tissue necrosis and rapid bone loss interproximally. This condition may be localized or sometimes even generalized type is observed after a severe drop in the CD4+ cell count. The bone is exposed which results in its necrosis and sequestration. Necrotizing ulcerative periodontitis is very painful at the start and hence warrants immediate treatment.

In a few cases, the necrotizing lesions may undergo spontaneous resolution which leaves deep craters interproximally which are painless and difficult to clean hence leading to conventional periodontitis. The treatment of NUP is scaling and root planning, local debridement, and irrigation with antimicrobial rinses like chlorhexidine gluconate or povidone-iodine in the office. Additionally, the home regimen includes meticulous maintenance of oral hygiene along with the use of antimicrobial rinses. Severe cases of NUP may warrant the administration of antibiotics. But it should be prescribed with caution in HIV-positive individuals to prevent serious opportunistic infections like localized candidiasis or candidal septicemia. Metronidazole is the drug of choice in patients requiring antibiotics. It is administered at a dose of 250 mg with 2 tablets administered immediately followed by consumption of 2 tablets 4 times a day for 5-7 days. Prophylactic prescription of systemic or topical antifungals is advocated in cases where antibiotic is used [3].

Abscesses of the Periodontium

Gingival Abscess

It is an acute inflammatory condition presenting as a localized, red, smooth, and fluctuant swelling which may have associated pain. It occurs as a result of microbial plaque infection, foreign body impaction or trauma (Fig. **25**).

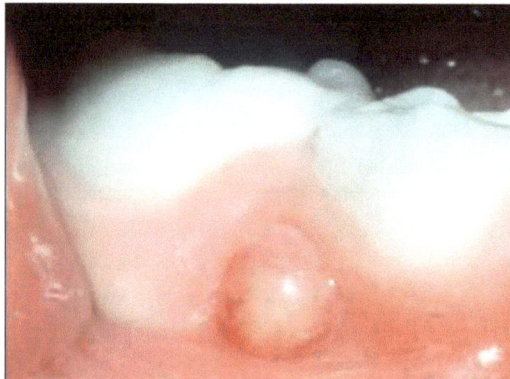

Fig. (25). Gingival abscess.

Periodontal Abscess

It is a localized purulent inflammation of the periodontal tissue. Also called *parietal abscess* or *lateral abscess*. A *gingival abscess* is confined to the gingiva without the involvement of supporting structures resulting usually from any injury to the outer surface of the gingiva. It may occur in the presence/absence of a pocket. The formation of periodontal abscess occurs as follows:

i. The infection from a pocket extends into deeper parts of the periodontium and the suppurative process is localized along the lateral portion of the root.
ii. Inflammation is extended laterally from the inner surface of the pocket into the connective tissue of the pocket wall. Impairment of drainage into pocket space results in an abscess.
iii. Formation in a pocket with tortuosity around the root. The abscess may form in a cul-de-sac whose deep portions are cut off from the surface.
iv. Incomplete removal of calculus while treating pockets. There will be shrinkage in the gingival wall which occludes the pocket orifice hence leading to abscess formation in the sealed area of the pocket.
v. Lateral wall perforation during root canal treatment or traumatic injury to tooth cause formation of periodontal abscess in the absence of periodontal disease.
    Periodontal abscesses are classified according to location as follows:
      i. Abscess in the *supporting periodontal tissue* along the lateral portion of the root. In this case, the sinus forms in the bone that extends laterally from the abscess to the external surface.
      ii. Abscess involving *soft tissue wall* of a deep pocket.

Abscess shows the presence of several bacteria including gram-negative cocci, diplococci, spirochetes, and fusiform. Invasive fungi have also been demonstrated and were interpreted as "opportunistic invaders." Mostly gram-negative anaerobic rods are primarily implicated in periodontal abscesses.

Pericoronal Abscess

It occurs as a result of inflammation of the operculum which is the soft tissue covering present over the partially erupted tooth. Mandibular third molars most frequently present with this condition. This abscess occurs as a result of food impaction, trauma, or plaque retention in that region.

In conclusion, gingival and periodontal diseases are present universally irrespective of age right from childhood to old age. There exists a common myth that periodontal conditions are only restricted to adults, but the fact is that its inception may occur right from childhood. Incomplete knowledge regarding these conditions or ignorance of signs may jeopardize the periodontal status in adulthood.

CONCLUSION

Gingival diseases concerning children are plentiful and may make headway to endanger the periodontal condition of adults as well. Pediatric dentists are responsible for the early identification and judgement of gingival and periodontal conditions to adjust the treatment modalities. Children and adolescents are subjected to a wide array of gingival and periodontal diseases. Periodontal conditions among children are not given enough focus, which may be owing to the short life span of deciduous dentition. Early diagnosis is the mainstay of successful management hence periodontal examination must be conducted as part of routine dental visits.

Additionally, severe periodontal diseases may provide an early indicator of underlying systemic conditions. Medical evaluation should be done to ascertain the systemic causes in patients exhibiting severe periodontitis, especially if it is resistant to treatment.

CONSENT FOR PUBLICATION

Not applicable.

CONFLICT OF INTEREST

The authors declare no conflict of interest, financial or otherwise.

ACKNOWLEDGEMENT

Declared none.

REFERENCES

[1]   Pradhan S, Mohanty S, Acharya S, Shukla M, Bhuyan S. Gingival Diseases in Children and Adolescents. Indian J of Forensic Medi Toxicol 2020; 14(4): 8932-7.

[2]   Ilango P, Subbareddy V, Katamreddy V, Parthasarthy H. Gingival diseases in childhood–A review. J Clin Diagn Res 2014; 8(10): ZE01-4.
[PMID: 25478471]

[3]   Califano JV, Rees TD, Cutler C, Damoulis P, Fiorellini J, Giannobile W, *et al.* Periodontal diseases of children and adolescents. Pediatr Dent 2009; 31(6): 255-62.
[PMID: 16541922]

[4]   Wyrębek B, Orzechowska A, Cudziło D, Plakwicz P. Evaluation of changes in the width of gingiva in children and youth. Review of literature. Med Wieku Rozwoj 2015; 19(2): 212-6.
[PMID: 26384125]

[5]   American Academy of Pediatric Dentistry. Classification of Periodontal Diseases in Infants, Children , Adolescents , and Individuals with Special Health Care Needs. Pediatr Dent 2019.

[6]   Murakami S, Mealey BL, Mariotti A, Chapple ILC. Dental plaque-induced gingival conditions. J Periodontol 2018; 89 (Suppl. 1): S17-27.
[http://dx.doi.org/10.1002/JPER.17-0095] [PMID: 29926958]

[7]   Omar R. Puberty Associated Gingival Enlargement: Clinical Case Report and Periodontal Management. Journal of Dental Science Research Reviews & Reports 2020; 2(1): 1-3.
[http://dx.doi.org/10.47363/JDSR/2020(2)103]

[8]   Tevatia S. Puberty Induced Gingival Enlargement. Biomed J Sci Tech Res 2017; 1(1): 103-4.
[http://dx.doi.org/10.26717/BJSTR.2017.01.000126]

[9]   Barbosa TS, Gavião MBD, Mialhe FL. Gingivitis and oral health-related quality of life: a literature review. Braz Dent Sci 2015; 18(1): 7-16.
[http://dx.doi.org/10.14295/bds.2015.v18i1.1013]

[10]   Yaacob M, Han TM, Ardini YD, *et al.* Periodontal diseases in children and adolescent with diabetes mellitus. Mater Today Proc 2019; 16: 2292-301.
[http://dx.doi.org/10.1016/j.matpr.2019.06.124]

[11]   Hasan S, Khan N, Reddy LB. Leukemic gingival enlargement: Report of a rare case with review of literature. Int J Appl Basic Med Res 2015; 5(1): 65-7.
[http://dx.doi.org/10.4103/2229-516X.149251] [PMID: 25664273]

[12]   Agrawal AA. Gingival enlargements: Differential diagnosis and review of literature. World J Clin Cases 2015; 3(9): 779-88.
[http://dx.doi.org/10.12998/wjcc.v3.i9.779] [PMID: 26380825]

[13]   Farook FF. M. Nizam MN, Alshammari A. An Update on the Mechanisms of Phenytoin Induced Gingival Overgrowth. Open Dent J 2020; 13(1): 430-5.
[http://dx.doi.org/10.2174/1874210601913010430]

[14]   Holmstrup P, Plemons J, Meyle J. Non-plaque-induced gingival diseases. J Clin Periodontol 2018; 45 (Suppl. 20): S28-43.
[http://dx.doi.org/10.1111/jcpe.12938] [PMID: 29926497]

[15]   George AK, Anil S. Acute herpetic gingivostomatitis associated with herpes simplex virus 2: report of a case. J Int Oral Health 2014; 6(3): 99-102.
[PMID: 25083042]

[16]   Hanisch M, Hoffmann T, Bohner L, *et al.* Rare Diseases with Periodontal Manifestations. Int J Environ Res Public Health 2019; 16(5): 867.
[http://dx.doi.org/10.3390/ijerph16050867] [PMID: 30857312]

[17]   Scalioni FAR, Carrada CF, Martins CC, Ribeiro RA, Paiva SM. Periodontal disease in patients with Down syndrome. J Am Dent Assoc 2018; 149(7): 628-639.e11.
[http://dx.doi.org/10.1016/j.adaj.2018.03.010] [PMID: 29779565]

[18]   Triantafyllia V, Georgios T. Periodontal Diseases in Children and Adolescents Affected by Systemic Disorders - A Literature Review. International Journal of Oral and Dental Health 2018; 4(1): 1-10.
[http://dx.doi.org/10.23937/2469-5734/1510055]

CHAPTER 11

Maintenance of Oral Hygiene in Infants & Children

Mousumi Goswami[1,*] and **Sakshi Chawla**[2]

[1] *Professor and Head, Department of Paedodontics and Preventive Dentistry, I.T.S Dental College, Hospital and Research Centre, Greater Noida, Uttar Pradesh, India*

[2] *Research Officer, Department of Paedodontics and Preventive Dentistry, I.T.S Dental College, Hospital and Research Centre, Greater Noida, Uttar Pradesh, India*

Abstract: Infant oral care is the foundation on which motivation and education for oral hygiene and various preventive dental care must be relied upon to augment the possibility of a life free of preventable dental ailments. Dental assessments and evaluations for children during their first year of life have been recommended by various organizations such as the American Academy of Paediatric Dentistry and the American Association of Paediatrics. A comprehensive infant oral health care program may include risk assessments at regular dental visits. Preventive approaches include topical fluoride application, sealants, parental education on the correct methods to clean the infant's mouth and establishing a dental home. Infant oral health is an integral part of the general well-being of an infant as they grow. It encompasses the care of the oral cavity and monitoring of the teeth' development. Unfortunately, many expecting mothers, parents and caregivers of infants often do not receive timely and accurate education about preventive oral and dental health care. This chapter discusses the importance of infant oral health care and its clinical implications. The transition required to maintain oral health as an infant progress to early childhood is highlighted. Appropriate use of topical and systemic fluoride providing timely and appropriate oral hygiene instructions is encouraged and discussed.

Keywords: Brushing technique, Dental home, Infant oral care.

INTRODUCTION

The period of infancy is defined as the first year of life of the newborn after birth. Sound oral health is not only the product of dental care of the infant, but measures taken by the mother way before the child's birth. Expectant mothers are unaware of the implications of poor oral health on their pregnancy and the unborn child.

* **Corresponding author Mousumi Goswami:** Professor and Head, Department of Paedodontics and Preventive Dentistry, I.T.S Dental College, Hospital and Research Centre, Greater Noida, Uttar Pradesh, India; E-mail: mousumi_leo@yahoo.co.in

Satyawan Damle, Ritesh Kalaskar & Dhanashree Sakhare (Eds.)

Identifying and educating mothers with poor oral health about the consequences on their health and the unborn child's health can help change the trajectory of oral care.

This chapter will highlight the measures to maintain oral health from infancy through childhood.

- Prenatal Care
- Perinatal Care
- Postnatal Care
    1. Oral care in infancy
    2. Oral care in childhood

PRENATAL AND PERINATAL CARE

The first trimester of intrauterine life marks the development of the primary dentition. Thus, strengthening the developing dentition during this phase is of utmost importance. The maternal blood transports calcium, phosphorous and other minerals required during odontogenesis to the child's body. Hence a balanced nutritious diet with adequate supplementation of vitamins and minerals for expectant mothers must be prescribed by the treating doctor and other necessary minerals. Fluoride is one such element that must be supplemented to the mother in the dosage of 0.25-1 mg daily for proper odontogenesis and bone formation.

Mother's health in the first trimester is of paramount importance for sound primary dentition. An important risk factor for early involvement of primary dentition leading to advanced childhood caries is the usage of substances such as alcohol, tobacco and other addictive drugs becoming increasing popular in adulthood, also seen amongst expectant mothers [1]. A cohort study of 5.4 million participants noted that maternal substance usage before or during pregnancy doubles the risk of early childhood caries compared to no substance use [2]. To the pregnant mother, prescribing medications such as tetracycline and anti-epileptic drugs should be avoided. It has been shown to cause discoloration and developmental defects of the primary teeth.

The perinatal period starts around the 20th to 28th week of gestation and completes one to four weeks after birth. An inability to sustain and initiate enough respiration just after delivery is known as perinatal asphyxia. This impairment of gaseous exchange after delivery impacts the development of primary teeth. Many environmental factors such as substance use during pregnancy, infant birth weight and height, gestational age, nutritional status of the child, and infant feeding method have been significant determinants for the eruption and development of primary teeth [3, 4]. Delay in tooth emergence is seen in infants with low birth weight and conditions like hypothyroidism.

In contrast, accelerated tooth eruption has been reported with childhood obesity, diabetes mellitus and maternal smoking [5]. Acquisition of micro-organisms primarily from mother to infant can occur *via* maternal saliva. Transfer of maternal antibodies to infants can also affect the colonization of *S. mutans* in the infant's mouth. This crucial time is essential for the oral and overall health of the newborn child.

Health care professionals such as physicians, paediatricians and nurses are more likely to interact and see expectant mothers during this phase. They can guide them to seek dental care whenever necessary (Fig. **1**). Therefore, these providers should be educated about the most commonly occurring dental anomalies and associated risk factors to make appropriate timely referrals.

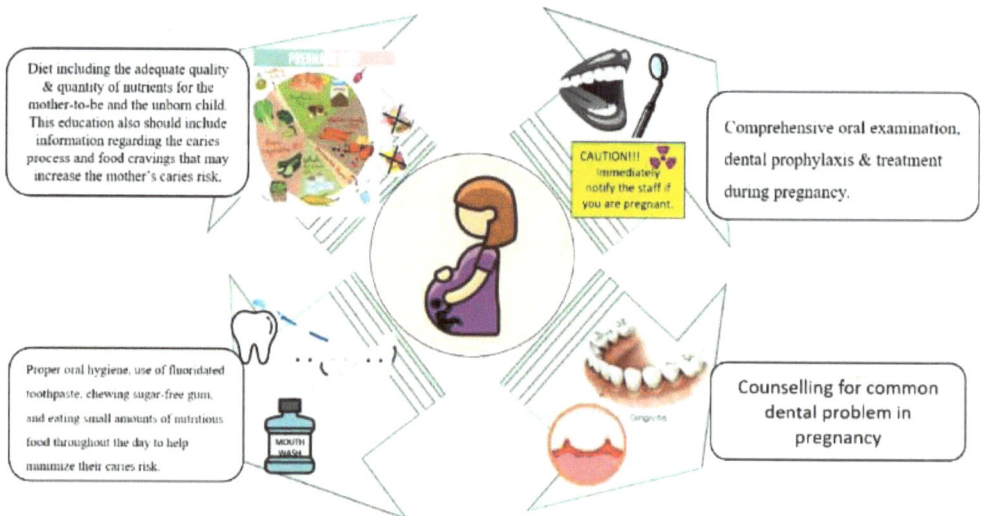

Fig. (1). Oral care during pregnancy.

POSTNATAL CARE

Infant Oral Health Care

The edentulous alveolar arches of the newborn after birth are known as gum pads. It is advisable to use clean wet cloth/gauze wrapped around the index finger for cleaning the gum pads after every feed. Wiping the gum pads also massages it, which soothes the child during teething (Fig. **2**). At six months of age, the first primary teeth erupt in the oral cavity, and the primary dentition completes by 33 months.

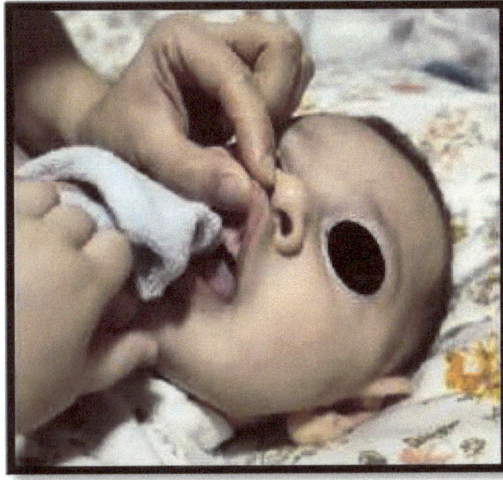

Fig. (2). Gum pad cleaning.

The primary teeth are more prone to dental decay than their permanent counterparts due to poor hygiene habits, increased sugar consumption, poor crystallinity, and lesser enamel thickness.

Mutans Streptococci act as the principal bacteria for the initiation of dental caries. Early colonization and growth of S. mutans due to high sucrose diet, prolonged breastfeeding, and nursing, putting the infant to bed at night or at nap time with a bottle increases the probability of early involvement of primary teeth. Therefore, measures such as oral hygiene methods modification of diet to a non-cariogenic habit should be established early in infancy. Dietary Guidelines Advisory Committee (2020) suggests no added sugar to be given to any child until two years [6].

This primary prevention level can be taught with the health promotion model and specific protection by individualized and community approach. The American Academy of Paediatric Dentistry (AAPD) has given the following recommendations on infant oral health care [7]:

Oral Health Risk Assessment

Evaluates patient's risk of developing oral diseases, including caries risk assessment. Caries risk assessment is performed by evaluating diet, feeding and oral hygiene practices.

Establish a Dental Home

The dental home is a comprehensive concept of delivering oral health care right from birth with the interaction of the patient, parents, dentists, dental professionals, and non-dental professionals. AAPD supports the policy of establishment of a dental home for all infants, children, adolescents, and persons with special health care needs. The policy states that a dental home should be established as early as six months of age or soon after the first tooth erupts and no later than 12 months of age. It should provide a place for children to be treated in case of emergency, where parents can feel comfortable and not worry about managing their child's oral emergencies (Fig. **3**).

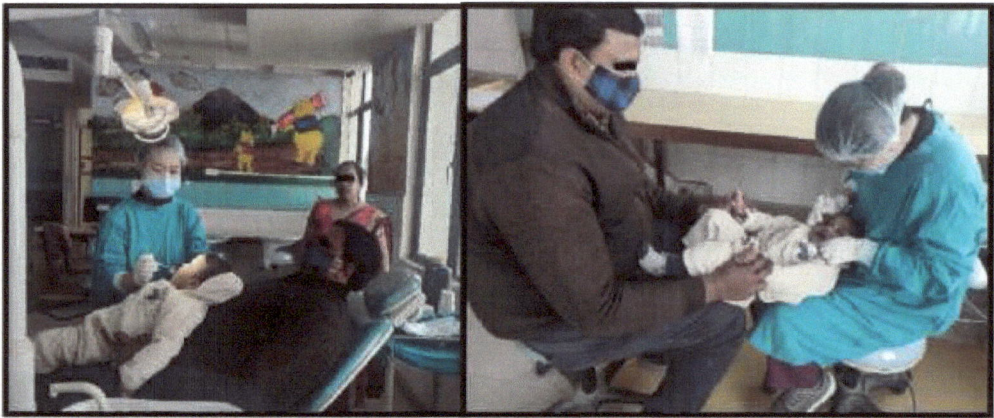

Fig. (3). Examination of infant (with parent and lap to lap examination).

The establishment of the dental home is initiated by the identification and interaction of these individuals, resulting in a heightened awareness of all issues impacting the patient's oral health.

- Comprehensive, continuous, accessible, family centred, coordinated, compassionate, and culturally appropriate care for children, as modelled by the American Academy of Pediatrics (AAP).
- Comprehensive, evidence-based dental care, including emergent, acute care and preventive services in accordance with AAPD periodicity schedules.
- Comprehensive assessment for oral diseases and conditions.
- Individualized preventive oral health program based on caries and periodontal disease risk assessment.
- Anticipatory guidance for growth and development.
- Therapeutic management of acute/chronic oral pain and infection.
- Management and adequate long term follow up for acute dental trauma.

- Information for proper care of the child's teeth, gingivae, and other oral structures. This would include the prevention, diagnosis, and treatment of diseases of the supporting and surrounding tissues and, therefore, aiding in the maintenance of health, function and aesthetics of these structures and tissues.
- Dietary counselling.
- Referrals to dental specialists when care cannot directly be provided within the dental home.
- Adequate education regarding future referral to a dentist knowledgeable in adult oral health issues for continuing dental care.

Teething

Teething is the process by which teeth erupt from the overlying gums. Teething is a physiological process that can be very discomforting for some children. It can be associated with red and swollen gums, anxiety, and grumbling, change in nutritional habits, decreased appetite, difficulty in sleeping. Commonly localized areas of irritability and excessive salivation are also seen. Often parents' resort to over the counter (OTC) soothing gels, teething rings, and homoeopathic alternatives. Food and Drug Administration (FDA) warns against using any topical medication to treat pain during teething in children, including prescription or OTC creams and gels or homoeopathic teething tablets [8].

At times, newborns are present with a tooth-like structure in the oral cavity or can experience such a finding in the first 30 days of infancy. These newly erupted teeth are referred to as natal and neonatal teeth, respectively (Table **1**).

Table 1. Type of teeth present in a newborn.

Natal Teeth	Neonatal Teeth	Precociously Erupted Teeth
Teeth present at the time of birth (Fig. 4)	Teeth erupting within the first 30 days of life.	Primary teeth erupting prematurely are known as congenital teeth/ foetal teeth / Dentition Precox.

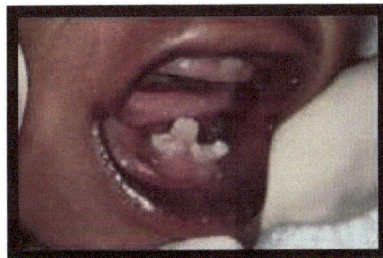

Fig. (4). One day old with natal teeth.

Children with special health care need also use rings/teething jewellery for sensory stimulation. AAP recommends and FDA supports rubbing infants' gums with a clean finger or providing a teething ring (Fig. **5**) made of firm rubber to chew on.

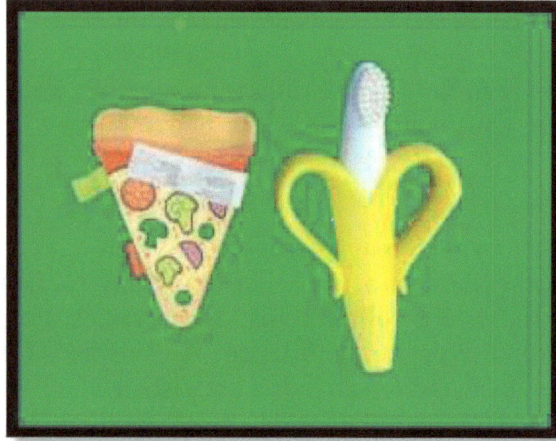

Fig. (5). Teething rings.

Classification [9]

A. Based on the degree of maturation, Spouge and Feasibly classified natal and neonatal teeth as:
   1. A mature natal or neonatal tooth is or fully developed.
   2. Immature natal or neonatal tooth with incomplete or substandard structure.
B. Based on the appearance, natal teeth can be classified into the following categories:
   ○ Category 1: A shell-like crown structure not rigidly attached to the alveolus by a rim of the oral mucosa, without any root.
   ○ Category 2: A solid crown poorly attached to the alveolus by gingivae with little or no root structure.
   ○ Category 3: The incisal edge of the crown recently erupted through the gums.
   ○ Category 4: A palpable unerupted tooth with mucosal swelling.

Riga-Fede Disease

- Antonio Riga first described Riga-Fede disease in 1881.
- Neonate and infants frequently presenting with natal and neonatal teeth often show chronic traumatic ulceration on the ventral surface of the tongue.
- *The site involved:* Tongue, lips, and buccal mucosa.
- *Lesion presentation:* Erythema surrounding a centrally removable, yellow, fibrinopurulent membrane. Adjacent to ulceration, a white hyperkeratotic border

is observed (Fig. **6A and B**). Lesions filled with granulation tissue have a raised exophytic appearance clinically like pyogenic granuloma.

• *Treatment:* Constant trauma and ulceration can hamper the infant's nutrition. Application of cellulose film or other protective dental

appliance, smoothening the incisal edges, adding a small increment of restorative material, oral disinfectant, corticosteroids, teething ring, extraction of the offending tooth may be considered [10].

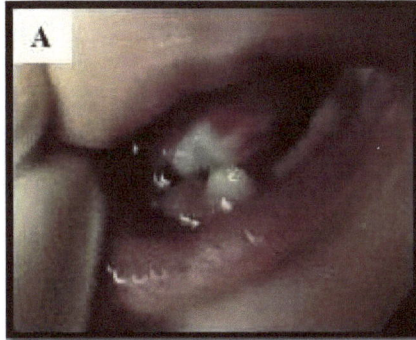

Fig. (6). (A): Ulceration of the tongue associated with natal teeth.

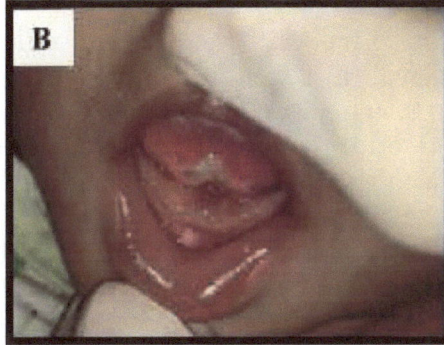

6(B) Improvements in the ulceration after removal of natal teeth followed up after three days.

Oral Hygiene

Most of the children are unable to clean their teeth effectively until 5-8 years of age. Total responsibility to perform and supervise brushing is the duty of a parent or caregiver in case of an infant, toddler, or young child. Infants' oral cavity should be cleaned once daily at least, and it is recommended to wipe the gum pads after every feed.

Diet Modification

Oral bacteria require a proper environment to cause dental caries. It is recommended to discontinue the nocturnal feeding practice after the first primary tooth eruption. When bottle-feeding is substituted with breastfeeding, it should simulate the natural nipple and breast with a broader base. The bottle should be withdrawn immediately after feeding, and the gum pads, as well as the teeth, should be cleaned.

Diet management also includes educating parents regarding the following facts:

a. Infants and children may need to eat more frequently than adults.
b. Between meals, snacks should consist of foods that have the least potential for promoting acid production. Snacks and retentive food high in sugar should be avoided.
c. Cookies, candies, cakes, and other potentially harmful foods should be offered at mealtimes than between meals.
d. The total amount of sugar consumed is not the key, it is the frequency of sugar intake, and the food's retentiveness is essential.

Fluoride

Fluoride has been proven to reduce the prevalence of dental caries and may be considered for children with a higher risk of caries. Infants living in fluoride deficient areas (less than 0.6 ppm F) should be supplemented with fluoride in their diet. Sources of dietary fluoride may include drinking water from home, day-care, and school; beverages such as soda, juice and infant formula, prepared food and even some toothpaste. The high risk of fluorosis has raised concerns regarding the concentrated infant formulas. Large consumption of such liquid in infancy and low body weight makes the child particularly susceptible to fluorosis. An evidence-based review highlights the increased risk of mild fluorosis with consumption of reconstituted infant formula but has recommended the continued use of fluoridated water [11].

Injury Prevention

Promoting safety and preventing injuries is a continuing task for parents during the first year of their child's life. Mindful awareness of developmental skills acquired by the infant, active supervision and intervention is required to ensure the safety of the developing child. Parents commonly underestimate their infant's motor skills while overestimating their infant's cognitive skills and judgment. Counselling in the primary care setting is essential to help parents understand the correct timing of the development. Education towards intentional and unintentional trauma (injuries like falls, fires and burns, poisoning, choking, animal bites, and drowning) must be done included in the visit. Each of these tragedies is preventable. Appropriate counselling can provide parents with the knowledge and strategies for reducing the likelihood of these injuries. The importance of establishing good habits begin in infancy, and parental counselling about the positive value of their behaviour as a role model for their child.

Advantage of Infant Oral Health

a. Intercept and modify detrimental feeding habits.
b. Assist parents in establishing snacking and dietary patterns favourable for dental health.
c. Educate parents regarding their role in cleaning teeth for their infants/toddlers.
d. Determine the fluoride status and recommend an optimum fluoridation program.
e. Introduce the child to dentistry in a pleasant, non-threatening manner.
f. Promote a positive image of dentist/dentistry.

8. Non-nutritive habits: The physiologic need of the infant thrives them towards non–nutritive sucking. This innate biological drive of sucking can be satisfied by nutritive breastfeeding and bottle-feeding options. Non-nutritive sucking objects such as digits, pacifiers, or toys, if prolonged, can lead to consequences in the development of orofacial structure and normal occlusion.

Furthermore, mothers should be educated about the importance of breastfeeding infants before 12 months of age to ensure the best possible health, developmental and psychosocial outcomes for infants. All primary health care professionals who serve mothers and infants should provide parent/caregiver education on the aetiology and prevention of early childhood caries. The infectious and transmissible nature of bacteria that cause early childhood caries and methods of oral health risk assessment, anticipatory guidance, and early intervention should be included in the curriculum of all medical, nursing, and allied health professional programs.

The Transition of Oral Hygiene Practice

Oral hygiene measure includes mechanical and chemical aids to maintain sound oral health. Mechanical aids include toothbrushes, floss, interdental cleaners, while chemotherapeutic agents such as mouth rinses and dentifrices are commercially available. The overall oral hygiene technique and aids adopted depends upon the child's manual dexterity, awareness, and oral condition. Gum pad cleaning is the first step towards the behavioural modification of the parents/caregivers. It continues in early childhood (6 months- 6 years.), where the parents assist or themselves brush their children's teeth due to their lack of motor control at a young age. Nevertheless, establishing good hygiene habits is valuable for present and future oral health (Table **2**).

Variety of toothbrushes present in the markets ranging from finger brushes, small head toothbrushes for toddlers and modifications such as adding new acrylic to the handle for moulding to the patient's handgrip can aid self-care for disabled patients (Fig. **7**). Electric toothbrushes are valuable as the automatic oscillating and rotating stroke motions require less effort for the individual or carer.

Table 2. Oral hygiene practices in children.

Gum Pad Cleaning	Fone's Method	Flossing
A wet clean cloth/gauze is wrapped around the index finger, and gum pads are massaged gently. Mothers are advised to clean both the gum pads after every feed and initiate toothbrushing with the eruption of first teeth.	Circular strokes are performed set of teeth where the brush is placed. The occlusal surface is cleaned by brushing in a back-and-forth motion. 	Eighteen inches (approximately) of floss is wrapped around the middle finger of the right hand, and the rest is secure to the middle finger of the left hand. The floss is passed over the tips of the thumbs and passed gently between each pair of teeth in a gentle swaying motion; it is then curved around the proximal surface of the tooth and rubbed up and down.

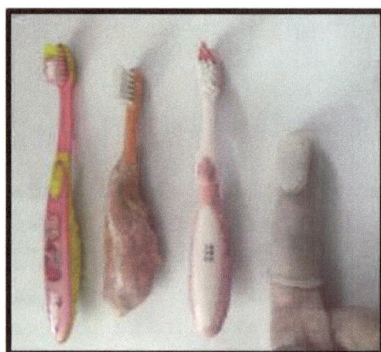

Fig. (7). Types of toothbrushes.

The toothbrushing technique also changes with the ever-changing toothbrush design as per the child's growth. The predominant methods are the Fones method, the Charters method, the horizontal scrubbing method, and the modified Stillman method. Also, an age-wise amount of toothpaste is recommended in the pediatric age group to prevent inadvertent ingestion (Fig. **8**).

1. Fones Method: Brush is placed in the centre of the maxillary and mandibular front teeth approximating each other and is moved in a circular direction on each set of teeth. The bristle covers the tooth and some parts of the gingiva—the gentle pressure massages the gingival tissue and mechanical cleansing of the teeth. The same motion is repeated for the buccal teeth, and the occlusal table is scrubbed in a back-and-forth motion.

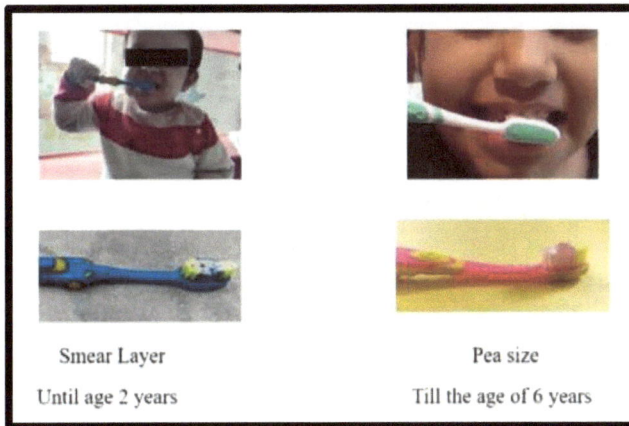

Smear Layer
Until age 2 years

Pea size
Till the age of 6 years

Fig. (8). Age-wise recommended toothpaste amount.

2. Charter's Method: The ends of the bristles are placed in contact with the enamel of the teeth and the gingiva, with the bristles pointed at about a 45° angle towards the plane of occlusion. Lateral and downward pressure is then placed on the brush, and the brush is vibrated gently back and forth a millimetre or so.

3. Horizontal Scrubbing Method: The brush is placed horizontally on buccal and lingual surfaces and moved back and forth with a scrubbing motion (Fig. **9**). Most commonly employed technique by young children newly adopting toothbrushing as a habit.

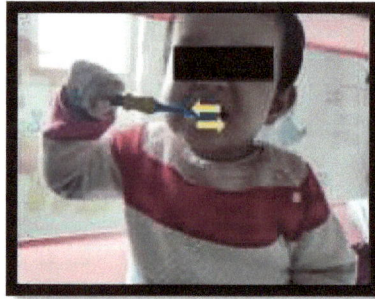

Fig. (9). Horizontal (scrub) technique brushing.

4. Modified Stillman Method: The modified Stillman method combines a vibratory action of the bristles with a stroke movement of the brush. Bristles are positioned partially on the cervical region of the teeth, partly on the gingiva and point apically.

Plaque Disclosing Agent

Disclosing agents can be used as an educational and motivational tool to improve the efficiency of plaque control procedures. These solutions stain bacterial deposits on the teeth, tongue, and gingiva (Fig. **10**). Solutions can be applied to teeth as concentrates on cotton swabs or diluted as rinses, and the wafer can be crushed between teeth and swished in the oral cavity for a few seconds and then spit out.

Mouth Rinse

Chlorhexidine 0.2% or Sodium fluoride (NaF) 0.05% for daily home care. AAPD policymakers advise home use prescription-strength 0.09% fluoride mouth rinse, and 0.5% fluoride gel/paste for its anti-caries effect. The activity should be supervised to avoid swallowing mouth rinse, especially in children with special health care needs and is not recommended for children under six years of age. In 1980, FDA approved neutral NaF rinses in concentrations of 0.05% or less for over-the-counter sales. Indian Dental Association further suggests vigorously swishing 10 ml of mouthwash between the teeth for 1 minute and then spit out for children older than six years (Table **3**).

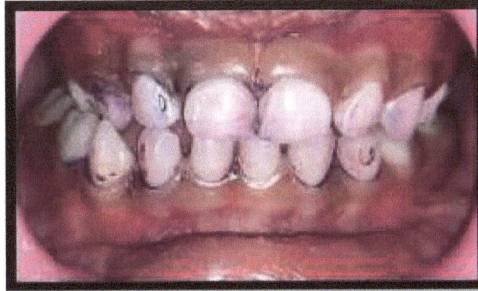

Fig. (10). Disclosing agent for oral hygiene education (Dye staining plaque retentive areas).

Table 3. Further Important Readings.

European Academy of Paediatric Dentistry (EAPD)	Guidelines on Prevention of Early Childhood Caries Guidelines on the use of fluoride in children
American Academy of Pediatric Dentistry (AAPD)	• Guideline on Caries-risk Assessment and Management for Infants, Children, and Adolescents • Guideline on Infant Oral Health Care • Guideline on Periodicity of Examination, Preventive Dental Services, Anticipatory Guidance/Counselling, and Oral Treatment for Infants, Children, and Adolescents
Nova Scotia Dental Association	Knee-To-Knee Training Video

CONCLUSION

Suggestive Infant Oral Program Checklist (By author) *
Patient History:
□ H/o preterm/normal/delayed delivery
□ H/o medical illness
□ H/o Ongoing medication
□ Nursing habits
□ Feeding Practice (use of bottles of milk or other sweet liquid while asleep, between meals food and drink exposure)
□ H/o Fluoride (water/supplements/topical)
□ Non-nutritive sucking habits (thumb/soother)
□ H/o Trauma/Cleft
Intra-oral Examination:
□ Knee-to-knee position
□ Examine dry teeth (wipe with gauze and use prop if required)
□ Evaluate White spots, caries, developmental anomalies, and trauma
□ Examine Soft tissue
Counselling:
□ Gum pad cleaning
□ Tooth brushing demonstration
□ Teething symptoms
□ Weaning

□ Weaning
□ Diet/Feeding/Nursing Modification
Preventive approach:
□ Oral prophylaxis
□ Topical fluoride application: 5% NaF fluoride varnish on the erupted/erupting teeth.
Treatment for an infant or a young child for severe early childhood caries (SECC) as soon as it is diagnosed:
□ White spot lesions (SECC) →Educate about oral health and diet, Apply Professional fluoride (varnish). Advise home use of a smear of fluoridated toothpaste twice daily.
□ Cavitated lesions in Maxillary Anterior→Interim therapeutic restoration (ITR) with glass ionomer as a preventive and therapeutic approach.
□ Large cavitated lesions: Advise full coverage restorations.
□ Extensive symptomatic disease: Definitive care by a specialist (Pulpal treatment/ Full coverage Crowns).
Recall
□ Periodic recall based on the assessment.
Source: *This suggestive checklist has been compiled by the author from policies and recommendations given by AAPD [7, 11].

Healthy primary teeth perform an incredibly essential role in the child's life as they help in eating, esthetics, phonetics, and maintaining space for permanent dentition. Unavailability of or inadequate dental care for children can negatively affect their physical and emotional health. These limitations negatively affect the children's growth and development, immune system, and overall health. Therefore, it is the responsibility of the pediatric dental surgeon and the parents to make sure the children receive adequate dental care and learn how to care for their teeth themselves. Infant oral health care can be understood as the foundation on which a lifetime of preventive education and dental care can be built up to enhance the opportunity of a lifetime of freedom from preventable oral diseases.

CONSENT FOR PUBLICATION

Not applicable.

CONFLICT OF INTEREST

The authors declare no conflict of interest, financial or otherwise.

ACKNOWLEDGEMENTS

To all the patients and their parents who cooperated and permitted their photographs

REFERENCES

[1]   Wu H, Chen T, Ma Q, Xu X, Xie K, Chen Y. Associations of maternal, perinatal and postnatal factors with the eruption timing of the first primary tooth. Sci Rep 2019; 9(1): 2645.
[http://dx.doi.org/10.1038/s41598-019-39572-w] [PMID: 30804498]

[2]   Auger N, Low N, Lee G, Ayoub A, Nicolau B. Prenatal substance use disorders and dental caries in children. J Dent Res 2020; 99(4): 395-401.
[http://dx.doi.org/10.1177/0022034520906820] [PMID: 32091957]

[3]   Żądzińska E, Sitek A, Rosset I. Relationship between pre-natal factors, the perinatal environment, motor development in the first year of life and the timing of first deciduous tooth emergence. Ann Hum Biol 2016; 43(1): 25-33.
[http://dx.doi.org/10.3109/03014460.2015.1006140] [PMID: 26065694]

[4]   Delgado H, Habicht JP, Yarbrough C, *et al.* Nutritional status and the timing of deciduous tooth eruption. Am J Clin Nutr 1975; 28(3): 216-24.
[http://dx.doi.org/10.1093/ajcn/28.3.216] [PMID: 804244]

[5]   Wu H, Chen T, Ma Q, Xu X, Xie K, Chen Y. Associations of maternal, perinatal and postnatal factors with the eruption timing of the first primary tooth. Sci Rep 2019; 9(1): 2645.
[http://dx.doi.org/10.1038/s41598-019-39572-w] [PMID: 30804498]

[6]   Dietary Guidelines Advisory Committee. Scientific report of the 2020 dietary Guidelines Advisory Committee: advisory report to the Secretary of Agriculture and the Secretary of Health and Human Services. Washington, DC: United States Department of Agriculture, Agricultural Research Service 2020.

[7]   American Academy of Pediatric Dentistry. Perinatal and infant oral health care The Reference Manual of Pediatric Dentistry. Chicago: American Academy of Pediatric Dentistry 2020; pp. 252-6.

[8]   [8] Food and Drug Administration (FDA) warns against using any sort of topical medication to treat pain during teething in children, including prescription or OTC creams and gels, or homeopathic teething tablets. 2018. Available https://www.fda.gov/news-events/press-announcements/fda-ta-es-action-against-use-otc-benzocaine-teething-products-due-serious-safety-risk-lack-benefit

[9]   Mhaske S, Yuwanati MB, Mhaske A, Ragavendra R, Kamath K, Saawarn S. Natal and neonatal teeth: an overview of the literature. International Scholarly Research Notices 2013.
[http://dx.doi.org/10.1155/2013/956269]

[10]   Kumari A, Singh PK. Diagnosis of Riga–Fede disease. Indian J Pediatr 2019; 86(2): 191.
[http://dx.doi.org/10.1007/s12098-018-2776-z] [PMID: 30191496]

[11]   American Academy of Pediatric Dentistry. Fluoride therapy The Reference Manual of Pediatric Dentistry. Chicago, Ill.: America Academy of Pediatric Dentistry 2020; pp. 288-91.

CHAPTER 12

Dental Materials Used in Pediatric Dentistry

Vidya Iyer[1,*] and **M. Vijay**[2]

[1] *Pedodontics and Preventive Dentistry, CSI Dental College and Research Centre, Madurai, Tamil Nadu, India*

[2] *Madura Dental Clinic, Madurai, Tamil Nadu 625001, India*

Abstract: The chapter describes various dental materials commonly used in Pediatric dental practice. Making an informed choice of the restorative material to be used in different clinical conditions is essential to ensure a successful and satisfactory restorative outcome. Knowledge of dental materials with their unique set of advantages and applications is an important determinant in the formulation of a treatment plan. Dental materials used for pulp therapies and full coverage restorations in primary teeth are exhaustive in their scope and as such, have been dealt with in depth in separate chapters.

Keywords: Alginate, Biodentin, Calcium hydroxide, Composite resins, Dental Materials, Elastomeric Impression Materials, Glass ionomer cement, Metapex, Mineral Trioxide Aggregate, Silver Amalgam, Zinc oxide eugenol.

INTRODUCTION

Dental caries is undoubtedly one of the most common chronic diseases of childhood. Its prevalence is higher than asthma and hay fever. Despite the innumerable advances in the field of preventive dentistry, restoration of teeth continues to be the mainstay of pediatric dental practice. Having said that, the clinical aspect of Pediatric dentistry has progressed in leaps and bounds in terms of the choices in restorative materials that are available today. Historically, pediatric dentists relied upon silver amalgam and stainless-steel crowns for restoring decayed posterior teeth; whereas, decayed anterior teeth were restored with silicate cement, acrylic, or other esthetically less-acceptable restorations.

The management of dental caries was originally based on the belief that caries is a progressive infectious disease that eventually leads to loss of teeth in the absence of a surgical/restorative intervention. However, it has now been established that

[*] **Corresponding author Vidya Iyer:** Pedodontics and Preventive Dentistry, CSI Dental College and Research Centre, Madurai, Tamil Nadu, India; E-mail: vidyaiyer04@gmail.com

dental caries is reversible in the initial stages of tooth demineralization shifting the focus on early intervention and prevention of decay. However, in case of cavitated lesions, restoring the form, function and esthetics of teeth using a biocompatible dental material is the standard practice.

SILVER AMALGAM

For decades, silver amalgam has been the gold standard for restorations in dentistry and has been the restorative material of choice for posterior teeth. The simplicity of its use, cost effectiveness and excellent mechanical properties has made silver amalgam one of the most dependable restorative materials. Its use in primary posterior teeth has resulted in successful long-term outcome. Amalgam contains a mixture of metals such as silver, copper and tin mixed with mercury. Silver amalgam restorations are generally recommended for Class I & II restorations in primary and permanent molar teeth and premolars [1]. In case of class II restorations in primary teeth, amalgam is suitable for preparations that do not extend beyond the line angles of teeth [2].

Composition

(Traditional low copper containing alloys)

Silver – 65 wt.%

Tin – 29 wt.%

Copper – 6 wt.% or less

High copper containing alloys (with copper content between 6 to 30 wt.%) possess superior physical properties as compared to the low copper alloys.

Classification

Silver Amalgam can be classified in various ways as shown in Table **1**.

Table 1. Classification of silver amalgam.

Based on alloy particle size and shape
Lathe cut alloys (irregularly shaped)
Spherical alloys (produced by atomizing the liquid alloy)
Admixed alloys (containing a mixture of lathe cut and spherical alloy particles)
Based on copper/zinc content in the alloy
Low copper alloys

(Table 1) cont.....

High copper alloys
Zinc containing alloys (Zinc content more 0.01%)
Zinc free alloys (alloys containing 0.01% or less zinc)
Based on addition of noble metals
1st generation – 3 parts silver + 1 part tin (original peritectic alloy)
2nd generation – original alloy + copper upto 4% + zinc upto 1%
3rd generation – Silver – copper eutectic alloy
4th generation – Alloy containing copper + silver + tin upto 29%
5th generation - Alloy containing silver, copper, tin + Indium
6th generation – Palladium + silver + copper eutectic alloy

Manipulation

Silver alloy powder and mercury are dispensed in a ratio of 1:1 (Eames technique). This minimal mercury technique is a good way of reducing mercury content, whereby 50% or less mercury will be present in the final restoration. For high copper alloys, a mercury-alloy proportion of 1:1 is recommended; whereas for low copper alloys, a 40:60 mercury-alloy ratio is advised. The process of mixing the silver alloy powder with mercury is termed as trituration and can be achieved by the following means:

a. Hand trituration –The specified quantity of silver alloy powder and mercury is dispensed in a glass/ceramic mortar and triturated into a homogenous mix with the help of a glass/ceramic pestle. After trituration, the excess mercury is squeezed out of the mix using a squeezing cloth. Following this the mix is mulled and condensed into the prepared cavity. As silver amalgam relies on mechanical retention, the GV Black's principles of cavity preparation should be strictly adhered to for clinical success of amalgam restoration (Fig. **1**).

b. Mechanical trituration – Pre-proportioned capsules containing alloy powder, mercury and a cylindrical metal or plastic piston is placed on a triturator/amalgamator and oscillated at the designated speed in order to obtain a more standardized mix as compared to the hand trituration method (Fig. **2**).

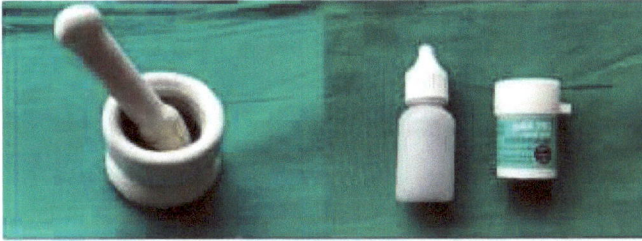

Fig. (1). Silver alloy powder and mercury along with mortar and pestle used for hand trituration.

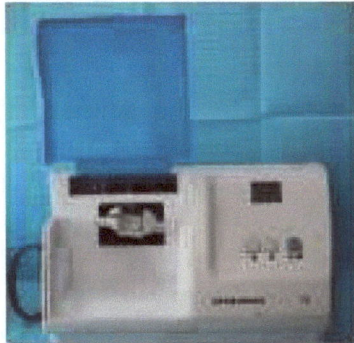

Fig. (2). Amalgamator used for mechanical trituration.

Restoration

The mixed amalgam is condensed in the prepared cavity in increments using an amalgam carrier. With the help of condensers, the amalgam is condensed beginning from the center of the cavity and progressing towards the walls in a stepping motion. The amalgam mix in smaller increments can also be mechanically condensed into the cavity using an automated device. With each increment being condensed, a mercury-rich amalgam layer is brought to the top of the increment being condensed so that successive increments bond together. The triturated amalgam should be condensed into the cavity within 4 minutes of mixing.

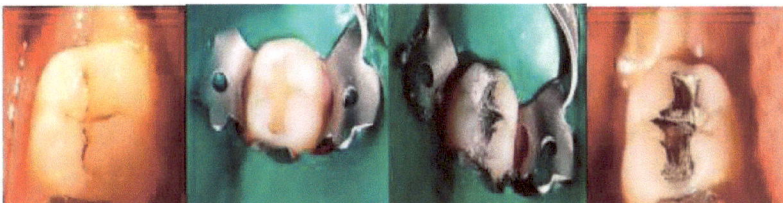

Fig. (3). a - Pit and fissure carious lesion in tooth 37; **b** - Class I cavity preparation; **c,d** - Finished and polished Class I amalgam restoration in 37.

Condensation of amalgam is followed by carving of the restoration to reproduce the tooth anatomy. The carved & finished restoration is burnished with the help of a ball burnisher. Burnishing is considered as a continuation of condensation and is carried out from the restoration towards the tooth surface. Burnishing is not recommended for fast setting high copper alloys. Some researchers also suggest that burnishing should not be done as it increases the mercury concentration on the surface margins of the restoration. Following condensation, occlusal adjustments are made as necessary, and the occlusion is re-checked using an articulating paper. The final finishing of restoration is carried out with the help of a rubber cup and polishing paste after at least 24 hours of restoration placement (Figs. **3a-d**).

Amalgam restorations are subject to tarnish and corrosion in the oral environment. Tarnish is surface discoloration or loss of brightness of metal due to the formation of a chemical film – usually sulfides or oxides. Tarnish is generally the forerunner of corrosion. Corrosion is the disintegration of metal caused by the action of moisture, acidic or alkaline solutions and other chemicals. Corrosion occurs at the interface between the tooth and restoration. A gradual build-up of the corrosion products (oxides and chlorides of tin) seals this interface, making amalgam a self-sealing restoration Fig. (**4**). The advantages and disadvantages of silver amalgam restoration are discussed in Table **2**.

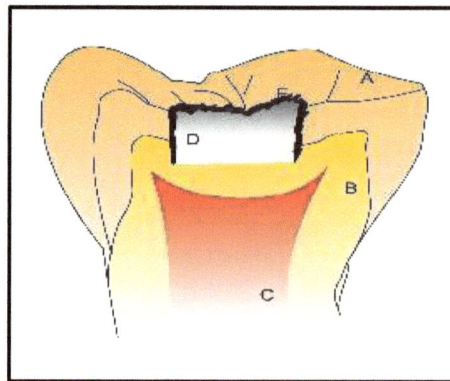

Fig. (4). Diagrammatic representation of Corrosion seen in Amalgam restoration. A-Enamel, B-Dentin, C-Pulp, D-Amalgam restoration, E-Corrosion products at restoration- tooth interface.

Table 2. Advantages and disadvantages of silver amalgam restoration.

Advantages	Disadvantages
✓ Ease of use - manipulation and placement	✖ Unesthetic appearance of the restoration
✓ Relatively cost effective	✖ Tarnish and corrosion leading to discoloration of tooth structure
✓ Excellent wear resistance	✖ Water – reaction medium
✓ Marginal leakage reduces after period due to deposition of corrosion products	✖ Initial marginal leakage leading to post-operative sensitivity
✓ Maintains anatomical form and function of the tooth	✖ Lack of chemical adhesion to the tooth structure
✓ Well condensed and triturated amalgam has good compressive strength	✖ Mercury toxicity
✓ Placement of amalgam restoration is relatively not technique sensitive	-

Mercury Toxicity

Concerns regarding mercury toxicity among dental professionals is one of the reasons for gradual decline in the use of silver amalgam. Another reason is the lack of esthetics thereby restricting its use to the posterior teeth. With the introduction of newer restorative materials having satisfactory physical properties as well as excellent esthetics, the use of silver amalgam has reduced.

Coombs' type IV hypersentivity or contact dermatitis has been reported in response to silver amalgam restorations. Dental surgeons, assistants, and other auxiliary personnel in the operatory are at a risk of mercury toxicity. Mercury can be absorbed through skin or inhaled as mercury vapors by the dental professionals. The maximum level of occupational exposure considered safe is 50 microgram of mercury per cubic meter of air. Long term exposure to mercury vapor can pose significant health risks [3]. Some of the methods to minimize mercury exposure and toxicity include:

1. Having a well-ventilated operatory
2. Freshly mixed amalgam contains free mercury and care should be taken to avoid skin contact or handling the mix with bare hands. If mercury comes in contact with skin, then the area of contact should be washed with soap and water.

3. All excess mercury, including waste, disposable capsules, and amalgam removed during carving should be collected and stored in a well-sealed container.
4. Mercury waste disposal should be according to the norms of bio-hazardous waste disposal to prevent environmental pollution.
5. Amalgam scrap, materials and instruments contaminated with mercury or amalgam should not be incinerated or subject to heat sterilization.
6. Spillage of mercury should be avoided. Should spillage occur, it should be cleaned as soon as possible.
7. Periodic monitoring of exposure levels in the operatory should be undertaken. Film badges, like the radiation exposure badges can be used by dental office personnel.

The Minamata Convention on Mercury

In October 2013, a new international binding treaty instrument called the Minamata Convention on Mercury opened for signature in Minamata City, Japan, the site of arguably the worst public health and environmental disaster involving mercury contamination. It is a global treaty to protect human and environmental health from adverse effects of mercury and its compounds. The treaty has proposed a worldwide reduction and ultimate elimination in the production and use of mercury containing products. The Convention called for a phasing down of dental amalgam use through greater emphasis on dental caries prevention, research into new dental materials, and best management practices. On 18th June 2018, India submitted its instrument of ratification, thereby becoming the 93rd country to ratify the Minamata convention proposal. As of January 2020, a total of 128 governments have pledged their support for curtailing the harmful effects of mercury on the environment by signing this treaty out of which 116 governments have ratified it [4].

Glass Ionomer Cement (GIC)

Glass ionomer cement (GIC) was first introduced in 1971 by McLean, Wilson, and Kent. GIC, also known as 'Polyalkenoate Cement,' is a salt formed by the reaction between calcium-alumino-fluorosilicate glass powder and an aqueous solution of polyacrylic acid. From being first introduced as a restorative material, GIC has a wide range of applications in today's dental practice [5].

Composition: GIC is either dispensed as powder and liquid or in capsule form to be used with a mechanical device like an amalgamator (Fig. **5a, b**). The composition of powder and liquid components of GIC are listed in Table **3**.

Table 3. Composition of glass ionomer cement.

Powder	Liquid
Silicon dioxide – 35-40%	Polyacrylic acid (copolymer with iticonic acid, maleic acid and tricarballylic acid –reduce viscosity and increase reactivity)
Aluminium oxide – 20-25%	Tartaric acid – improves handling characteristics, increases working time, and reduces setting time
Calcium fluoride – 15-20%	Water – reaction medium
Sodium fluoride – 4-10%	-
Aluminium phosphate – 4-15%	-

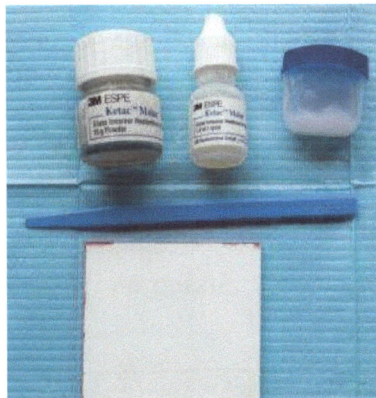

Fig. (5a). GIC powder and liquid with mixing pad, spatula, and Vaseline.

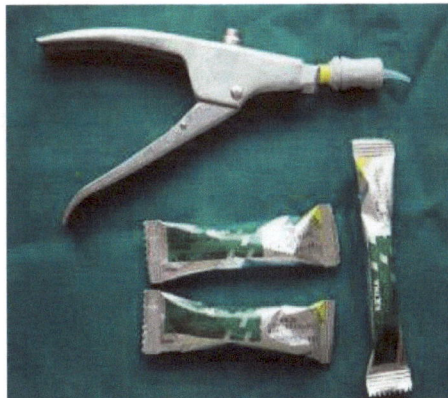

Fig. (5b). GIC premeasured capsule and applicator gun.

Glass ionomer cements are radio opaque and for this purpose strontium, barium, lanthanum, or zinc oxide are added to the powder. The powder and liquid are dispensed as per the proportion recommended by the manufacturer on an oil impervious mixing paper pad. The powder is incorporated into the liquid in 2 increments by means of a plastic mixing spatula in a folding motion until a homogenous mix is obtained. The folding mixing motion is important to preserve the gel structure of the mix. The manipulation of GIC should be completed within 45 seconds followed by its quick placement into the prepared cavity. The excess GIC is removed with the help of a carver and the occlusion is checked using an articulating paper. The GIC restoration is coated with Cocoa butter or petroleum jelly to prevent its dehydration.

Setting Reaction

Glass ionomer cement sets in two phases in the form of a diffusion-controlled process. The initial set occurs within 2-3 min of mixing by means of an acid-base reaction. The hydrated protons from the polyacid react with the surface of the glass particles leading to the release of sodium, calcium, and aluminum ions. These ions interact with the polyacid molecules to form ionic crosslinks and the resultant salt forms the rigid framework for the set cement. As part of the secondary phase of setting reaction, a crosslinking of aluminum ions takes place beginning from 10 mins of cement mixing and progresses slowly for about 24 hours [6].

Water is an essential component of glass ionomer cement. Water is the solvent for the polymeric acid, serves as the medium in which the setting reaction takes place and lastly, it is also a component of the set cement. The unbound water can be lost from the surface of a newly placed GIC restoration leading to a chalky white appearance and microscopic cracks developing on the surface of the restoration. Hence, it is recommended to protect the newly placed GIC restoration with petroleum jelly, cocoa butter, or varnish. Fig. (**6**) Based on its uses, GIC is classified into 9 types (Table **4**).

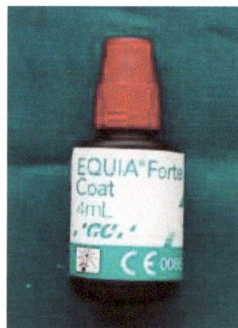

Fig. (6). Protective coat for application over GIC restorations.

Table 4. Classification of glass ionomer cement.

TYPE GLASS IONOMER CEMENT
I Luting
II Restoration
III Liners and Bases
IV Pit & Fissure Sealants
V For orthodontic brackets & band cementation
VI For core buid-up
VII Fluoride releasing
VIII High viscosity GIC used for ART
IX GIC used for primary teeth

Modifications of Glass Ionomer Cement

Modified versions of Glass Ionomer Cement were introduced primarily to overcome the disadvantages of the traditional GIC. Some of the clinically successful modified GICs include:

- Water settable GIC (Anhydrous GIC) – The polyacrylic liquid component is incorporated in the GIC powder in a freeze-dried form in one bottle and water or water with tartaric acid is supplied in another bottle. When the powder is mixed with water in the designated proportion, the freeze-dried acid dissolves to reconstitute the liquid acid. The setting reaction further proceeds in a manner like the conventional GIC. These cements have a longer working time and shorter setting time.
- Metal modified GIC – silver alloy admixed, cermet – The mechanical properties of the conventional GIC was found to be inferior to silver amalgam and hence metal reinforcement of GIC was attempted. This led to an increase in strength of the cement as well as provided radio-opacity to the restoration but compromised on the esthetics of the restoration.

Aluminium, chromium, nickel-aluminum alloy, and silver-tin alloy particles incorporated in GIC powder was introduced as 'Miracle mix' in 1983. In an alternate approach, silvery alloy particles were fused with the glass particles of GIC to form 'Cermet' (derived from ceramic and metal). However, low viscosity of the conventional GIC was not overcome by the addition of metal and further modifications in the composition of GIC was brought about to increase viscosity and improve the workability [7].

- High viscosity GIC – developed specifically for atraumatic restorative treatment (ART) – A higher powder liquid ratio in high viscosity GIC formulations results in improved mechanical properties like wear resistance, compressive strength, and marginal adaptability.
- Resin modified GIC (RmGIC) – Resin modified GIC is obtained by the addition of monomer to the liquid component of GIC along with an associated initiator (camphoroquinone). The setting of RmGIC involves the twin processes of acid-base reaction as well as polymerization by light curing. In the case of RmGICs, even in the presence of resins, they retain the properties of GIC. Addition of resin improves the binding strength, tensile & compressive strengths as well as reduces the solubility in an aqueous environment. Despite having better mechanical properties than conventional GIC, RmGICs restorations release lesser amounts of fluoride and are less biocompatible than GIC due to the release of hydroxy ethyl methacrylate (HEMA) mainly during the first 24 hours of placement [6]. RmGICs are used mainly in Class I, Class II, Class III & Class V restorations in primary teeth. Its other uses include – liners and bases, fissure sealants and bonding of orthodontic brackets.
- Compomers were introduced in 1993 and have been used extensively in the field of Pediatric dentistry since then. They are described as poly acid modified composite resins indicating that their chemical composition closely resembles composite resins as compared to GIC. Compomers contain ion-leachable glass particles and acidic polymerizable monomer molecules. The main feature of compomers is the absence of water and the subsequent lack of an acid-base reaction for which the presence of water is indispensable. The setting reaction is light activated and bonding to the tooth is dependent on acid etching and bonding mechanisms like composite resins. The fluoride release from compomer restorations is less as compared to GIC and additionally, compomer restorations do not act as fluoride reservoir due to lack of fluoride uptake.
- Nano particle reinforcement – Titanium dioxide, silver nano particles, alumina, zirconia, and hydroxyapatite nanoparticles *etc.* have been added to the conventional GIC powder to improve its compressive strength [8]. Incorporation of zirconia fillers (Zirconomer) reinforces the structural integrity of the restoration and imparts superior mechanical properties. The strength and durability of this restorative material is comparable to that of amalgam. Among organic nanoparticles, cellulose nanocrystals have shown promising results in improving the mechanical properties and biocompatibility of GIC [9].
- Fiber reinforced GIC – Attempts have been made to add alumina & carbon fibers to GIC powder to improve its flexural strength. When added at 25% volume, a significant improvement in the flexural strength of GIC was reported [10]. Glass fibers and cellulose microfiber reinforcements of conventional and resin modified GICs have also been considered as possible options for

improvement of mechanical properties.

GIC, along with its modifications is one of the most widely used dental restorative materials in Pediatric dentistry. Its advantages and disadvantages are listed in Table **5**.

Table 5. Advantages and disadvantages of GIC.

Advantages of GIC	Disadvantages of GIC
✓ **Chemical bond with enamel and dentin**	✗ Low strength
✓ **Good Biocompatibility**	✗ Short working time
✓ **Fluoride release and uptake from oral environment**	✗ Poor esthetics as compared to composite resin
✓ **Thermal expansion like that of dentin**	✗ Susceptibility to moisture during initial phase of setting
✓ **Better esthetics than Amalgam**	✗ Not suitable for Cl II, III and IV restorations
✓ **Less moisture sensitive than composite**	✗ Desiccation after setting and brittleness of restoration

Composite Resin

Composite resins are one of the most esthetically acceptable dental materials currently in use. Composite resins contain a monomeric or prepolymeric resin that is filled to various levels with glass or quartz. The glass particles are silanized to allow the hydrophilic filler particles to bond with the hydrophobic resin matrix. Good silanization is therefore essential for obtaining a stable material which is resistant to wear and homogenous in its composition [11] (Fig. **7**).

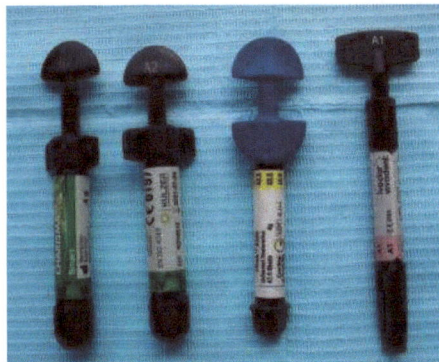

Fig. (7). Different shades of composite restorative material.

Composition

The composition and filler content of composite materials are important determinants of its clinical applications (Table **6**). Additionally, composites are classified based on the filler content and curing mechanism (Table **7**).

Table 6. Composition of composite resins.

RESIN MATRIX – Bis GMA or urethane Di methacrylate (UEDMA), tri-ethylene glycol Di methacrylate (TEGDMA)
FILLER – Quartz, colloidal silica, or heavy metal glasses
COUPLING AGENT – Coupling agents help the bonding of filler particles to the resin matrix. Organosilanes, titanates, zirconates are commonly used coupling agents
ACTIVATOR – Tertiary amines, Diketones
INITIATOR – Benzoyl peroxide (for chemically activated resins), Camphoroquinone (for light activated resins). Camphoroquinone has an absorption range between 400 to 600 nm, with 470 nm being the peak
INHIBITOR – 0.01% Butylated hydrotoluene is added to minimize spontaneous polymerization of monomer. The inhibitor readily reacts with free radicals to prevent spontaneous polymerization
OPTICAL MODIFIERS/ COLOR PIGMENTS – metal oxides
OPACIFIERS – Aluminium oxide, titanium dioxide are added so that the restoration matches the shade and translucency of natural teeth. To prevent discoloration due to exposure to ultraviolet light, UV light stabilizers are also added.

Table 7. Classification of composite resins.

Based on Filler Particle Size	Based on Curing Mechanism
Traditional composite/Macrofilled (8-12μm)	Thermal activated
Small particle filled composite (1-5 μm)	Chemically activated
Microfilled composite (0.04-0.4 μm)	Chemically activated
Hybrid composite (0.6-1.0 μm)	-

Placement of Composite Restoration

Shade selection is the preliminary step in achieving a good esthetic restoration. Based on the involvement of caries, more than one shade of composite resin may be necessary to simulate the dentin as well as the translucency of enamel. Good isolation using a rubber dam plays an important role in the success of composite restoration (Table **8**). Following caries removal, the cavity is etched using 37-50% orthophosphoric acid (Fig. **8a**). Acid etching is crucial for achieving micromechanical retention of the composite to the tooth structure. The etchant gel is applied for 60 sec in permanent teeth and 90 sec in primary teeth. The etchant is rinsed thoroughly using a stream of water and upon air-drying, the etched surface exhibits a chalky white frosted appearance.

Table 8. Indication and contraindications of composite resin.

Indications	Contraindications
Class I cavities in primary and permanent teeth	Teeth that cannot be adequately isolated to obtain moisture control
Class II restorations in primary teeth that do not extend beyond proximal line angles	Uncooperative child patients who are unlikely to sit through longer appointments necessary for composite resin restorations
Class II restorations in permanent teeth that extend approximately one third to one half the buccolingual intercuspal width of the tooth	High caries risk patients or children with poor oral hygiene and poor compliance with oral hygiene practices
Class IV & V restorations in primary and permanent teeth	-
Strip crowns in primary teeth	-

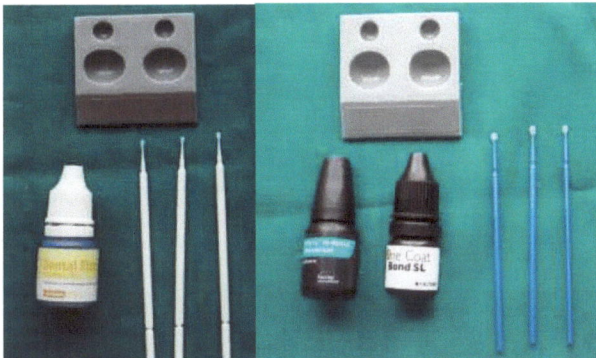

Fig. (8 a,b). Acid etchant and bonding agents with applicator tips and dispensing cup.

Etching is followed by application of bonding agent (low viscosity unfilled resin) which improves the wettability of the etched enamel (Fig. **8b**). The low viscosity of the bonding agent helps it to penetrate the micro-porosities created on the etched tooth surface leading to the formation of resin tags within the enamel. Unfilled resin when applied to the tooth structure, penetrated the primed enamel/dentin, and copolymerizes with the primer to form an intermingled layer of collagen and resin which is termed as the 'hybrid layer.' The bonding agent is cured using composite curing light source. The light source used could be halogen or LED based visible light. Protective eye wear for the operator, assistant and the patient is recommended as the visible light can cause vision impairment if looked at directly for an extended period (Fig. **9**).

After etching the tooth surface and application of bonding agent, the placement of composite resin is carried out in an incremental manner. An applicator tip or Teflon coated instruments are used to place the composite resin in increments of 2 mm to ensure adequate light penetration and complete curing of the increment (Fig. **10**). As the resin polymerizes, it tends to shrink towards the light source, affecting the tooth-resin bond interface. Researchers have recommended a slow rate of polymerization allows the resin polymer to flow adequately and dissipate the stress while maintaining a sufficient bond to the tooth structure. The pulse delay polymerization achieved using halogen lights ensures that the resin is not polymerized too quickly. A fast-setting rate of the resin leads to stress developing at restoration margins causing marginal fracture and/or post-operative sensitivity [12].

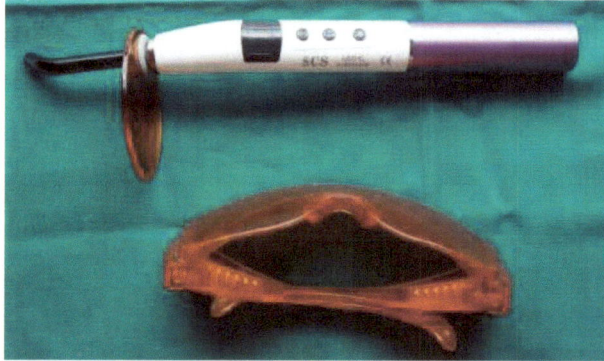

Fig. (9). LED curing light and protective glasses.

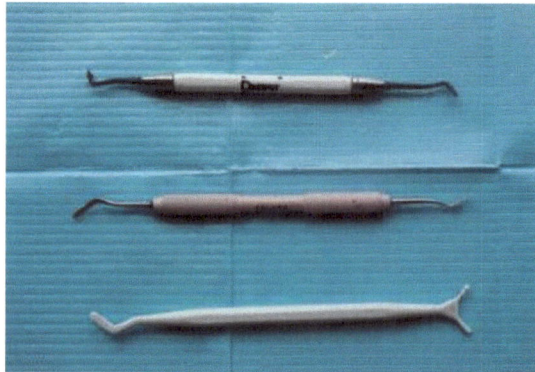

Fig. (10). Teflon coated and plastic instruments for placing and carving composite restorative material.

The composite restoration is completed in increments, following which the occlusion is checked and excess material, if any, is removed using rotary instruments. This is followed by polishing of the restoration using the polishing discs, and cups provided in the composite polishing kit. The final finishing of the restoration is done with the application of a thin layer of bonding agent over the restoration surface and curing it. As the resin shrinks towards the light source and away from the cavity walls during curing, the application of bonding agent helps to seal this marginal gap.

Flowable Composites

Flowable composites are low viscosity composite restorative materials which were developed to overcome the handling difficulties of traditional viscous paste-like composites. Flowable composites are available in a syringe which makes it easy to directly dispense the required quantity of material into the prepared cavity (Fig. **11**). Flowable composites have been mainly indicated for minimally invasive cavity preparations, for sealing pits and fissure and for treating abrasions and small cervical cavitated lesions. Clinical application of flowable composites in class I and II restorations has been limited due to lack of adequate strength attributable to low filler content. However, addition of nano fillers to flowable composites is said to improve the physical properties of flowable composites at par with those of conventional composites.

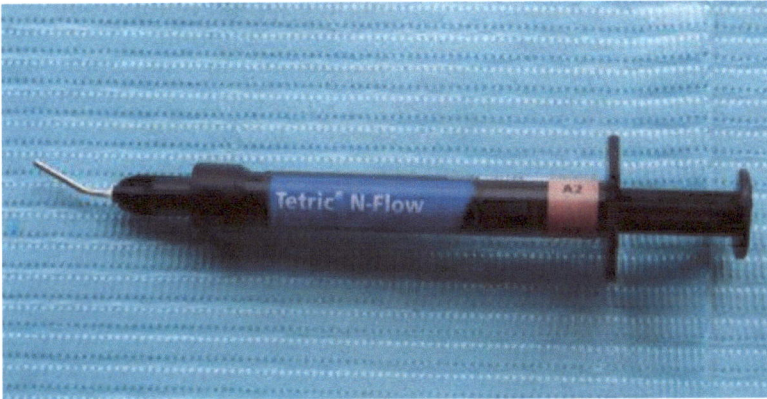

Fig. (11). Flowable composite resin.

Liner and Bases

Liners and bases act as a buffer layer sealing the dentinal tubules and thereby reducing post-operative sensitivity. Contact of dissimilar metals, desiccation of the cavity during preparation and thermal conductivity of the restorative material are possible causes of post-operative sensitivity. The presence of an intermediary material between the tooth and the restoration minimizes post-operative discomfort. Clinical considerations for using liners and bases beneath a restoration is based upon the remaining dentin thickness (RDT) separating the restoration and the pulp tissue. A liner/base offers chemical, thermal, electrical, and mechanical protection to the pulp and may additionally act as pulpal medication [13].

Liners

Cavity liner is a suspension of calcium hydroxide in an organic solvent applied as a thin layer for protecting the pulp. The objective of using a liner is to seal the dentinal walls and floor of the cavity from ingress of oral bacteria and irritants from restorative procedure. Upon application, the aqueous or resin carrier solution of the liner evaporates, leaving behind a thin layer of calcium hydroxide on the cavity walls. The alkaline pH of 11 of calcium hydroxide is helpful in neutralizing the damage caused by acidic restorative materials and in counteracting the acidic byproducts of bacteria entering the tooth-restoration interface by way of microleakage. Additionally, being an irritant to pulp, the alkalinity of calcium hydroxide stimulates the formation of reparative dentin [14, 15] (Fig. **12**).

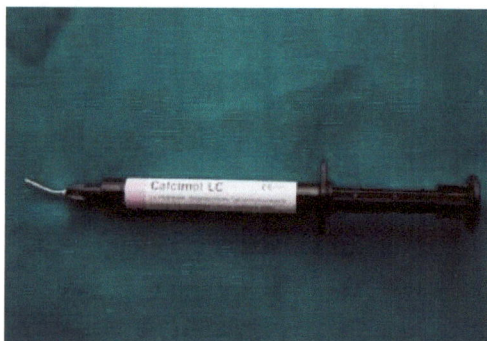

Fig. (12). Light cured, radio-opaque calcium.

Other than calcium hydroxide-based cavity liners, low viscosity zinc oxide eugenol (Type IV) and glass ionomer liners (both powder-liquid and light cured GIC liners) can also be used [12]. Glass ionomer cavity liners (Type III GIC) is used under composite restorations placed near the pulp. In this case, the glass ionomer liner acts as an intermediary bonding material between the tooth structure and the resin restoration. The placement of GIC liners beneath composite restoration is known as the **'Sandwich technique'** and it utilizes the desirable qualities of the glass ionomer cement; and at the same time, provides the esthetics of composite restoration. Sandwich technique is particularly recommended for class II composite restorations in both primary and permanent teeth.

Compared to the bonding agents essential for micromechanical retention of composite resin restoration, the use of GIC liners has additional advantages of chemical bonding with the tooth, reduced technique sensitivity and an established anticariogenic mechanism by virtue of fluoride release. After the glass ionomer liner sets, the surface of the liner is etched, rinsed followed by application of bonding agent on the liner as well as the walls of the cavity and the adjacent beveled enamel surfaces. This is followed by placement of composite resin restoration in the usual manner. However, if light cured GIC is used as the liner, then its surface is not etched. After application of bonding agent to the liner surface and walls of the cavity, composite resin is placed in increments and cured in the usual manner.

Bases

As opposed to liners, bases are thicker protective layers of cements placed underneath the restorative material to prevent thermal and chemical injury to the underlying pulp. The base material should be strong enough to support the restorative material during placement and function, as well as provide protection from galvanic activity. Dycal, a two-paste system containing calcium hydroxide has been in use since long as a base to protect the pulp tissue beneath deep carious lesions (Fig. **13**).

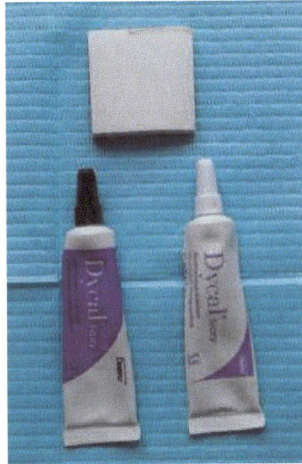

Fig. (13). Dycal – calcium hydroxide paste in 2 paste system.

Type II zinc oxide eugenol cement is used as an insulating base material. Zinc oxide eugenol cement is known to be the least irritating of all dental materials. The powder is composed of 69% by weight zinc oxide along with white rosin (29.3%), zinc stearate (1%), zinc acetate (0.7%) and magnesium oxide. The liquid component is eugenol which is derived from clove oil. The mixed zinc oxide eugenol cement has a pH of about 7 and has a sedative effect on the pulp. However, in high concentrations, eugenol can be toxic to the pulp (Fig. **14a**).

The use of zinc oxide eugenol cement as a liner or base beneath composite resin restorations is contraindicated as eugenol interferes with resin polymerization. Zinc oxide eugenol can be used as a sub-base beneath zinc phosphate base for silver amalgam restorations in instances where the base of the cavity is near the pulp [16].

Other useful applications of zinc oxide eugenol cement include root canal filling of primary teeth following pulpectomy, as a temporary/interim restoration (Fig. **14b**) placed prior to placement of final restorations, indirect pulp capping, temporary luting of crowns and its use as a periodontal surgical dressing.

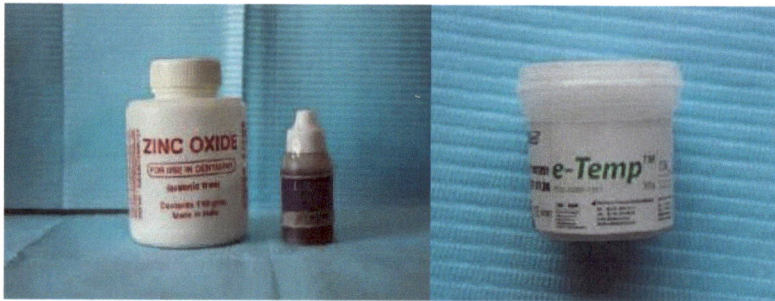

Fig. (14). (a) Zinc oxide powder and eugenol liquid; **(b)** Temporary restoration material.

Zinc phosphate cement (also known as zinc orthophosphate cement) is a powder-liquid system with the powder containing 90% zinc oxide, 8.2% magnesium oxide, 1.4% silica and 0.1% bismuth trioxide. The liquid is composed of 38.2% phosphoric acid, 36% water, 16.2% Aluminium phosphate and 7.1% zinc. Attempts have been made to modify zinc phosphate cements with the incorporation of stannous fluoride, cuprous and cupric oxides. Addition of fluoride confers an anti-cariogenic property but leads to a decrease in strength and increase in the solubility of zinc phosphate cement. Addition of oxides of copper makes zinc phosphate cements bacteriostatic. It is mainly used as a thermal insulating base under silver amalgam restorations, and its other uses include luting of orthodontic bands and as an intermediate restoration. As a base, zinc phosphate is mixed to produce a thick, dry, putty-like consistency. This ensures a strong, hard base and a shorter setting time. An additional advantage of a thick mix will be less free liquid available to act as an irritant. But with the declining use of silver amalgam, the use of zinc phosphate cement as a base has also reduced.

Varnish

Cavity varnish consists of one or more resins (from natural gum, synthetic resins, or rosin) in an organic solvent like acetone, chloroform, or ether. Like cavity liners, cavity varnish is also applied as a thin layer to the walls of the prepared cavity. Upon evaporation of the solvent, the remaining solute seals the tubules. Cavity varnish provides a protective barrier against irritants from the restorative materials and from the oral fluids penetrating the dentin. Varnish is recommended beneath silver amalgam restorations because freshly placed amalgam shrinks on setting, allowing microleakage to occur. Application of cavity varnish seals the tooth-amalgam interface till the amalgam starts to corrode and seals the interface. The cavity varnish also prevents the corrosion by-products from leaching into the enamel and staining the tooth. Cavity varnishes do not possess adequate mechanical strength and they have minimal film thickness, thus are unsuitable to be used as a cavity base. The use of cavity varnish is not recommended for composite restorations because the solvent in the varnish may soften the resin and the varnish coating prevents proper wetting of the prepared cavity by the bonding agents. Cavity varnish is also contraindicated under glass ionomer cement restorations as the varnish would interfere with the chemical bonding between GIC and the tooth. Some of the difficulties faced with the use of cavity varnish include uneven film, lack of thermal insulation, lack of chemical adhesion with dentin and solubility over time. As an alternative to varnish application, the application of dentin bonding agent is said to provide a better sealing ability.

Materials Used in Pediatric Endodontic Therapy

Mineral Trioxide Aggregate (MTA)

In 1824, Joseph Aspdin, a British stone mason, obtained a patent for a cement he formulated in his kitchen. The inventor heated a mixture of finely ground limestone and clay and ground the mixture into a powder creating a hydraulic cement (one that hardens with the addition of water). Aspdin named the product Portland cement because the set cement resembled a stone quarried on the Isle of Portland off the British coast. Aspdin had no way of knowing that roughly 170 years after his discovery this same product would form the backbone of a new class of calcium and alumina silicate based so-called "bioactive" dental materials, one of which was mineral trioxide aggregate (MTA). The constituents of MTA are derived from a Portland cement parent compound. Although these compounds are similar in some respects, Portland cement and MTA are not identical.

MTA has mainly replaced calcium hydroxide in its use for vital pulp therapies in both primary and permanent teeth. A very practical advantage of MTA is that unlike many other dental materials, MTA sets in a moist environment. When it is in contact with moisture, it is main component calcium oxide converts into calcium hydroxide, resulting in a high pH microenvironment exhibiting antibacterial effects. Unlike calcium hydroxide, however, this material has very low solubility and maintains its physical integrity after placement [17].

In the early 1990s, Torabinejad and colleagues began testing and experimenting with an MTA compound they developed at Loma Linda University that was essentially a modified Portland cement. They found it had significantly better sealing abilities than conventional endodontic materials when used as a root end sealer and in the repair of furcation and lateral root perforations. This was due, in part to the fact that MTA sets and functions well in the inherently moist environment in and around a tooth in an *in vivo* situation. In fact, just as water is an essential component in the setting of Portland cement, it is also required in and enhances the setting of MTA.

MTA is a non-resorbable material with an alkaline pH of 10.2 which increases to 12.5 after 3 hours of mixing. Compared to calcium hydroxide, MTA has shown a remarkable improvement in promoting healing of pulp and peri radicular tissues (Table **9** and **10**). MTA is either available as a fine ash colored powder (grey MTA) or white MTA (Fig. **15**). When mixed with distilled water, a colloidal gel is formed which sets in approximately 3-4 hrs. The mixed MTA is carried to the desired tooth surface with the help of an MTA carrier (Fig. **16**), or an amalgam carrier.

Table 9. Composition of MTA.

Composition of MTA
Tricalcium silicate
Dicalcium silicate
Tricalcium aluminate
Gypsum
Tetracalcium aluminoferrite
Bismuth oxide

Table 10. Advantages, disadvantages and uses of MTA.

Advantages of MTA	Disadvantages of MTA
✓ Promotes the formation of a thicker dentinal bridge and at a faster rate	✖ Expensive
✓ Material of choice for apexification of pulpally involved permanent teeth with immature apices	✖ Technique sensitive
✓ Good sealing ability and prevents bacterial leakage	✖ Long setting time

(Table 10) cont.....

Advantages of MTA	Disadvantages of MTA
✓ **Effective even in moist environment and does not mandate a dry field of action**	✖ Tooth discoloration with grey MTA
✓ **Excellent biocompatibility**	✖ High solubility prior to setting
USES OF MTA	DISADVANTAGES OF MTA (As a pulp capping material)
✓ **Pulp capping in primary and permanent teeth and for apexogenesis**	✖ Layering of MTA with zinc oxide eugenol or glass ionomer cement has been shown to affect the setting of the material
✓ **For apexification of young permanent teeth**	✖ An extended setting time of 140 - 170 minutes and high solubility while setting hampers its sealing ability
✓ **Repair of perforation in furcation areas, and root perforations.**	✖ Zinc is taken up by MTA from the adjacent zinc oxide cement and retards the hydration further
✓ **Repair of resorptive perforation, if not too extensive**	✖ Poor Handling characteristics due to granular consistency, slow setting time

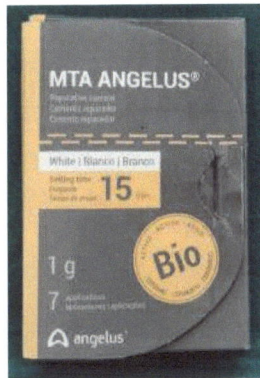

Fig. (15). White Mineral trioxide aggregate.

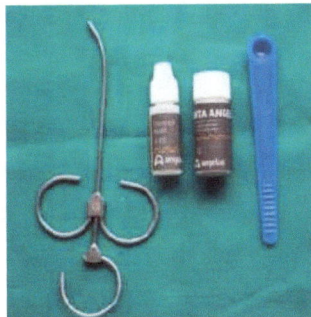

Fig. (16). MTA powder, distilled water, scoop, and MTA carrier.

Metapex

Calcium hydroxide cement has been used extensively for pulp therapy of primary and permanent teeth. The rate of resorption of calcium hydroxide is either faster or similar to the physiological root resorption. In particular, the addition of iodoform to the traditional calcium hydroxide composition (Vitapex/Metapex) has yielded good results in primary teeth pulpotomies and as a root filling material in primary tooth pulpectomy (Table **11**). It can also be used for stimulating root end closures in apexogenesis and to induce a mechanical bridge formation at the root apex during apexification procedure. As an interim intracanal medicament during root canal therapy, Metapex has shown excellent antimicrobial properties and peri apical healing.

Table 11. Composition and advantages of MTA.

Composition of Metapex	Advantages of Metapex
Iodoform – 40.4%	✓ Easy To use
Calcium hydroxide – 30.3%	✓ Radiopaque
Silicone – 22.4%	✓ Rate of resorption is faster than the primary root
-	✓ Does not produce any toxic effects on erupting permanent successors

Metapex is a viscous mixture of calcium hydroxide and iodoform in a syringe. The disposable tips have stoppers for accurate placement of the material at the apex of the tooth (Fig. **17**).

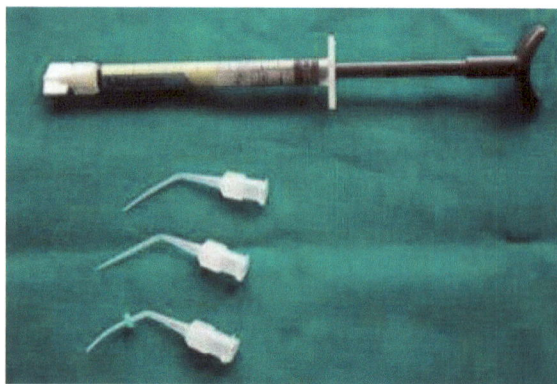

Fig. (17). Metapex syringe with applicator tips.

Impression Materials

Alginate

Alginate is one of the most commonly used impression materials in dentistry. It is extracted from marine algae and has been in use since 1947. The word alginate is derived from 'Algin' – a mucous extract obtained from algae. Factors like ease of manipulation, adequate hard and soft tissue reproducibility for preliminary impression purposes and relatively low cost have ensured its continued use over the past several decades. Also known as irreversible hydrocolloids, alginates form a viscous sol when mixed vigorously with water. In the presence of calcium sulphate, this aqueous alginate forms an insoluble calcium alginate gel which constitutes the set mass of an alginate impression (Table **12**) [18, 19].

Table 12. Composition of alginate.

Composition of Alginate
Potassium alginate (Soluble alginate) – 15% by weight
Calcium sulphate (Reactor) – 16% by weight
Zinc oxide (Filler) – 4% by weight
Potassium titanium fluoride (Accelerator) – 3% by weight
Diatomaceous earth (Filler) – 60% by weight
Sodium phosphate (Retarder) – 2% by weight

Alginate impression material is available as individually sealed pouches with sufficient powder pre-weighed for an individual impression, or in bulk form in a can. Plastic scoops are provided to dispense alginate powder along with plastic measuring cylinder for water. Alginate should be stored in tightly sealed containers as its shelf life is affected by storage temperature and moisture levels in the ambient air.

The measured quantity of alginate powder is dispensed in a flexible rubber mixing bowl and incorporated into the measured quantity of water. A stiff bladed spatula is used to mix alginate with water in a figure of eight motion (Fig. **18**). A mixing time of 45 sec to 1 minute produces a creamy, smooth mix that does not drip off the spatula blade. Reducing the temperature of the water used for mixing improves the working time. The prepared mix is loaded on a perforated metal or plastic trays for recording the impression. A minimum alginate thickness of 3 mm between the tray and the tissues ensures adequate strength of the set impression. The impression should be rinsed carefully with water, disinfected, and poured immediately using dental stone. If any delay in pouring the impression is anticipated, then the impression should be wrapped in a paper towel, saturated with water, and placed in a closed container to create a 100% humid environment.

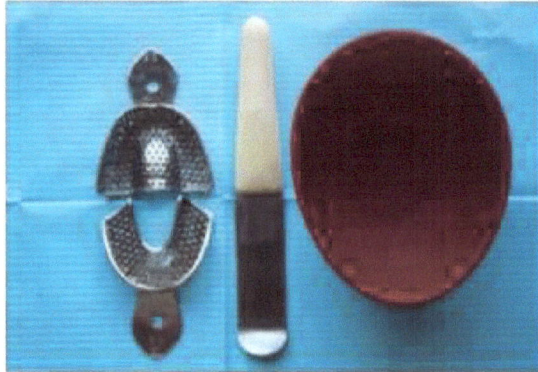

Fig. (18). Flexible rubber bowl, stiff bladed spatula and perforated trays used for alginate impression material.

Newer Alginate Materials

Alginates have been introduced in various flavors (Mint, strawberry *etc.*) to increase patient acceptability especially among the pediatric age group. Chromatic alginates are also well accepted by pediatric patients especially since there is an observable change in color of the alginate mix as per the phase of setting. The color change of the chromatic alginates also serves as a reference guide for the operator and indicates the time for retrieval of the impression from the oral cavity. Dust-free alginates were introduced to prevent the hazardous effects of inhalation of the fine airborne silica particles during mixing of alginate. Dust free alginate contains glycerin which helps in agglomeration of the fine powder dust and makes the powder dust-free (Fig. **19**).

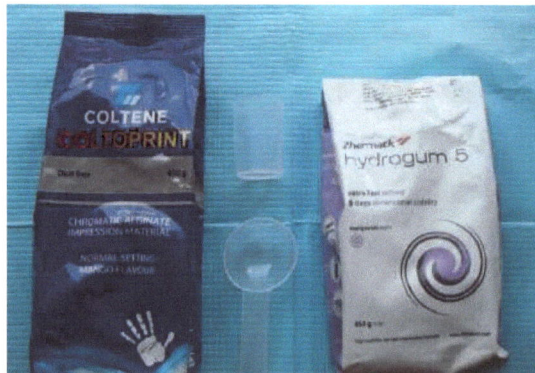

Fig. (19). Chromatic and dust-free alginate impression materials.

Impression Compound

Impression compound is composed of a mixture of waxes, thermoplastic resins, a filler, and coloring agent. Since the waxes tend to be brittle, plasticizers such as shellac, stearic acid and gutta percha are added to improve the plasticity and workability of impression compound [19]. The impression compound (also known as modeling plastic) is mainly used for recording a preliminary impression of edentulous arches using non perforated steel trays. The working model obtained from this preliminary impression is used for the fabrication of custom-made tray to be used with other impression materials for recording the final impression. The impression compound is softened over a flame (stick compound) or immersing it in a hot water bath. While it is still in the plastic state, it is placed on the tray and the impression is recorded. After the cast is poured and the plaster sets completely, it is removed from the impression compound by immersing it in warm water to allow the compound to soften sufficiently to permit easy separation from the cast.

Among pediatric patients, impression compound has limited uses. It is sometimes used for recording the primary impression in neonates with cleft palate, with utmost precaution to not let the softened material flow in undercut areas. A custom-made tray is used to record the final impression for the fabrication of feeding plates or obturators.

Elastomeric Impression Materials

Elastomeric impression materials are irreversible but highly elastic impression materials that can be stretched and yet rapidly recover to their original dimensions (Table **13**). Commonly used elastomeric impression materials include – polysulfide, addition & condensation silicones, and polyether. Elastomeric materials are supplied as 2 component systems – base and catalyst pastes that are available in light, medium, heavy, and putty consistencies. Same lengths of the 2 pastes are dispensed on a glass slab or a mixing pad. The base paste is scraped up with a spatula and spread over the catalyst paste and mixed uniformly. While using the putty, equal scoops of the base and catalyst component is dispensed and kneaded using fingers until a uniform color is obtained (Fig. **20 a,b**).

Table 13. Advantages and disadvantages of elastomeric impression materials.

Advantages	Disadvantages
✓ Long working time	✗ High cost as compared to the other impression materials
✓ High tear resistance	✗ Polysulfides have an unpleasant odor

(Table 13) cont.....

Advantages	Disadvantages
✓ **Excellent reproducibility of hard and soft tissue details**	✖ Condensation silicone impressions must be poured immediately
✓ **Good elasticity and minimal distortion of impression during removal from undercuts**	✖ Polysiloxanes are hydrophobic and hence may not flow adequately in moist sulcus
✓ **Polysiloxanes allow for same impression to be poured multiple times**	-
✓ **Vinyl polysiloxane impressions can be poured upto 1 hour after recording**	-

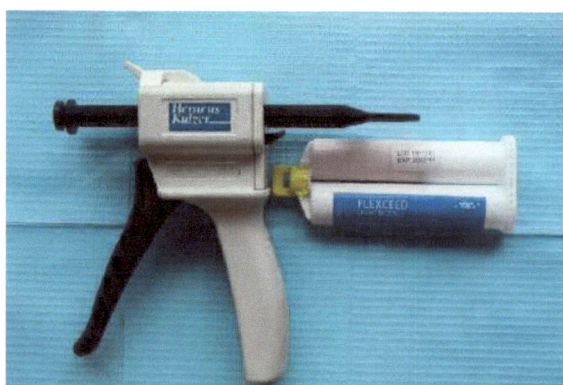

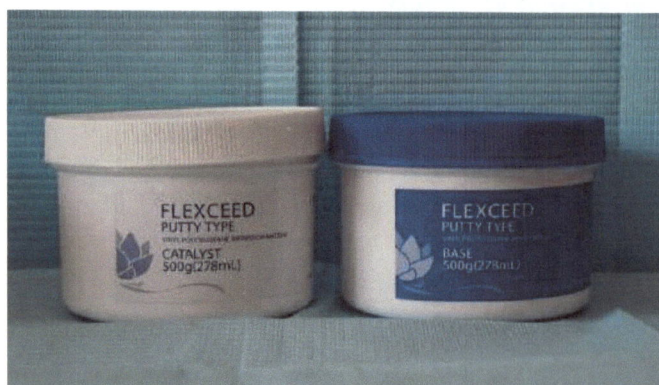

Fig. (20 a,b). Light body (with dispensing gun) and Putty elastomeric impression material.

Gypsum Products

Gypsum products like dental plaster and dental stone are widely used in dentistry for preparation. Dental plaster and stone are produced by the method of calcination of gypsum (calcium sulphate dihydrate) at temperatures ranging between 110-130ºC. Upon mixing with water, the dental plaster or stone powder, the process of calcination is reversed, and gypsum is formed. This setting reaction is an exothermic reaction and the heat evolved is equivalent to the heat used originally during calcination.

During the setting reaction, the growth and subsequent impingement of the dehydrate crystals causes an outward thrust leading to setting expansion. Accelerators and retarders added to the plaster/stone powder decrease and increase the setting time, respectively. However, both accelerators and retarders reduce the setting expansion of gypsum products (Fig. **21 a,b**). The types of gypsum products are enumerated below. Impression Plaster (Type I) is a dental plaster with modifiers to regulate setting time and setting expansion can be used for recording impressions. However, with the introduction of more state-of-the-art impression materials, impression plasters are rarely used nowadays (Table **14**).

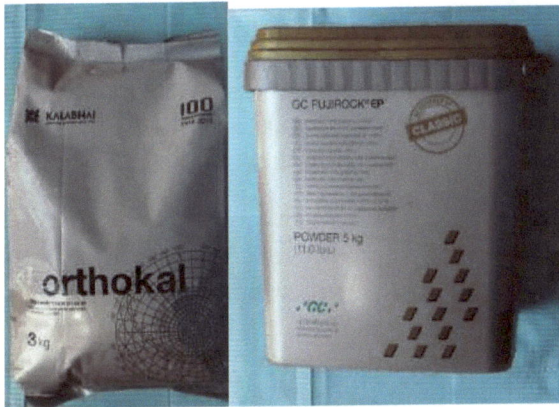

Fig. (21 a,b). Type III & Type IV Dental stone.

Table 14. Classification and uses of gypsum products.

Classification of Gypsum Products	Uses of Gypsum Products
TYPE I – Impression Plaster	✓ Making study models for diagnosis and record keeping
TYPE II – Model plaster	✓ Making working models for fabrication of removable appliances, space maintainers
TYPE III – Dental stone	✓ Carrying out space analysis
TYPE IV – Dental stone with high strength	✓ Fabrication of prosthetic appliances
TYPE V – Dental stone with high strength, high expansion	✓ As dental investment material during casting of appliances in laboratory

Mixing

Dental plaster/stone is mixed with water using a rubber bowl and stiff bladed straight spatula. A mixing time of about one minute is necessary for incorporating the plaster/stone powder into water resulting in a smooth mix. Mechanical mixing requires about 20 to 30 sec of mixing time. If the mix is overmixed, the formed gypsum crytals are broken up and the strength of the final mix is adversely affected. The mix is tapped or vibrated gently to facilitate the removal of air entrapped in the mix. Thereafter, a working time of 3 minutes is utilized to pour the impression. The set plaster has a porous structure, and the porosity increases with an increase in the water powder ratio [19].

Bio Smart Dental Materials

Traditionally, dental materials were developed to play a passive and inert role in the oral environment. For decades, the success of a restorative material was based on its non – reactive nature inside the oral cavity. The phenomenon of 'fluoride release' by certain materials when exposed to saliva presented a unique opportunity to utilize the properties of these materials for them to play a more active role as a restoration.

Smart dental materials possess properties that can be altered in a controlled manner by stimuli such as a change in temperature, pH, moisture, stress, electric field *etc*. More importantly, the smart materials return to their original state upon the removal of the stimuli. Smart dental materials exhibit a dynamic behavior and react in a reliable, and usually reproducible manner to an external stimulus [20]. In recent years, the focus of restorative dental procedures has shifted towards not only providing a long-term functional restoration but also to use materials that promote remineralization of tooth structure and help in hard and soft tissue repair and regeneration.

Nickel-Titanium Smart Alloys

Nickel-Titanium (NiTi) alloys or shape-memory alloys have been in use as orthodontic wires since their introduction by Beuhler *et al* in Maryland. NiTi wires possess 'superelasticity' and 'shape memory' due to its ability to undergo a phase change in response to a change in temperature or under mechanical stress. NiTi arch wires are preferred over stainless-steel wires as the NiTi wires exert continuous but gentle force on the teeth for a longer period.

In the field of Endodontics, the use of 'NitiNOL' (55 wt.% and 45 wt% Ti) has revolutionized root canal treatment procedure. Beginning from handheld Niti files to rotary cleaning and shaping files, their application has also extended to pediatric dentistry with these files being used for biomechanical preparation of primary and permanent teeth in children. The super elastic property of these files gives them the ability to undergo mechanical stress during chemo-mechanical preparation of root canals without exhibiting permanent deformation. This provides an improved access to curved root canals and allows a more centered canal preparation without much exertion of lateral force.

Glass Ionomer Cements with Bio Active Glass: Bioactive Glass (BAG) has been added to the Glass Ionomer cement to improve its bioactivity and tooth regeneration capacity in addition to its property of fluoride release and acting as a fluoride reservoir. BAG was first introduced by Larry Hench in 1969 and is composed of silicon, sodium, calcium, and phosphorus oxides. BAG was initially introduced as a replacement to osseous tissue as it forms a strong bond with bone through production of hydroxyapatite and is not rejected by the body. It also integrates the hydroxyapatite with collagen tissue present in bone and dentin. BAG have been added to the conventional GIC as well as the resin modified GIC with the bioactive component making its use effective in case of the sandwich technique where the restoration is likely to be near the pulp tissue, and for the treatment of root caries [21].

Other uses of BAG include repair of osseous bone defects post oral and maxillofacial surgery, osseointegration of dental implants and repair of periodontal bone loss. Recently, bio glass has been used in the treatment of dentin hypersensitivity. Fine particles of bio glass have been incorporated in dentifrice using an aqueous vector. When the dentifrice is used, bio glass particles act on exposed dentinal surfaces to rapidly produce hydroxycarbonapatite layer which seals the dentinal tubules and relieves sensitivity and pain.

Smart Composites: Amorphous calcium phosphate (ACP) can be used as a filler in bioactive polymeric composites. The ACP is added in an encapsulated form within a polymer binder. Sustained release of calcium and phosphate ions have been reported, having a potential for dentin repair. In the presence of dental plaque and acidic oral environment, ACP containing composites have been shown to release calcium and phosphate ions into the saliva, contributing towards a cario protective action. In addition to excellent biocompatibility, the inorganic ions released by smart composites are deposited on the tooth structure as an apatite mineral like hydroxyapatite [20, 22].

Bio Dentine

Bio dentine is a calcium-silcate based material manufactured by Septodont, St.-Maur-des-Fossés. This calcium silicate-based cement uses synthetically created raw materials mainly consisting of tricalcium silicate [$3CaOSiO_2$] and dicalcium silicate [2CaOSiO$_2$] as the main bulk of the material, calcium carbonate [CaCO$_3$] as filler for enhancing mechanical properties and accelerating the hardening of the cement and zirconium dioxide [ZrO$_2$] as a radio pacifier. The liquid consists of calcium chloride [CaCl$_2$.H$_2$O], a setting accelerator, a hydro soluble polymer functioning as a water reducing agent, and water. It has a positive effect on vital pulp cells and stimulates tertiary dentin formation and releases calcium [Ca^{2+}] and hydroxide [OH$^-$] ions making it suitable for pulp capping. Bio dentine, when applied directly onto pulp, induces reparative dentine formation resulting in complete dentin bridge formation, absence of an inflammatory pulp response and layers of well-arranged odontoblasts and odontoblast-like cells observed after 6 weeks. The antibacterial property is like MTA and can be attributed to the high alkaline pH of Biodentin. Biodentin has been shown to promote hard tissue regeneration and has shown to not evoke any adverse reactions from dental pulp.

In contrast to MTA, which uses only distilled water for setting, bio dentine uses a mix of distilled water, calcium chloride and a hydro soluble polymer. Calcium chloride acts as an accelerator of the setting reaction. The hydro soluble polymer reduces the necessary water of the reaction. With these improvements in its composition, the initial setting time of Bio dentine (12 min) is much lower than that of MTA (180 min). Biodentin has superior sealing ability as compared to MTA due to penetration into the dentin tubules forming tag-like structures, lower setting time and better handling characteristics. It does not cause discoloration like MTA and hence can be used safely as pulp capping agent. Compared to MTA, it has few disadvantages like low radio opacity which reduces further over the period; and low shear bond strength to restorative material like composites (Fig. **22**).

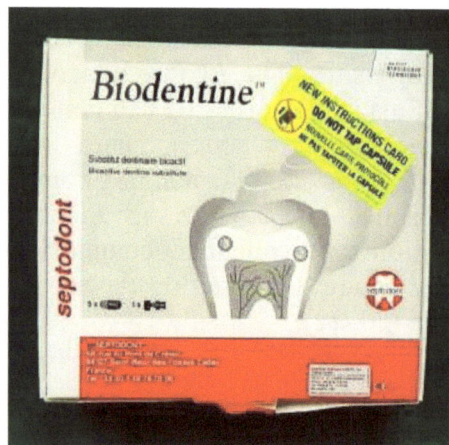

Fig. (22). Biodentin.

Bio dentine™ offers the advantage of good mechanical properties with excellent biocompatibility as well as a bioactive behavior. Bio dentine is being marketed as the first all-in-one bioactive and biocompatible dentine substitute based on unique Active Bio silicate Technology™ designed to treat damaged dentine both for restorative and endodontic purposes [23]. Bio dentine is available in the form of a powder in a capsule and liquid in a pipette (Fig. **23a**), (Table **15**).

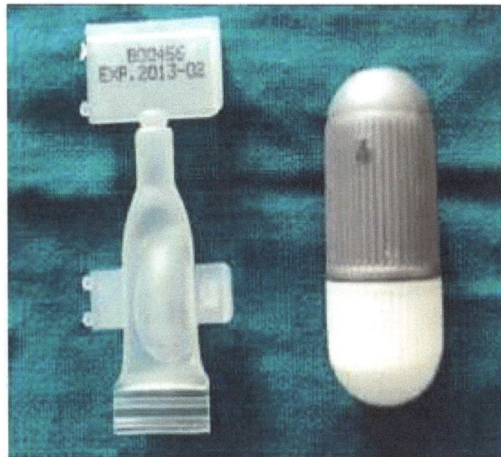

Fig. (23a). Capsule of bio dentin with pipette containing the liquid.

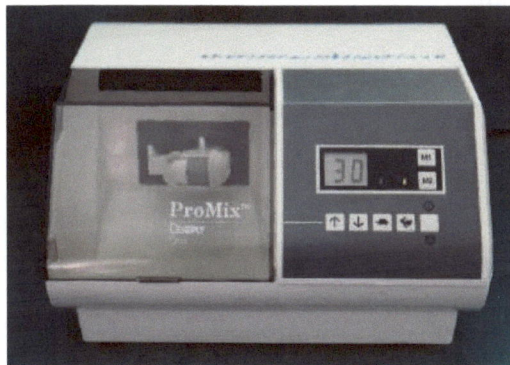

Fig. (23b). Mechanical device for mixing bio dentin capsule.

Table 15. Composition of biodentin.

Composition of Biodentin
The powder contains Tricalcium and dicalcium as well as calcium carbonate
Zirconium dioxide as contrast medium.
The liquid consists of calcium chloride in aqueous solution with an admixture of polycarboxylate

Manipulation

5 drops of liquid is dispensed in the capsule containing the powder. The capsule is placed in an amalgamator and mixed at a speed of 4000–4200 rotations/min for 30s (Fig. **23b**). The mix is then carried to the prepared tooth surface using an amalgam carrier and is condensed evenly using a plastic filling instrument. Bio dentine allows a working time of 5–6 min and sets in approximately 12 min. Bio dentine application is followed by an interim or final restoration.

TheraCal

TheraCal [Bisco Inc, lot. 603-189-A] is light-curable pulp-capping material consisting of a single paste containing CaO, calcium silicate particles [Type III Portland cement], Strontium glass, fumed silica, barium sulphate, barium zirconate and a resin containing Bis-GMA and PEGDMA. TheraCal has better marginal sealing property compared to MTA and biodentin and better shear bond strength when layered with composite or RMGIC. It also has the advantage of immediate setting as it can be light cured unlike MTA and biodentin. Significant disadvantages of Theracal include low release of calcium ions from the cement due to resin component. It is less well tolerated by pulp fibroblasts and studies have shown lower quality calcific barrier formation, extensive inflammation, and less favourable odontoblastic layer formation. Hence, this material at present can be recommended for indirect pulp capping only [24].

ACTIVA BioACTIVE

ACTIVA BioACTIVE-BASE/LINER [Pulpdent, USA] was launched in 2014 as a "light-cured resin-modified calcium silicate" [RMCS] combining attributes of both composite and glass ionomers [GI]. It sets by 3 mechanisms: self-cure, light cure, and an acid base reaction like GIC. It is said to have, aesthetics and physical properties of composites and increased release and recharge of calcium, phosphate, and fluoride in comparison with glass ionomer [GI]. The bioactive properties of ACTIVA BioACTIVE products are based on a mechanism whereby the material responds to pH cycles and plays an active role in releasing and recharging of significant amounts of calcium, phosphate, and fluoride. These ions stimulate the hard tissue formation [25]. However, insufficient literature is available regarding the effectiveness of ACTIVA BioACTIVE for vital pulp therapy in primary teeth.

Propolis

Propolis is collected from trees and shrubs by honeybees. The main chemical classes present in propolis are flavonoids, phenolics and other various aromatic compounds. Flavonoids are well-known plant compounds which have antioxidant, antibacterial, antifungal, antiviral, and anti-inflammatory properties. Propolis is composed of 50% resin and vegetable balsam, 30% wax, 10% essential and aromatic oils, 5% pollen and 5% other various substances, including organic debris. Propolis to known to stimulate the production of transforming growth factor [TGF] Beta 1 which is important for the differentiation of odontoblasts. It also induces the synthesis of collagen by dental pulp cells. The mechanism of action of propolis includes increase in cell membrane permeability of microbes and reduction of ATP production by microorganisms, decreasing bacterial mobility and enhancing the body's immune system [26].

In animal studies using propolis, no pulpal inflammation and necrosis was seen, and induction of high-quality tubular dentin production has been reported [27]. So direct pulp capping with propolis containing flavonoids, in contrast to propolis without flavonoid and zinc oxide, delay the pulp inflammation and stimulate dentin reparative formation.

CONCLUSION

The field of dental materials has progressed rapidly in the past few years. With the pediatric dentist being presented with such a wide range of materials, a clear understanding of the characteristics, advantages, disadvantages, and applications of each material is necessary for a successful clinical outcome. With continued improvements in the existing dental materials and the introduction of newer materials, the use of these materials is likely to become more user friendly with the added advantage of enhanced physical properties, esthetics, and patient acceptance. Although the traditional concepts of restorative dentistry are still extremely relevant, newer materials allow for modifications to be made during treatment planning ensuring high levels of patient and operator satisfaction.

CONSENT FOR PUBLICATION

Not applicable.

CONFLICT OF INTEREST

The authors declare no conflict of interest, financial or otherwise.

ACKNOWLEDGEMENT

Declared none.

REFERENCES

[1]   Kateeb ET, Warren JJ. The transition from amalgam to other restorative materials in the U.S.

predoctoral pediatric dentistry clinics. Clin Exp Dent Res 2019; 5(4): 413-9.
[http://dx.doi.org/10.1002/cre2.196] [PMID: 31452952]

[2]   Fuks AB. The use of amalgam in pediatric dentistry: new insights and reappraising the tradition. Pediatr Dent 2015; 37(2): 125-32.
[PMID: 25905653]

[3]   Tibau AV, Grube BD. Mercury Contamination from Dental Amalgam. J Health Pollut 2019; 9(22): 190612.
[http://dx.doi.org/10.5696/2156-9614-9.22.190612] [PMID: 31259088]

[4]   Balaji SM. Mercury, dentistry, minamata convention and research opportunities. Indian J Dent Res 2019; 30(6): 819.
[http://dx.doi.org/10.4103/ijdr.IJDR_924_19] [PMID: 31939353]

[5]   Berg JH. The continuum of restorative materials in pediatric dentistry--a review for the clinician. Pediatr Dent 1998; 20(2): 93-100.
[PMID: 9566012]

[6]   Sidhu S, Nicholson J. A review of glass-ionomer cements for clinical dentistry. J Funct Biomater 2016; 7(3): 16.
[http://dx.doi.org/10.3390/jfb7030016] [PMID: 27367737]

[7]   Baig MS, Fleming GJP. Conventional glass-ionomer materials: A review of the developments in glass powder, polyacid liquid and the strategies of reinforcement. J Dent 2015; 43(8): 897-912.
[http://dx.doi.org/10.1016/j.jdent.2015.04.004] [PMID: 25882584]

[8]   Gjorgievska E, Nicholson JW, Gabrić D, Guclu ZA, Miletić I, Coleman NJ. Assessment of the impact of the addition of nanoparticles on the properties of glass-ionomer cements. Materials (Basel) 2020; 13(2): 276.
[http://dx.doi.org/10.3390/ma13020276] [PMID: 31936253]

[9]   Menezes-Silva R, de Oliveira BMB, Fernandes PHM, *et al.* Effects of the reinforced cellulose nanocrystals on glass-ionomer cements. Dent Mater 2019; 35(4): 564-73.
[http://dx.doi.org/10.1016/j.dental.2019.01.006] [PMID: 30711272]

[10]   Tanaka CB, Ershad F, Ellakwa A, Kruzic JJ. Fiber reinforcement of a resin modified glass ionomer cement. Dent Mater 2020; 36(12): 1516-23.
[http://dx.doi.org/10.1016/j.dental.2020.09.003] [PMID: 33010942]

[11]   Yadav R, Kumar M. Dental restorative composite materials: A review. J Oral Biosci/ JAOB, Jpn Assoc Oral Biol 2019; 61(2): 78-83.
[http://dx.doi.org/10.1016/j.job.2019.04.001] [PMID: 31109861]

[12]   Donly KJ, García-Godoy F. The use of Resin – based composite in children. Ped Dent 2015; 37(2): 136-43.
[PMID: 25905655]

[13]   Hilton TJ. Sealers, Liners, and Bases. J Esthet Restor Dent 2016; 28(3): 141-3.
[http://dx.doi.org/10.1111/jerd.12218] [PMID: 27178665]

[14]   Arandi NZ, Rabi T. Cavity Bases Revisited. Clin Cosmet Investig Dent 2020; 12: 305-12.
[http://dx.doi.org/10.2147/CCIDE.S263414] [PMID: 32801924]

[15]   Arandi N. Calcium hydroxide liners: a literature review. Clin Cosmet Investig Dent 2017; 9: 67-72.
[http://dx.doi.org/10.2147/CCIDE.S141381] [PMID: 28761378]

[16]   Dutra-Correa M, Bezerra CP, Campos CF, *et al.* On the understanding of zinc-oxide eugenol cement use prior to etch-rinse bonding strategies. Indian J Dent Res 2019; 30(3): 424-7.
[http://dx.doi.org/10.4103/ijdr.IJDR_302_16] [PMID: 31397420]

[17]   Torabinejad M, Parirokh M, Dummer PMH. Mineral trioxide aggregate and other bioactive endodontic cements: an updated overview - part II: other clinical applications and complications. Int

Endod J 2018; 51(3): 284-317.
[http://dx.doi.org/10.1111/iej.12843] [PMID: 28846134]

[18] Cervino G, Fiorillo L, Herford A, *et al.* Alginate materials and dental impression technique: a current state of the art and application to dental practice. Mar Drugs 2018; 17(1): 18.
[http://dx.doi.org/10.3390/md17010018] [PMID: 30597945]

[19] Anusavice S. Rawls Phillip's Science of Dental Materials. 12th ed., Elsevier 2013.

[20] Journal TSW. Corrigendum to "biosmart materials: breaking new ground in dentistry". ScientificWorldJournal 2020; 2020: 1.
[http://dx.doi.org/10.1155/2020/7291341] [PMID: 32395088]

[21] Najeeb S, Khurshid Z, Zafar M, *et al.* Modifications in glass ionomer cements: nano-sized fillers and bioactive nanoceramics. Int J Mol Sci 2016; 17(7): 1134.
[http://dx.doi.org/10.3390/ijms17071134] [PMID: 27428956]

[22] Khan AS, Syed MR. A review of bioceramics-based dental restorative materials. Dent Mater J 2019; 38(2): 163-76.
[http://dx.doi.org/10.4012/dmj.2018-039] [PMID: 30381635]

[23] Kaur M, Singh H, Dhillon JS, Batra M, Saini M. MTA *versus* biodentine: Review of literature with a comparative analysis. J Clin Diagn Res 2017; 11(8): ZG01-5.
[http://dx.doi.org/10.7860/JCDR/2017/25840.10374] [PMID: 28969295]

[24] Jain B, Tiku A. A comparative evaluation of shear bond strength of three different restorative materials to biodentine and TheraCal LC: An in-vitro study. IJADS 2019; 5(2): 426-9.

[25] Karabulut B, Dönmez N, Göret CC, Ataş C, Kuzu Ö. Reactions of Subcutaneous Connective Tissue to Mineral Trioxide Aggregate, Biodentine, and a Newly Developed BioACTIVE Base/Liner. Scanning 2020; 6570159.

[26] Przybyłek I, Karpiński TM. Antibacterial Properties of Propolis. Molecules 2019; 24(11): 2047.

[27] El-Tayeb MM, Abu-Seida AM, El Ashry SH, El-Hady SA. Evaluation of antibacterial activity of propolis on regenerative potential of necrotic immature permanent teeth in dogs. BMC Oral Health 2019; 19(1): 174.

CHAPTER 13

Minimal Intervention Dentistry

Arthur M. Kemoli[1,*], **Vidya Iyer**[2] and **Sheeba Saini**[3]

¹ Department of Paediatric Dentistry & Orthodontics, University of Nairobi, Nairobi, Kenya

² Department of Pediatric and Preventive Dentistry, CSI College of Dental Sciences, East Veli Street, Madurai, Tamil Nadu, India

³ Himachal Institute of Dental Sciences, Paonta Sahib, Himachal Pradesh 173025, India

Abstract: Minimally invasive treatment of dental caries is an approach that uses conservative management strategies focusing on maximum preservation of tooth structure. Unlike the principles enumerated by GV Black, which advocated maximal excavation of carious tooth structure, Minimal Invasive Dentistry (MID) conserves as much tooth structure as possible and provides a conducive environment for the affected tooth tissue to self-heal. This chapter enumerates the various modalities of Minimal Intervention Dentistry or Minimally Invasive Dentistry (MID) and discusses Atraumatic Restorative treatment (ART) in detail.

Keywords: ART, Air Abrasion, Chemomechanical Caries Removal, MID, Microdentisry, Ozone Therapy.

INTRODUCTION

Despite the innumerable advances in dental materials, prevention methods and techniques, dental caries remain a scourge that is yet to be eradicated. It has long been recognized that the traditional treatment of dental caries involving cavity preparation and restoration with silver amalgam involves unnecessary removal of healthy tooth tissues, thereby weakening the tooth structure. This "extension for prevention" approach was necessary earlier on, given the understanding of dental caries at that time, its high prevalence among populations, the limitations of dental materials available, and the lack of proven alternative treatment options. The difficulty in diagnosing dental caries in its initial stages; before the stage of cavitation, also contributed to clinical decisions involving surgical intervention rather than attempts at remineralization & monitoring of carious lesions.

---

[*] **Corresponding author Arthur M. Kemoli:** Department of Paediatric Dentistry & Orthodontics, University of Nairobi, Nairobi, Kenya; E-mail: musakulu@gmail.com

However, with a greater understanding of the dynamics of dental caries, coupled with recent multifold developments of adhesive and biomimetic restorative materials, a paradigm shift has occurred towards 'Minimally invasive dentistry(MID). This MID approach for the management of dental caries incorporates the science of detecting, diagnosing, intercepting and treating dental caries at a microscopic level. Also known as 'Microdentisty,' the MID approach also includes non-surgical modalities based on the concept that, to a certain extent, dental caries is a 'reversible' infectious disease [1].

Components of Minimal Interventional Dentistry

The components of MID are listed in Fig. (**1**).

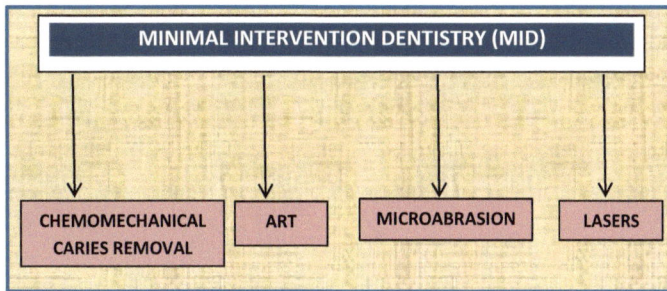

Fig. (1). Components of Minimum Intervention Dentistry.

Goals of Minimal Intervention

Minimal intervention dentistry focuses on arresting and reversing the progression of dental caries as compared to aggressive surgical intervention (removal of carious tooth tissue and replacing it with a dental restorative material), which has been the norm. The objective of MID is to defer operative/surgical intervention of dental caries for as long as possible and to conserve demineralized, non-cavitated enamel and dentin. This can be achieved through early detection of dental caries, evaluation of individual caries-related patient factors (caries risk assessment), interception of the process and finally, the treatment for any lesions already evident, with the aim of maximal preservation of tooth tissue and facilitation of self-repair of the tooth.

The principles of MID have been enumerated by Tyas *et al.* [2] as being as follows:

Early Caries Diagnosis

Besides early caries diagnosis, the operator must also evaluate the caries activity using caries activity tests, as an adjunct to clinical and radiographic examination.

Newer caries diagnostic methods like diagnosis, quantitative laser fluorescence *etc.*, can also help in the early diagnosis of caries.

Classification of Caries Depth and Progression

The use of the International Caries Detection and Assessment System (ICDAS) can serve as a good guide regarding the extent of the carious lesion. Digital radiography with low radiation exposure, diagnostic lasers and dental operative microscopes are other means to gain clarity on the caries lesion depth.

Assessment of Individual Caries Risk

Low Risk – Patients without caries in the past year, coalesced or sealed pits and fissures, good oral hygiene, appropriate fluoride use and regular dental visits.

Moderate Risk – Patients with a carious lesion in the past year, deep pits and fissures, fair oral hygiene, white spots or interproximal radiolucency, inadequate fluoride exposure, irregular dental visits and/or undergoing orthodontic treatment.

High Risk – Patients with two or more carious lesions in the past year, past smooth surface caries, deep pits and fissure, no/little fluoride exposure, elevated S. mutans count, poor oral hygiene, frequent sugar intake, inadequate salivary flow rate, irregular dental visits and prolonged bottle-feeding or nursing (infants).

Reduction of Cariogenic Bacteria To Decrease the Risk of Further Demineralization and Cavitation

Since demineralization of enamel and dentin is not a continuous irreversible process, the operator must utilize the tooth's capacity to self-heal (in case of a non-cavitated carious lesion) by altering the oral environment to favour remineralization. Proven preventive methods like diet modification and good plaque control measures at the dental office and at home should be emphasized, as they help reduce the bacteria population and improve oral health.

Arrest of Active Carious Lesions

Periodic topical fluoride application is necessary for ensuring increased availability of fluoride ions for the formation of fluorapatite, thereby increasing the resistance of teeth to demineralization. Other ways to intervene and convert an active carious lesion into an arrested lesion include the application of silver diamine fluoride, resin infiltration *etc.*

Remineralization and Monitoring of Non-cavitated Arrested Lesions

The arrested carious lesions should be monitored and evaluated for signs of caries progression, cavitation and secondary caries. MID measures can succeed only if carried out in conjunction with regular use of various preventive techniques and repeated patient education.

Examples of MID for Teeth with Cavitated Lesions

Cavitated carious lesions generally act as a nidus for food and plaque accumulation and make plaque control extremely difficult. Hence, the MID approach relies on the removal of infected tissue followed by the placement of a suitable restorative material. Adhesive restorative materials allow for a conservative cavity preparation using air abrasion, lasers, chemomechanical methods of caries removal, Atraumatic restorative procedure, resin infiltration, Hall's technique *etc.* which helps in maximum conservation of natural tooth structure.

Air Abrasion

This technology can be used to both diagnose early dental caries as well as treat them with a minimalistic cavity preparation. Air abrasion utilizes the kinetic energy of certain abrasive particles, like aluminium oxide, directed against the tooth surface to be prepared. When narrow, powerful stream abrasive particles hit the tooth surface, the tooth is abraded and a shallow cavity is prepared without the production of heat, vibration or noise. The resultant cavities tend to have more rounded internal contours than those prepared with rotary burs. Air abrasion can prove to be a highly effective way of performing a minimum intervention for the restoration of decayed teeth [3].

Lasers

Lasers can be an invaluable asset for a dental surgeon as they permit the selective removal of carious tissue, leaving behind healthy enamel and dentin. Different lasers like erbium:yttrium-aluminium garnet, erbium, chromium:yttrium-scandium-garnet lasers have been tried. Lasers can be used for both soft and hard tissue procedures and facilitate a painless, high precision cavity preparation with no vibration, little or no noise, no sensitivity and no numbness associated with anaesthesia. Cavity preparations are shallow and rounded and are suitable for placement of adhesive materials like GIC, RmGIC, composites *etc.*

Resin Infiltration

Deemed as a micro-invasive procedure, the resin infiltration method is advocated for the management of smooth surface and proximal non-cavitated lesions. It involves the superficial sealing and arrest of white spot lesions by infiltration of the porous decalcified areas with resorcinol-formaldehyde resins. The infiltration using a low viscosity resin creates a diffusion barrier within the lesion, thereby either delaying the placement of a restoration. The enamel surface is prepared by the application of 15% hydrochloric acid or 37% phosphoric acid before infiltration. This method offers several advantages – it is non-invasive, can be completed in a single visit, arrest/retard the lesion progression, no postoperative pain or sensitivity and improves esthetics as the resin infiltration masks the white spots on the labial surfaces of teeth, high patient acceptance [4].

Hall's Technique

This technique, introduced by Dr. Norna Hall, involves the placement of a preformed stainless-steel crown over a carious tooth, without local anaesthesia, caries removal or tooth preparation. An appropriate-sized stainless-steel crown is selected and cemented over the carious primary molar using glass ionomer cement. Any biofilm microflora remnants sealed under the crown change into a less carious one and retards the progression of dental caries. The seating and cementation of the crown are carried out with the operator's finger pressure or the biting force of the patient. This technique is useful in the restoration of multi-surface carious lesions in children. The initial open bite associated with the technique usually self-resolves within a few weeks. Hall's technique is associated with good patient acceptance as this technique does not necessitate the use of local anaesthesia and rotary instruments. This technique has been discussed in greater detail in another chapter of this book [5].

Conservative Cavity Preparation

Using high-speed rotary handpiece and burs, the cavity is prepared conservatively, focusing only on carious tissue removal and retaining as much sound tooth structure as possible. Modifications such as tunnel preparation, minibox or slot preparations can be utilized wherever possible. In case of tunnel preparation, the infected dentin of an interproximal carious lesion is accessed from the occlusal surface, leaving the marginal ridge intact. For the inexperienced operator, the tunnel preparation can prove challenging because of the limited access, poor visibility and minimal amount of tooth structure removed. The use of magnification loupes during cavity preparation can aid in better visualization. Tunnel preparations can help preserve the marginal ridge and the proximal surface enamel when prepared appropriately.

A saucer-shaped or a shallow box-shaped cavity called the minibox or slot preparation involves the removal of the marginal ridge of the tooth. It is indicated in interproximal caries, which minimally/do not involve the occlusal surface of the tooth. The slot preparation is typically confined to the proximal surface with the inclusion of the adjacent marginal ridge. However, slot preparation is generally not extended to the pits and fissures of the tooth.

Enameloplasty

Followed by pit and fissure sealant application is a commonly practised MID technique. Deep pits and fissures are either cleaned with pumice or are re-shaped using rotary instruments. The prepared pits and fissures are filled with flowable composites or sealants. Enameloplasty and sealant application are measured as capable of preventing dental caries by the minimalistic intervention of the occlusal surface of susceptible teeth.

Preventive Resin Restoration (PRR)

In instances where small cavitation of an occlusal pit or fissure has taken place, then such a tooth can be treated conservatively with the help of a round bur and a slow-speed handpiece. The cavitated pit or fissure is slightly widened; enough to permit caries excavation. This minimalistic cavity is then restored using composite resin, followed by pit and fissure application to include the rest of the pits and fissures. Preventive Resin Restoration helps in the repair of the carious lesion as well as protects the tooth from future attacks of dental caries.

Chemomechanical Caries Removal

This method of caries removal involves chemical softening of the carious dentine prior to its removal through gentle excavation using a spoon excavator or other hand instruments. It is a slow and non-invasive method of caries removal, which is perceived as a non-threatening procedure by pediatric patients as well as highly apprehensive adult patients. The use of hand instruments alone for caries excavation ensures a conservative cavity preparation. Following caries excavation, the cavity is restored using the appropriate dental material. The commonly used agents for chemomechanical caries removal methods include Carisolv and Papacarie [6].

Atraumatic Restorative Treatment (ART)

This method advocates the use of hand instruments to remove the soft carious tissue, followed by restoration using glass ionomer cement. ART is ideal for communities where there is no electricity, running water or proper dental equipment and healthcare facilities (Fig 2). ART restorations have good survival rates for single-surface restorations in both primary and permanent dentitions.

However, for multi-surface cavities, ART has shown a lower survival rate. (For more information, see the next section of this chapter).

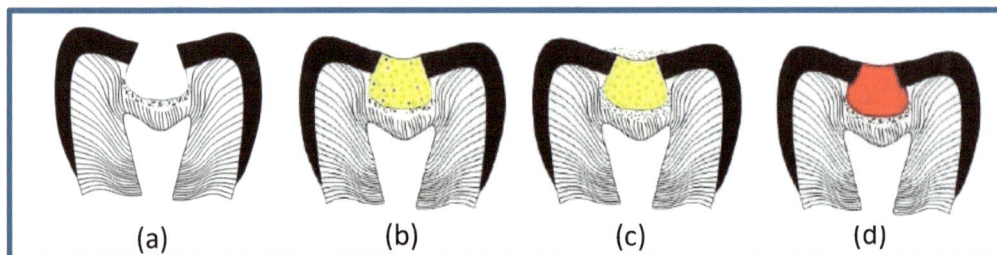

Fig. (2). (a) Pit & fissure caries **(b)** Caries removal **(c)** GIC restoration **(d)** Post restoration fluoride release and healing.

Ozone Therapy (ART)

This is one of the most minimally invasive treatment methods causing no discomfort or pain. Ozone has been known to kill bacteria, fungi and viruses by the destruction of the cytoplasmic membrane of the cells. Ozone application opens up dentinal tubules, thereby promoting the diffusion of calcium and phosphorus ions and enhancing the remineralization of teeth. The bactericidal action of ozone takes place at a concentration of 0.3 to 0.9 ppm. However, the bactericidal concentrations of ozone have been reported to be close to the permissible limit for human exposure. Ozone therapy has the potential to arrest dental caries and can be used in conjunction with fluorides to promote remineralization. Ozone inhalation can have toxic effects on the lungs. Other side effects of ozone include epiphora, rhinitis, upper respiratory tract infection, cough, headache, occasional nausea and vomiting [7].

1. ***Repair, rather than replacement of defective restorations*** – Whenever possible, attempts should be made to repair fractured or faulty restorations instead of replacing them. Each time a restoration is replaced, there is an inevitable extension of the existing cavity leading to a greater loss of tooth structure, endangering pulpal health.
2. ***Assessing disease management outcomes at pre-established intervals with regular recall and follow-ups*** – As with all intervention procedures, it is imperative that the tooth treated using the MID method be assessed periodically for signs of progression of dental caries. Regular follow-up is crucial for the success of MID. Additionally, changes in the patient's caries risk status, caries activity levels, oral hygiene practices, compliance with diet modifications *etc.*, should also be evaluated.

ATRAUMATIC RESTORATIVE TREATMENT

Introduction and Historical Background

The burden of dental caries is experienced more in developing countries and places that lack access to proper oral healthcare. Early and regular visits to the dentist can not only slow down the onset of dental caries in children but also result in fewer subsequent treatment visits and treatment costs. It appears that the prevailing methods of caries prevention and treatment that are effective in developed countries are either unaffordable or unavailable in low-income countries.

With the changing paradigms of treatment approach leaning towards minimal intervention and maximum conservation of tooth structure, techniques such as the Atraumatic Restorative Treatment (ART) have gained importance. ART is an invaluable tool to reduce the aerosol-generating treatment procedures while proving to be a good therapeutic as well as a preventive treatment in primary and permanent teeth [8]. Since its development as part of a community-based primary health program carried out in Tanzania in the mid-1980s, the ART technique has emerged as a viable alternative to the more invasive conventional restorative treatment. This method of treating dental caries without using a drill, water or electricity was presented and accepted at the headquarters of the World Health Organization, Geneva, on World Health Day, April 7, 1994 [9]. The ART technique can be made available to the remotest, most deprived and underprivileged population, resulting in increased levels of care and improved oral health for this population. The benefits of ART are enumerated in Table **1**.

Table 1. Advantages of ART with its simple equipment and materials.

Benefits and Applications of ART
• Electrically driven equipment is not required
• Local anaesthesia is generally not necessary
• Removal of only decalcified tissue and conservation of sound tooth structure
• Chemical adhesion of the restorative material to the tooth
• Causes less anxiety to the patients
• Low cost
• Combination of preventive and curative treatment in a single procedure
• Fluoride release from restorative material offers additional protection against recurrent or secondary caries
• ART can be practised along with various school health programs. Using ART, a comprehensive oral health education, prevention and treatment plan can be delivered to the children.

The use of ART is no longer restricted to underprivileged populations but also had application in the underserved populations in developed countries, where affordability and access to oral health care may be a constraint. It seems to be the preferred technique [10] in situations such as:

1. Introducing oral care to very young children, not previously exposed to dental treatment
2. For patients with extreme fear or anxiety of dental treatment
3. For mentally and/or physically challenged patients
4. For home-bound elderly patients or those living in nursing homes
5. In high caries-risk patients, an intermediate therapeutic restoration (ITR), is to be replaced by a more definitive restoration in due course of time

ART Technique

As with any other procedure, the case selection for ART is of paramount importance. Due to its reliance on handheld instruments for caries excavation, ART is best suited for single surface carious lesions (Class I and Class V lesions). The armamentarium required for ART includes those shown in Fig. (3), Table **2**.

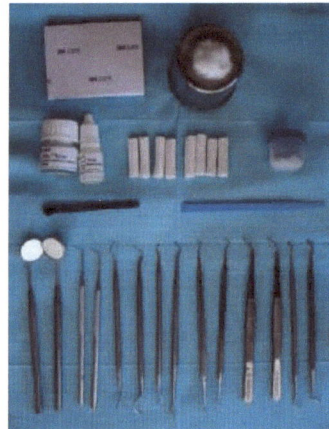

Fig. (3). Instruments required for ART.

Table 2. The materials that are used when using the ART technique.

INSTRUMENTS
Mouth mirror
Explorer
Pair of tweezers
Dental hatchet

(Table 2) cont.....

INSTRUMENTS
Spoon excavator – small/medium/large
Applier/Carver

Method

A proper operator-patient position is established before starting treatment. In a community or school setting, the child patient should be made to lie down in a supine position on a flat surface like a (Table **3** and Fig. **4**).

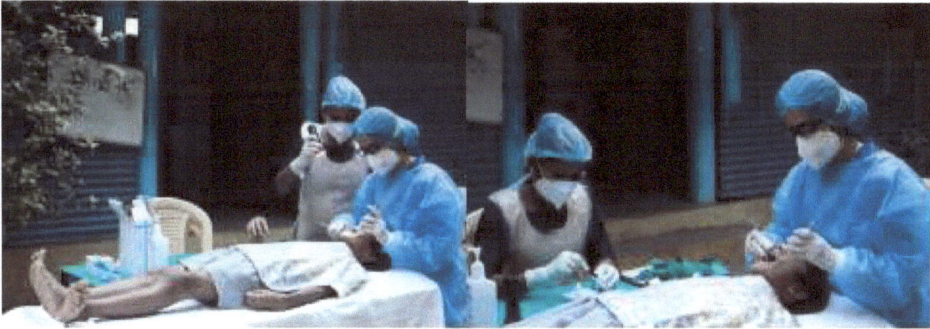

Fig. (4). Position of Operator, Patient and Assistant during ART.

A small, cushioned headrest can make the patient feel more comfortable during treatment [9]. The operator is seated at the head end of the table, and the technique of ART is performed.

1. ***Identification and isolation*** - With the help of natural daylight or a battery-powered headlamp, an oral examination is carried out and the tooth/teeth to be restored are identified. The teeth to be restored are isolated using cotton wool rolls. The materials applied when using the technique are listed in Table **3**.
2. ***Cleaning of the tooth to be treated*** - Using a wet cotton pellet, the tooth surface to be restored is cleaned. This helps in the removal of food debris and plaque and improves the visibility of the tooth surface. The adjacent pits and fissures are also cleaned using a dental probe and wet cotton pellets.
3. ***Widening the entrance of the lesion*** – A dental hatchet is used to widen the entrance of the cavity. The working tip of the hatchet is placed at the entrance of the lesion and rotated backwards and forwards. For opening up very small cavities, the angle or corner of the working tip is placed in the cavity first and rotated. All unsupported enamel is removed, and the cavity is made wide enough to be excavated with a spoon excavator.
4. ***Caries removal & Conditioning of the cavity*** – depending upon the size of the

cavitated lesion, a small/medium or large spoon excavator is used to remove the soft carious dentin. The amount of carious tissue that should be removed depends mainly on the cavity depth. In cavities of shallow and medium depth, carious tissue is removed up to the affected dentine, which feels firm upon probing. In deep or very deep cavities, in which there is no sign of pulp exposure, pulp inflammation and/or history of spontaneous pain, some soft dentine can be left in the pulpal floor/wall to avoid pulp exposure. The prepared cavity and adjacent pits and fissures are conditioned using a 15-second application of the conditioning agent. The dentin conditioner has 20% polyacrylic acid and 3% aluminium chloride hexahydrate. The conditioner removes the smear layer and dentinal debris and improves the bonding of the GIC cement with the tooth structure. It also seals dentinal tubules and reduces post-treatment sensitivity, if any. The conditioned dentin surfaces are cleaned thoroughly using wet cotton pellets and dried using dry cotton pellets.

5. *Restoration of the cavity* – The glass ionomer cement powder and liquid are dispensed by the powder-liquid ratio specified by the manufacturer. If an assistant is available, then the assistant helps the operator in mixing the GIC powder and liquid; leaving the operator free to concentrate on the isolation of the tooth and conditioning of the cavity, *etc.* After mixing, the cement is placed in the prepared cavity and the adjacent pits and fissures using an applicator. During the application of the cement, the operator must ensure that no air entrapment and subsequent voids are created in the restoration. The cavity is slightly overfilled and using a gloved finger coated with petroleum jelly, the restoration is pressed down gently for a few seconds. This constitutes the 'press-finger technique', which helps in pushing the restorative material into the deeper parts of the cavity, pits and fissures. Before the cement sets completely, the excess restorative material is removed with a carver.

6. *Checking the bite* – Using an articulating paper, the bite is checked, and the occlusion is adjusted accordingly by carving the restoration and removal of excess restorative material, if any. The restoration is coated with another layer of petroleum jelly or varnish and the patient is instructed not to eat for an hour. (Fig. **5 (a, b,c, d, e, f, g)**) shows the different steps taken when preparing and filing the dental cavity using the ART approach, and, Fig. (**6**) shows the pre- and post-operative treatment with the use of ART.

Table 3. The materials that are used when using the ART technique.

Materials	Other Equipment
Cotton wool rolls	Examination gloves
Cotton wool pellets	Mouth mask
Clean water	Operating light

(Table 3) cont.....

Materials	Other Equipment
Glass ionomer restorative material-liquid, powder & measuring spoon	Operation bed/headrest extension
Glass ionomer cement mixing pad and spatula	Stool for the operator and auxiliary personnel
Dentin conditioner	Methylated alcohol
Petroleum jelly	Pressure cooker for steam sterilization
Wedges	Instrument forceps
Mylar strips	Soap & towel
Articulation paper	Sharpening stone

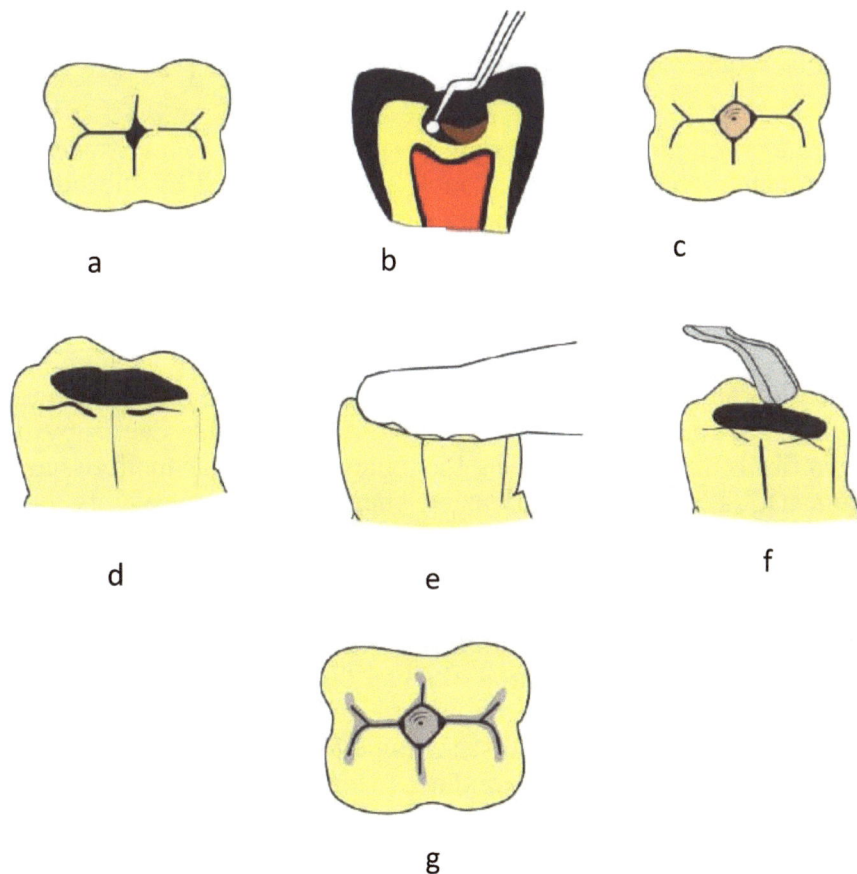

Fig. (5). (a) – Class I carious lesion. (b) – Removal of dental caries using a spoon excavator. (c) – Prepared cavity. (d) – Cavity slightly over-filled with Glass ionomer cement. (e) – Restoration pressed into the cavity using the press-finger technique. (f) – Removal of excess restorative material using a carver. (g) – Filled cavity and sealed fissures. Adapted from – Frencken J et al 1996 [9].

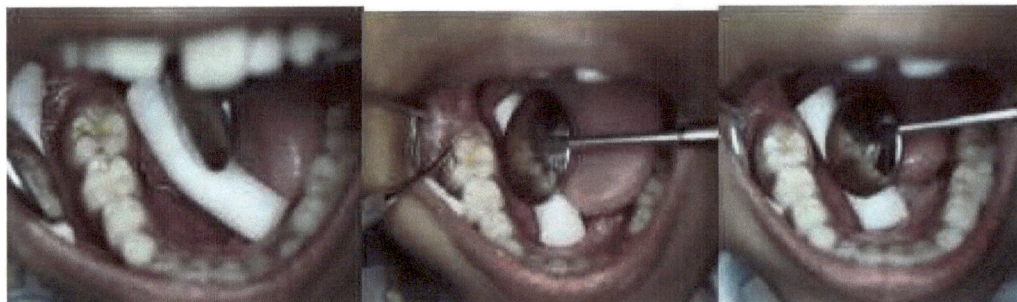

Fig. (6). (a) - Class I cavity in tooth 85,46 pre-operative photograph; **(b)** - Removal of unsupported enamel using a dental hatchet; **(c)** - Restoration of 85,46 with glass ionomer cement.

Modified ART (mART)

The principles of the original ART technique have been modified to be carried out in places where traditional dental equipment is available [11].

1. *Use of rotary equipment*- either slow-speed rotary burs or high-speed diamond burs and handpiece to open the tooth cavity, followed by the normal ART procedure in cleaning and restoring the cavity. This combination of rotary equipment and hand excavation has been said to save time & energy, provide better visualization of the lesion, minimize operator fatigue and decrease patient discomfort.

2. *Use of chemo-mechanical means of caries removal* – ART technique can be practised in conjunction with chemo mechanical caries removing agents like Carisolv, Papacarie gel, *etc.* These gels dissolve carious dentin by breaking collagen fibrils, thereby facilitating the removal of carious tooth tissue by hand instruments. The advantages of using chemo-mechanical agents along with ART include the reduction of pressure applied for caries removal during hand instrumentation and the subsequent minimization of pain or discomfort experienced.

3. *Silver Diamine fluoride application followed by ART* – After caries removal with hand instruments, application of silver diamine fluoride can be beneficial in arresting caries in the remnants of infected dentin, if any. Application of silver diamine fluoride for 30-60 sec is to be followed by the restoration of the prepared cavity using glass ionomer cement as per the tenets of the conventional ART technique.

Despite the numerous advantages, the ART method has a few limitations, as listed in Table **4**.

Table 4. Limitations of ART.

Limitations
• Limited applicability of ART to small and single surface carious tooth surfaces
• Not suitable for deep carious lesions, pulpal-involved teeth
• Poor wear resistance of glass ionomer cement can lead to loss of restoration over some time
• Operator fatigue resulting from the use of hand instruments
• Hand mixing of the glass ionomer restorative material may result in a relatively unstandardized mix

SMART

A 'Simplified and Modified Atraumatic Restorative Treatment' to remove caries followed by minimal cavity preparation using only hand instruments can be applied to the restorative treatment of primary teeth. This method using GIC as the restorative material can achieve comparable clinical results to composite resin and amalgam restorations, without inducing fear in children. It is a slow and gentle technique that is well tolerated by the most fearful patients. It is more comfortable than standard techniques using rotary instruments. No injections or powered drills are needed. Young children respond and tolerate SMART very well.

Research and Updates

Different aspects of the ART technique, especially, the material used for restoring teeth following ART, have been the subject of research for many years. The short-term survival of ART restorations is comparable to silver amalgam restorations. Single surface ART restorations (Class I & V) have a good short-term success rate of 80-90%, as compared to Class II (55-75%) or multi-surface ART restorations (35-55%) [12]. The survival rates of single surface ART restorations using resin-modified GIC in primary and permanent posterior teeth have been reported to meet the ADA specifications for quality restorations. Generally, a good marginal seal is obtained when the glass ionomer cement is placed using the 'press finger technique;' however, the restoration can still fail due to inadequate cleaning of pits and fissures, poor tooth isolation before placement of restoration and the low compressive strength of the GIC restorative material. The durability of ART restorations using GIC in cavities involving proximal surfaces is known to be significantly lower than the durability of GIC on occlusal surfaces. The common causes of failure in proximal surface restorations include cervical marginal gaps, total or partial loss of restorations and gross marginal defects [13, 14].

To address these issues, the use of resin-modified GIC cement is recommended for ART use. Glass ionomer cement has also been specifically designed for the ART technique, for example, high viscosity GIC – type VIII (Ketac Molar Easymix, 3M ESPE, Seefeld Germany). The high viscosity GIC is known to possess a high powder-liquid ratio which improves its mechanical properties like wear resistance, compressive strength and marginal adaptability. The survival rates of high viscosity GIC did not differ significantly from those of compomers & composite resin. Other materials like resin-modified GIC, compomers, *etc.*, have also been used for performing ART restorations.

Despite the advances in restorative materials, class III & class IV ART restorations usually fail due to loss of restoration. Loss of restoration is also seen in sealed occlusal pits & fissures. The probable reason for this could be the difficulty in achieving adequate bulk of restoration in these areas using ART hand instruments alone. Due to similar reasons, ART restorations are usually restricted to class V restorations in anterior teeth.

According to a randomized controlled trial carried out by Arrow P and Forrest H [15], the use of ART and Hall's technique enabled timely dental treatment of very small and uncooperative children who would otherwise be treated under general anaesthesia. Hence, they suggest that ART and other modalities of minimal intervention dentistry should be among the treatment options considered instead of recommending treatment under general anaesthesia as a protocol for pre-cooperative pediatric patients.

Fluoride release is considered an additional advantage of the dental materials used for ART restorations and is helpful in the prevention of secondary or recurrent caries. Based largely on *in-vitro* studies, Kumari *et al.* discussed the fluoride-releasing ability of various dental materials used for ART restorations – Glass ionomer cement and resin-modified GIC. The initial burst of fluoride release from glass ionomer cement seen within the first 24 hrs of restoration is essential for tooth remineralization as well as for the reduction of viable microorganisms that may have been left behind after hand instrumentation. Furthermore, the fluoride uptake & re-release capability of glass ionomer cement following exposure to fluoridated products such as toothpaste, mouthwash and, fluoride varnish/gel *etc.*, add to the cario-protective role of the cement. This phenomenon is seen less in resin-modified glass ionomer cement due to the presence of the resin matrix. Kumari *et al.* [16] have also suggested the incorporation of neem extract (Azadirachta indica) in modified glass ionomer cement meant for ART use so that additional antimicrobial properties of the neem extract can be utilized for bacteriocidal/bacteriostatic effects on cariogenic oral microflora.

The simplicity of the ART technique should not preclude proper operator training and following all steps meticulously with attention to detail. Operator skill and the type of restoration undertaken for ART are the 2 main factors influencing the clinical success of ART. As regards patient acceptance of the ART technique, most of the studies have concluded that hand instruments elicit minimum pain, thereby eliminating the use of local anaesthesia for ART procedures. Due to these factors, very good patient acceptance for ART has been reported over the years.

The practice of ART is the successful culmination of efforts to provide comprehensive oral health care, offering preventive and restorative treatment to disadvantaged populations simultaneously. After the proven success of ART restorations, several countries have now included ART in their oral health policy guidelines. Despite its various limitations, ART is perceived as a non-threatening procedure by child patients and has been therefore well received by them. The conservative cavity preparation resulting from the use of hand instruments alone is by tenets of biologic cavity preparation. Other benefits of ART, such as little/no pain during the procedure, reasonable cost-benefits, and sustainable out-reach applicability in rural & semi-rural scenarios, make this procedure an invaluable tool in the armamentarium of a pediatric dentist. The ART restorative method is indicated for treating single-surface cavities in primary and permanent teeth, and in multiple-surface cavities in primary teeth. Insufficient information is available to conclude its use for treating multiple-surface cavities in permanent teeth. It is safe to say that a judicious selection of cavities to be restored, use of the appropriate restorative material, and good operator training have resulted in saving numerous teeth that would have otherwise been extracted. Given the guidelines emphasizing the reduction in aerosol-generating procedures in the post-Covid-19 era, the ART technique will be especially relevant in clinical as well as field and community settings.

CONCLUSION

Minimally invasive dentistry is based on the caries risk assessment and control of the infectious component of dental caries. It is a concomitant application of preventive and interceptive techniques to avoid cavitation and deter disease progression in a tooth. The decision to restore a tooth with early signs of demineralization is delayed until it is evident that the tooth surface is likely to become cavitated despite all practical preventive and remineralization efforts. The successful remineralization and prevention of cavitation in a tooth are a highly rewarding outcome of MID. As has been summarized by Dr. Miles Markley, the loss of even a part of the human tooth should be considered a serious injury; and the goal of dentistry should be to preserve healthy, natural tooth structure [17].

CONSENT FOR PUBLICATION

Not applicable.

CONFLICT OF INTEREST

The authors declare no conflict of interest, financial or otherwise.

ACKNOWLEDGEMENT

Declared none.

REFERENCES

[1]   Murdoch-Kinch CA, McLEAN ME. Minimally invasive dentistry. J Am Dent Assoc 2003; 134(1): 87-95.
[http://dx.doi.org/10.14219/jada.archive.2003.0021] [PMID: 12555961]

[2]   Tyas MJ, Anusavice KJ, Frencken JE, Mount GJ. Minimal intervention dentistry — a review. Int Dent J 2000; 50(1): 1-12.
[http://dx.doi.org/10.1111/j.1875-595X.2000.tb00540.x] [PMID: 10945174]

[3]   Rainey JT. Air abrasion: an emerging standard of care in conservative operative dentistry. Dent Clin North Am 2002; 46(2): 185-209.
[http://dx.doi.org/10.1016/S0011-8532(01)00011-8] [PMID: 12014032]

[4]   Anand V, Arumugam SB, Manoharan V, Kumar SA, Methippara JJ, Methippara JJ. Is resin infiltration a microinvasive approach to white lesions of calcified tooth structures?: a systemic review. Int J Clin Pediatr Dent 2019; 12(1): 53-8.
[http://dx.doi.org/10.5005/jp-journals-10005-1579] [PMID: 31496574]

[5]   Altoukhi DH, El-Housseiny AA. Hall technique for carious primary molars: a review of the literature. Dent J 2020; 8(1): 11.
[http://dx.doi.org/10.3390/dj8010011] [PMID: 31963463]

[6]   Moimaz SAS, Okamura AQC, Lima DC, Saliba TA, Saliba NA. Clinical and microbiological analysis of mechanical and chemomechanical methods of caries removal in deciduous teeth. Oral Health Prev Dent 2019; 17(3): 283-8.
[PMID: 31209448]

[7]   Sen S, Sen S. Ozone therapy a new vista in dentistry: integrated review. Med Gas Res 2020; 10(4): 189-92.
[http://dx.doi.org/10.4103/2045-9912.304226] [PMID: 33380587]

[8]   Al-Halabi M, Salami A, Alnuaimi E, Kowash M, Hussein I. Assessment of paediatric dental guidelines and caries management alternatives in the post COVID-19 period. A critical review and clinical recommendations. Eur Arch Paediatr Dent 2020; 21(5): 543-56.
[http://dx.doi.org/10.1007/s40368-020-00547-5] [PMID: 32557183]

[9]   Frencken JE, Pilot T, Songpaisan Y, Phantumvanit P. Atraumatic restorative treatment (ART): rationale, technique, and development. J Public Health Dent 1996; 56(3): 135-40.
[http://dx.doi.org/10.1111/j.1752-7325.1996.tb02423.x] [PMID: 8915958]

[10]   Saber A, El-Housseiny A, Alamoudi N. Atraumatic restorative treatment and interim therapeutic restoration: a review of the literature. Dent J 2019; 7(1): 28-38.
[http://dx.doi.org/10.3390/dj7010028] [PMID: 30866534]

[11]   Massara MLA, Bönecker M. Modified ART: why not? Braz Oral Res 2012; 26(3): 187-9.
[http://dx.doi.org/10.1590/S1806-83242012000300001] [PMID: 22641436]

[12]   Faustino-Silva DD, Figueiredo MC. Atraumatic restorative treatment—ART in early childhood caries in babies: 4 years of randomized clinical trial. Clin Oral Investig 2019; 23(10): 3721-9.
[http://dx.doi.org/10.1007/s00784-019-02800-8] [PMID: 30666480]

[13]   Granville-Garcia AF, de Medeiros Serpa EB, Clementino MA, Rosenblatt A. The effect of atraumatic restorative treatment on adhesive restorations for dental caries in deciduous molars. J Indian Soc Pedod Prev Dent 2017; 35(2): 167-73.
[http://dx.doi.org/10.4103/JISPPD.JISPPD_98_16] [PMID: 28492197]

[14]   Ortiz-Ruiz AJ, Pérez-Guzmán N, Rubio-Aparicio M, Sánchez-Meca J. Success rate of proximal tooth-coloured direct restorations in primary teeth at 24 months: a meta-analysis. Sci Rep 2020; 10(1): 6409-23.
[http://dx.doi.org/10.1038/s41598-020-63497-4] [PMID: 32286461]

[15]   Arrow P, Forrest H. Atraumatic restorative treatments reduce the need for dental general anaesthesia: a non-inferiority randomized, controlled trial. Aust Dent J 2020; 65(2): 158-67.
[http://dx.doi.org/10.1111/adj.12749] [PMID: 32040875]

[16]   Kumari PD, Khijmatgar S, Chowdhury A, Lynch E, Chowdhury CR. Factors influencing fluoride release in atraumatic restorative treatment (ART) materials: A review. J Oral Biol Craniofac Res 2019; 9(4): 315-20.
[http://dx.doi.org/10.1016/j.jobcr.2019.06.015] [PMID: 31334004]

[17]   Markley MR. Restorations of silver amalgam. J Am Dent Assoc 1951; 43(2): 133-46.
[http://dx.doi.org/10.14219/jada.archive.1951.0192] [PMID: 14850207]

CHAPTER 14

Molar Incisor Hypoplasia (MIH)

Priyanka Bhaje[1,*], **Vidya Iyer**[2] and **Abdulkadeer Jetpurwala**[3]

[1] *Rungta College of Dental Sciences and Research, Bhilai, Chhattisgarh 490024, India*

[2] *Pedodontics and Preventive Dentistry, CSI Dental College and Research Centre, Madurai, Tamil Nadu, India*

[3] *Department of Pediatric Dentistry, Nair Hospital Dental College, Mumbai, India*

Abstract: Developmental defects of enamel a commonly encountered condition in both primary and permanent teeth enamel. Ameloblasts being highly specialized cells are highly sensitive to a host of environmental factors. As a result, a large number of factors can cause hypomineralization. Of the various hypoplastic and hypomineralization defects affecting the enamel, this chapter focuses on a distinct condition of hypomineralization involving mainly the molar and incisor teeth.

Keywords: Cheese molars, Hypoplasia, Idiopathic enamel opacities, Internal enamel hypoplasia, MIH, Non-endemic mottling of the enamel, Post eruptive breakdown.

INTRODUCTION

Enamel hypomineralization is a condition with the decreased mineral content of the enamel which is associated with a clinical presentation of well-demarcated chalky-white opacities. A disturbance during the late maturation and mineralization phase of amelogenesis leads to enamel defects. A commonly encountered pattern of such hypomineralization is seen as enamel defects in first permanent molars with or without the involvement of permanent incisors and has been termed as 'Molar Incisor Hypomineralization (MIH)' (Figs. **1** and **2**). MIH has also been observed in primary molars, in which case it is referred to as hypomineralized second primary molars (HSPMs). More importantly, HSPM is considered as a predictor for MIH [1].

---

* **Corresponding author Priyanka Bhaje:** Rungta College of Dental Sciences and Research, Bhilai, Chhattisgarh 490024, India; E-mail: priyanka22bhae@gmail.com

Satyawan Damle, Ritesh Kalaskar & Dhanashree Sakhare (Eds.)

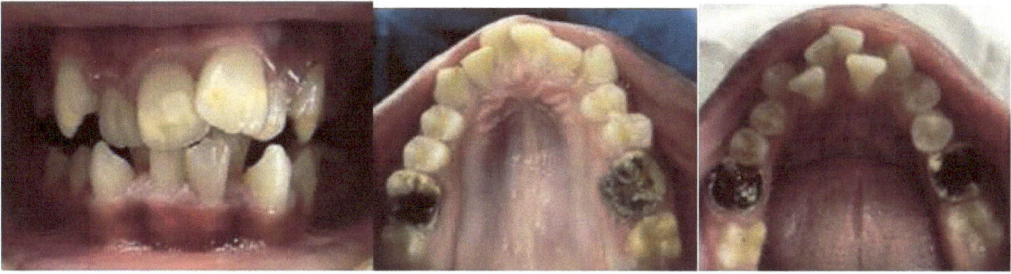

Fig. (1). MIH affecting permanent maxillary central incisors and all 4 first permanent molars.

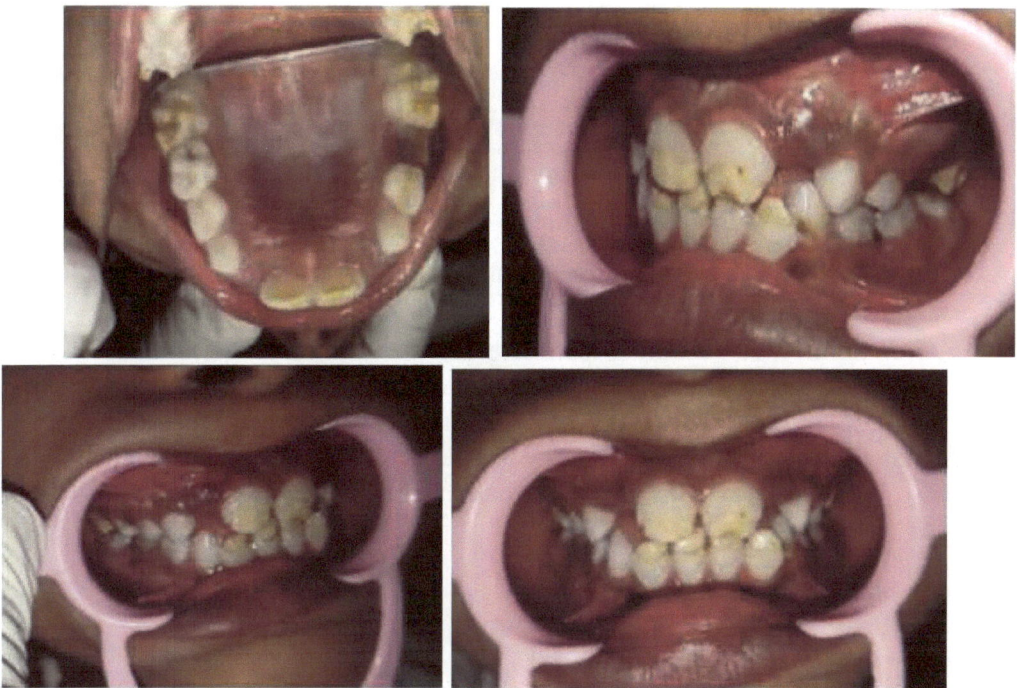

Fig. (2). MIH affecting maxillary 1st permanent molars along with maxillary and mandibular incisors, incisal tips of mandibular canine.

The term Molar Incisor Hypomineralisation (MIH) was first introduced by Weerheijm *et al* in 2001; and is defined as a developmentally derived dental defect that involves hypomineralisation of 1 to 4 permanent first molars, frequently associated with similarly affected permanent incisors. MIH is also known as *nonfluoride enamel opacities, internal enamel hypoplasia, nonendemic mottling of enamel, opaque spots, cheese molars, idiopathic enamel opacities, enamel opacities, and idiopathic enamel hypomineralization.* Hypomineralized enamel has higher porosity and less strength to withstand occlusal forces. The characteristics of MIH-affected teeth are mentioned in Table **1**. There have been reports of a greater incidence of dental caries and post-eruptive breakdown (PEB) in teeth affected by MIH. Often the teeth affected by MIH become sensitive to thermal changes and the breakdown of tooth structure makes it difficult to maintain oral hygiene, further increasing the risk of caries [2].

Table 1. Criteria for diagnosing MIH as enumerated by Weerheijm (2001).

Criteria	Definitions
Opacity	A defect involving an alteration in the translucency of the enamel, variable in degree. The defective enamel is of normal thickness with a smooth surface and can be white, yellow, or brown in color. The border of the lesions is demarcated
Post Eruptive Breakdown (PEB)	A defect that indicated deficiency of the surface after eruption of the tooth. This may be caused by such factors as trauma and attrition.
Atypical restoration	The size and shape of restoration do not conform to typical restorative characteristics. In most cases, restorations will be extended to the buccal or the palatinal smooth surface. At the border of the restoration, opacity may be noticed.
Extraction due to MIH	Absence of a molar should be related to the other teeth of the dentition. Absence of a first permanent molar in a sound dentition is suspected to have been an MIH molar.

Various epidemiological studies estimate the prevalence of MIH to be ranging from 2.8 to 40.2%. Currently, it is estimated that MIH affects one in six children worldwide [3]. Initially, MIH was described as a developmental qualitative defect of enamel affecting the permanent first molars and permanent incisors. But currently, MIH is known to affect primary molars as well as other permanent teeth.

Etiology and Diagnostic Criteria for MIH

The exact etiology of MIH is unclear. The localized and asymmetrical lesions seen in MIH probably suggest a systemic origin with the subsequent disruption of amelogenesis [4]. Many factors are known to be contributing to MIH; however, the threshold levels of these factors needed to cause enamel defects during the sensitive stages of amelogenesis not accurately known. Children with poor general health, those suffering from upper respiratory diseases, asthma, otitis media, tonsillitis, chicken pox, measles, and rubella. During the first 4 years of their life may exhibit MIH. Certain systemic conditions such as nutritional deficiencies, brain injury and neurologic deficits, cystic fibrosis, syndromes of epilepsy and dementia (Kohlschutter-Tonz syndrome), nephrotic syndrome, atopia, lead poisoning, repaired cleft lip and palate, radiation treatment, rubella embryopathy, epidermolysis bullosa, ophthalmic conditions, celiac disease, and gastrointestinal disorders also have been associated with MIH. Pre-term birth as well as the presence of polychlorinated dibenzo-p-dioxins (PCDDs) in breast milk known to have a positive correlation to enamel defects such as enamel hypoplasia and hypomineralization in the permanent dentition [5].

Examination for MIH should be undertaken on clean wet teeth bearing in mind that the clinical presentation of MIH can vary from creamy white opacities to yellowish brown lesions with either symmetrical or asymmetrical. Histopathologically, hypomineralization in cases of MIH begins at the dentino-enamel junction (DEJ), unlike other types of enamel defects that generally affect the surface enamel. In mild instances of MIH, the innermost layer of enamel is affected whereas the enamel surface remains intact. In moderate to severe MIH cases, the entire enamel layer is hypomineralized. Along with reduced mineral content, the affected enamel also exhibits higher protein content as compared to normal enamel. As a result, the enamel exhibits a soft, porous structure and is highly susceptible to dental caries and enamel breakdown soon after eruption of the tooth. In severely affected teeth, the cusps and occlusal surface of the tooth rapidly disintegrate leading to the rapid progression of caries [6]. Affected teeth also exhibit hypersensitivity, loss of restorations and secondary caries. MIH affected anterior teeth may also have a significant psychological impact on the child patient.

The European Academy of Pediatric Dentistry (EAPD) in 2003 proposed judgement criteria for MIH that include demarcated opacities, post-eruptive enamel breakdown, atypical restorations, and extraction due to MIH (Table 2). The clinician is expected to record the severity of MIH as mild or severe. In mild cases, there are demarcated enamel opacities without enamel breakdown, occasional sensitivity to external stimuli, *e.g.,* air/water but not to brushing. The patients generally report mild esthetic concerns regarding the discolored incisors. However, in severe cases, demarcated enamel opacities are seen with enamel breakdown, caries, persistent/spontaneous hypersensitivity affecting function, *e.g.,* during brushing and also pressing esthetic concerns may have socio-psychological impact on the child if left untreated.

Table 2. Judgement criteria for MIH proposed by EAPD (2003).

Criteria	Features
Teeth Involved	One to all four permanent first molars shows hypomineralization of the enamel. Simultaneously, the permanent incisors can be affected. The defects can also be seen in second primary molars, incisors, and the tips of canines. To diagnose MIH, at least one primary molar has to be affected

(Table 2) cont.....

Criteria	Features
Demarcated Opacities	The affected teeth show clearly demarcated white, creamy, or yellow to brownish opacities at the occlusal and buccal parts of the crown. The defects may vary in size and extent. It is recommended that defects less than 1 mm not be reported
Post Eruptive breakdown (PEB)	The degree of porosity of the hypomineralized opaque areas varies. Severely affected enamel subjected to masticatory forces soon breaks down, leading to unprotected dentin and rapid caries development
Atypical Restorations	FIRST PRIMARY MOLARs and incisors with restorations revealing similar extensions as MIH are recommended to be judged as affected
Tooth Sensitivity	The affected teeth may be reported frequently as sensitive, ranging from a mild response to external stimuli to spontaneous hypersensitivity; these teeth are usually difficult to anaesthetize
Extracted Teeth	Extracted teeth can be defined as having MIH only in cases where there are notes in the records or demarcated opacities on the other FIRST PRIMARY MOLAR. Otherwise, it is not possible to diagnose MIH

Differential Diagnosis of MIH

MIH should be differentiated from other conditions that have a similar clinical presentation such as

a. ***Dental fluorosis*** – Fluorosis affected teeth display diffuse, linear, and confluent opacities that do not have a clear demarcation from sound enamel. Fluorosis is also invariably associated with a history of fluoride ingestion during enamel formation; generally due to consumption of drinking water having high levels of fluoride. Fluorosis affects teeth in a bilateral and symmetric pattern unlike MIH which can have a unilateral and asymmetric presentation.

b. ***Enamel hypoplasia*** – Idiopathic enamel hypoplasia is a quantitative defect of the enamel with the borders of the hypoplastic lesion being smooth. MIH on the other hand is a qualitative defect of enamel with the lesion displaying sharp and irregular margins due to post-eruptive wearing off of the enamel. Hypoplastic lesions of enamel are seen in the form of pits, grooves, or a generalized lack of surface enamel.

c. ***Amelogenesis Imperfecta*** – Amelogenesis imperfecta is a genetic condition presenting with a generalized hypoplastic and hypomineralized enamel generally affecting both primary and permanent dentition. A family history generally shows other family members with a similar condition.

d. ***White spot lesion*** – White spot lesions are the earliest clinical sign of dental caries and appear as chalky white areas that are opaquer to the adjacent sound enamel. These areas of demineralization are generally seen near areas of opaque build-up like the cervical margins of the teeth, around orthodontic brackets, *etc.* White spot lesions become more evident upon drying of the tooth surface since drying heightens the difference in refractive index between sound enamel and adjacent demineralized enamel. Examination for MIH is however carried out on wet teeth surfaces.

e. ***Traumatic hypomineralization*** – Traumatic hypomineralization is seen in instances of chronic periapical infection associated with a traumatized primary tooth. Long-standing periapical infection in primary teeth can disturb the process of mineralization of the underlying permanent tooth germ. Such traumatic hypomineralization is often limited to a single tooth with a positive history of trauma to the primary predecessor tooth.

Treatment

The treatment of teeth affected by MIH can be challenging due to the rapid progression of dental caries and the associated sensitivity with such teeth. Repeated marginal breakdown of restorations is an additional factor to be considered prior to treatment planning. As compared to the management of affected permanent incisors and primary molars; the management of 1st permanent molars is crucial and deserves special attention (Table **3**). Identifying children at risk for MIH can ensure a timely and conservative management of the condition. Children at risk for MIH are those with poor general health during early childhood and/or those with HSPMs.

Table 3. Management of 1st Permanent Molar affected by MIH.

Risk Identification	Assess medical history to identify etiological factors
Early Diagnosis	Examine at risk molars on radiograph if possible Monitor these teeth during eruption
Remineralization And Desensitization	Topical fluoride application Minimum intervention techniques like resin infiltration etc.
Prevention Of Dental Caries And Peb	Institute thorough home care program for oral hygiene maintenance Appropriate diet modifications Placement of pit and fissure sealants
Restorations And Extractions	Placement of intracoronal (resin composite restoration) bonded with self-etching primer adhesive or extracoronal restorations (stainless steel crowns) Consider orthodontic management postextraction
Maintenance	Monitor margins of restorations for PEB Consider full coronal coverage restorations in the long-term

Considering the young age of children affected by MIH, it is imperative that preventive modalities and minimum intervention techniques be zealously implemented; failing which, other restorative or surgical options can be explored. Simultaneously, it is important to address the esthetic concerns of the patients due to the involvement of anterior teeth. The comprehensive treatment planning for molars and incisors affected by MIH can be summarized as follows [7]:

Preventive Management

Intensive prevention strategies should be implemented as soon as MIH is diagnosed, or as soon as a child at risk for MIH is identified. Affected children and their parents should be advised regarding appropriate dietary modifications.

- Topical fluoride application in the form of professionally applied fluoride gels & varnishes along with use of dentifrices containing a minimum of 1450 ppm fluoride help in reducing caries risk and tooth sensitivity.
- Desensitizing toothpaste can be prescribed for symptomatic relief.
- Daily application of casein phosphopeptides-amorphous calcium phosphate (CPP-ACP) formulation as part of home care can prove helpful in remineralization of incipient carious lesions especially in the newly erupted teeth. The use of CPP-ACP increases the bioavailability of calcium and phosphate ions in saliva thereby facilitating remineralization as well as desensitization of affected teeth. CPP-ACP has the ability to bond with the biofilm present on the tooth surface and therefore the calcium, phosphate and fluoride ions penetrate the subsurface carious lesions and remineralize the body of the lesion. Whereas fluoride application alone achieves remineralization of only the surface layer of the carious lesion. The combined use of CPP-ACP and fluoride is known to give enhanced results as compared to the use of either product alone [3].
- Use of resin-based pit and fissure sealants combined with an adhesive bonding agent can help in better retention of the sealant. Application of de-proteinising agents like 5% sodium hypoclorite or papacarie gel for 60 sec after *etc*hing can enhance the bond strength of the sealant. In cases of partially erupted molars, or molar teeth displaying PEB and hypersensitivity, glass ionomer cement can serve as a temporary sealant. Following application, all sealants must be regularly monitored and replaced when lost.

Restoration

- Cavity margin placement – Enamel affected by caries is removed keeping in mind the need for conservative cavity preparation. Only the very porous enamel is removed, until good resistance to a probe or tip of the bur is felt.

- GIC restorations – Due to its various advantages like adhesive capability to both enamel and dentin and long-term fluoride release, conventional GIC or resin modified GICs (RMGIC) are recommended for an intermediate restoration. However, considering the poor mechanical properties of GIC and its inability to withstand occlusal forces in stress bearing areas, the interim restorations should be followed by full coverage restoration of the affected molar teeth.
- Composite resin restorations – Composite resins possess good handling characteristics and improved stability compared to other restorative materials. Additionally, the polyacid modified resin composites exhibit fluoride uptake and release. These polyacid modified resin composites display tensile and flexural strength properties superior to GIC and RMGIC, but inferior to that of resin composite and therefore their use in permanent teeth is restricted to nonstress-bearing areas. The use of composite resin infiltration to strengthen the affected tooth is also advocated in cases of teeth affected by incipient caries.
- Full coverage restoration – In case of molars having moderate to severe post-eruptive breakdown, restoration using preformed stainless-steel crowns (SSCs) is the treatment of choice. Full coverage restoration helps prevent further tooth breakdown, and progression of tooth decay, minimizes tooth sensitivity, establishes correct interproximal contacts and occlusal relationships. Other advantages of stainless-steel crowns are that they are not as technique sensitive or costly as cast restorations and require little time to prepare and insert. When used judiciously, stainless steel crowns can protect and preserve the integrity of MIH-affected 1st permanent molars until cast restorations are feasible. However, if not placed properly, stainless steel crowns may cause an open bite, gingivitis, or both.
  - Partial or full coverage using cast crown and onlays can also be used for teeth affected by MIH. Compared to SSCs, cast restorations require minimal tooth reduction, provide high strength for cuspal overlays, and maintain periodontal health due to their supragingival margins.
- Extraction and orthodontic consideration – Despite the best preventive and interventional care, at times the MIH-affected tooth may not be salvageable. Extraction of such teeth may be considered in instances of severe hypomineralization, severe sensitivity or pain large multi surface lesions, questionable restorability of crown, behavior management problems preventing restorative treatment, apical pathosis, orthodontic space requirements (extraction of MIH affected primary molars), crowding distally in the arch and third permanent molars reasonably positioned, financial considerations precluding other forms of treatment *etc.*
  - Difficulty in anesthetizing MIH affected molars is well documented in the literature. To overcome this, use of anesthetic adjuncts such as intraligamental, intraosseous and palatal anesthesia can be considered. Inhalational sedation

using nitrous oxide can be helpful in increasing the pain threshold and ensuring patient cooperation during both restorative procedures as well as extraction, if necessary [8].

CONCLUSION

Teeth affected by MIH need immediate attention as MIH predisposes teeth to dental caries. A higher incidence of caries has been reported in teeth affected by MIH as compared to developmentally sound teeth. A multidisciplinary approach to management of MIH is necessary with a greater emphasis on preventive aspects such as controlling dietary factors, improving oral hygiene and periodic fluoride application; and combining the preventive measures with minimal intervention techniques and attempts at remineralization of incipient carious lesions.

CONSENT FOR PUBLICATION

Not applicable.

CONFLICT OF INTEREST

The authors declare no conflict of interest, financial or otherwise.

ACKNOWLEDGEMENT

Declared none.

REFERENCES

[1]   Garot E, Denis A, Delbos Y, Manton D, Silva M, Rouas P. Are hypomineralised lesions on second primary molars (HSPM) a predictive sign of molar incisor hypomineralisation (MIH)? A systematic review and a meta-analysis. J Dent 2018; 72: 8-13.
        [http://dx.doi.org/10.1016/j.jdent.2018.03.005] [PMID: 29550493]

[2]   Abdalla HE, Abuaffan AH, Kemoli AM. Molar incisor hypomineralization, prevalence, pattern and distribution in Sudanese children. BMC Oral Health 2021; 21(1): 9.
        [http://dx.doi.org/10.1186/s12903-020-01383-1] [PMID: 33407385]

[3]   Almuallem Z, Busuttil-Naudi A. Molar incisor hypomineralisation (MIH) – an overview. Br Dent J 2018; 225(7): 601-9.
        [http://dx.doi.org/10.1038/sj.bdj.2018.814] [PMID: 30287963]

[4]   Biondi AM, Córtese SG, Babino L, Toscano MA. Molar incisor hypomineralization: Analysis of asymmetry of lesions. Acta Odontol Latinoam 2019; 32(1): 44-8.
        [PMID: 31206574]

[5]   Vieira AR, Kup E. On the etiology of molar-incisor hypomineralization. Caries Res 2016; 50(2): 166-9.
        [http://dx.doi.org/10.1159/000445128] [PMID: 27111773]

[6]   Negre-Barber A, Montiel-Company JM, Catalá-Pizarro M, Almerich-Silla JM. Degree of severity of molar incisor hypomineralization and its relation to dental caries. Sci Rep 2018; 8(1): 1248.

[http://dx.doi.org/10.1038/s41598-018-19821-0] [PMID: 29352193]

[7]   Baroni C, Mazzoni A, Breschi L. Molar incisor hypomineralization: supplementary, restorative, orthodontic, and esthetic long-term treatment. Quintessence Int 2019; 50(5): 412-7.
[PMID: 30957114]

[8]   Patel N, Rao MH, Aluru SC, Bandlapalli A, Patel N. Molar incisor hypomineralization. J Contemp Dent Pract 2016; 17(7): 609-13.
[http://dx.doi.org/10.5005/jp-journals-10024-1898] [PMID: 27595731]

CHAPTER 15

Restoration of Carious Teeth in Children

Vidya Iyer[1,*], M. Vijay[2], Dhanashree Sakhare[3] and **Parag D. Kasar[4]**

[1] *Pedodontics and Preventive Dentistry, CSI Dental College and Research Centre, Madurai, Tamil Nadu, India*

[2] *Madura Dental Clinic, Madurai, Tamil Nadu 625001, India*

[3] *Founder, Lavanika Dental Academy, Melbourne, Australia*

[4] *Deep Dental Clinic, Navi Mumbai, Maharashtra 400706, India*

Abstract: Restorative procedures involving primary teeth constitute a major segment of clinical pediatric dentistry. Anatomic and histological differences between primary and permanent dentitions necessitate modifications of cavity preparation in primary teeth. Cavities must also be prepared keeping in mind the needs for newer restorative materials currently in use. Meticulously adhering to the principles of cavity preparation is essential for the longevity of restoration.

Keywords: Cavity preparation, Class I restoration, Class II restoration, GV Black's classification, Matrix, Wedges.

INTRODUCTION

Restoration of teeth affected by dental caries continues to remain the mainstay of dental treatment. Especially in children, dental caries is a major health problem that causes significant pain and discomfort. Even though the basic tenets of restoration of primary and permanent teeth are same, management of dental caries in children poses unique challenges in terms of obtaining patient cooperation during the treatment. Beginning with aggressive caries removal and extensive cavity preparation methods, the treatment strategy of dental caries has gradually shifted towards a more biological and conservative approach [1]. Additionally, a greater emphasis is now being laid upon prevention of dental caries and remineralization of incipient carious lesions by pediatric dental surgeons worldwide. Currently, restorations are being advised only when carious lesions have advanced to obvious cavitation and where remineralisation techniques have reached their limits.

* **Corresponding author Vidya Iyer:** Pedodontics and Preventive Dentistry, CSI Dental College and Research Centre, Madurai, Tamil Nadu, India; E-mail: vidyaiyer04@gmail.com

Restoration of primary teeth is aimed at preserving the integrity and function of the deciduous dentition so that a healthy oral environment is maintained till the permanent teeth occupy their rightful places in the dental arch (Table **1**).

Table 1. Goals of restoration of teeth in children.

Goals of Restoration of Teeth
• Symptomatic relief
• Arresting the progression of dental caries
• Prevention of damage to pulp tissue
• Maintenance of function
• Maintenance of arch length
• Improving esthetics

Anatomy and morphology of the primary teeth differ from that of the permanent teeth in spite of the same function and superficial resemblance. As a result, the clinical presentation of dental caries may differ between the two dentitions.

Crown Morphology

Crowns of the primary teeth are more bulbous than that of the permanent teeth. Mesiodistal width is bigger than that of the occluso-gingival height in primary molars whereas the permanent molars are wider buccolingually. However, the dimensions of anterior is same in primary dentition. Narrow occlusal table is seen in primary molars which is narrower in primary first molar as compared to that of primary second molar. Cervically, the tooth is broader with a prominent cervical bulge seen on the bucco-cervical aspect of mandibular first primary molar. Isthmus part of the tooth where occlusal and proximal preparations meet is very narrow in the primary molars so extra care is to be exercised during cavity preparation because it is a common site for restoration failure due to occlusal forces.

Contact Areas

Contact areas between teeth are broad and flat in primary dentition when compared to that of the permanent dentition. Hence, the proximal box is made wider to get a proper cavosurface margin. As the contact area is broad, proximal caries is difficult to detect during initial stages of decay. Bitewing radiographs can help in detecting proximal caries. In cases of extensive decay involving both the approximal surfaces of a primary molar, cavity preparation may be too close to the pulp chamber. Additionally, matrix placement is challenging in such cases as cervical constriction leads to less tooth surface in the cervical area. In such a scenario, restoration of the tooth with stainless steel crown is the preferred treatment option.

Enamel Rods

In the cervical area, the enamel rods in primary dentition are directed occlusally; unlike in permanent dentition where the enamel rods are directed gingivally. Hence, the proximal box preparation in primary teeth for a class II amalgam restoration differs slightly from that of permanent teeth.

Pulp and Root Morphology

Pulp horns are placed higher and closer to the occlusal surface in primary teeth. Primary mandibular molars present with four pulp horns, whereas the primary maxillary molars have three prominent pulp horns. Caries excavation and preparation of cavity should be carried out with caution to avoid iatrogenic pulp exposure in deciduous teeth.

Due to these anatomic differences, the cavity preparation in deciduous dentition differs from that in permanent dentition (Table **2**).

Table 2. Differences between cavity preparation in primary and permanent teeth.

Cavity Preparation in Deciduous Teeth	Cavity Preparation in Permanent Teeth
Cavity preparation is smaller (due to smaller crown size), shallower (due to thin enamel) and narrower (due to narrow occlusal table)	Cavity preparation is comparatively larger due to larger crown size, deeper due to thicker enamel and wider due to a broad occlusal table
Pulpal floor is saucer shaped due to higher pulp horns	The pulpal floor is prepared flat
Occlusal walls of cavity are less convergent	Occlusal cavity walls are more convergent
The buccal and lingual walls of the proximal box of Class II cavity are more convergent occlusally	Buccal and lingual walls of proximal box of a Class II cavity are less convergent occlusally
Buccal and lingual retentive grooves are not indicated	Buccal and lingual retentive grooves can be provided for additional retention
In the gingival seat of Class II restoration, a Cavo surface bevel is not given as the enamel rods are oriented occlusally	A Cavo surface bevel is given at the gingival seat of a Class II restoration as enamel rods are directed cervically
Width of the isthmus is $1/3^{rd}$ the intercuspal distance	Width of the isthmus is $1/4^{th}$ the intercuspal distance

Preparation of cavity for placement of restoration is based on the anatomic area involved by dental caries as enumerated by Dr G.V Black in 1924 (Table **3**). The cavity preparation based on this classification was intended for silver amalgam restoration. With the declining use of silver amalgam in recent years, cavity preparation has undergone modifications keeping in mind the availability of newer restorative materials [2].

Table 3. Classification of dental caries based on anatomic location.

Class	Description	Illustration
Class I	Pit and fissure lesions on occlusal surface of posterior teeth and lingual pits of anterior teeth	
Class II	Caries affecting the proximal surfaces of molars and premolars	
Class III	Caries involving the proximal surfaces of anterior teeth without the involvement of incisal edge	
Class IV	Caries affecting the proximal surfaces of anterior teeth, also involving the incisal edge	
Class V	Caries affecting the gingival third of facial or lingual surfaces of anterior or posterior teeth	

(Table 3) cont.....

Class	Description	Illustration
Class VI	Caries affecting those surfaces deemed naturally resistant to caries *e.g.,* Cusp tips	

Characteristics of Cavity Preparation

The traditional principles of cavity preparation follow the concept of 'Extension for prevention' and were designated especially for silver amalgam restoration. The cavity preparation is accomplished through a series of systematic procedures.

Class I

All carious tooth structure is removed beginning from the pits and fissures, extending to a depth of 0.2-0.5 mm into the dentin. The outline form is dove tailed and includes all unsupported enamel and developmental grooves. In case of maxillary second deciduous molars, the cavity preparation must include only the nearest occlusal pit; the oblique ridge is not included in the preparation unless it is undermined by dental caries.

The cavity walls are kept parallel with a slight occlusal convergence with the greatest width at the pulpal floor. Cavity preparation is extended until the cavity margins lie on sound tooth structure which is self-cleansing and permit good finishing of the restoration margins. Tooth structure along the cuspal inclines and marginal ridges is preserved as much as possible (Fig. **1**). Important features of a class I cavity in primary teeth are:

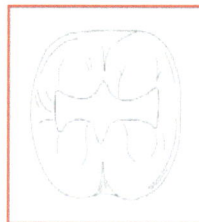

Fig. (1). Class I cavity preparation.

- Flat pulpal wall perpendicular to the longitudinal axis of the tooth
- External walls converged on occlusal
- Round internal angles

- Well-defined, sharp cavosurface angle Fig. (**1**): Class I cavity preparation

Class II

The occlusal part of cavity preparation is identical to the one described for class I cavity preparation. Preparation of proximal box in a class II restoration requires special attention. The isthmus is the common area of restoration failure, a narrow isthmus does not accommodate adequate amalgam bulk to resist fracture, and a wide isthmus compromises the tooth integrity by weakening the cusps [3]. Considering the broad and flat contact areas, the cavity outline is carried sufficiently into the embrasure area so as to remain easily cleansable (Fig. **2**). The use of matrix bands along with wedges is an indispensable aspect of a class II restoration. The salient features of a class II cavity include:

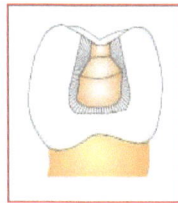

Fig. (2). Class II cavity preparation.

- Lingual and buccal walls having a slight occlusal convergence, following the contours of the external tooth surface
- Axiopulpal line angle should be gently rounded
- A sharp cavosurface angle
- The gingival seat should be placed beneath the point of contact without a bevel
- Flat gingival walls perpendicular to the longitudinal axis of the tooth

Class III & Class IV

Class III and IV cavities were prepared with a box like outline form for restoration using silver amalgam (Fig. **3**). Such restorations were at times placed in distal surface of canines when esthetics is not the prime consideration. However, with the proven clinical success of composite resins as a restorative material, the cavity preparation is limited to adequate removal of caries and bevelling the enamel margins of the cavity [4]. All unsupported enamel is included in the preparation and the external walls of the cavity are placed on sound tooth structure [5]. Placement of retention grooves or coves can provide additional retention for the bonded composite resins. Wherever possible, a lingual/palatal access is preferred rather than a facial access because:

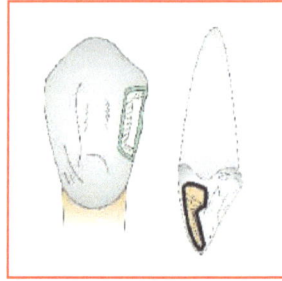

Fig. (3). Class III & IV Cavity preparations.

- The facial enamel can be conserved for esthetics
- Exact shade matching of the composite material is less crucial
- Discoloration or deterioration of the restoration is less visible

For large class IV cavities with significant involvement of dentine, additional retention features like retention grooves, increasing the width of the bevel to provide a greater surface area for etching, or full coverage of tooth with a crown may be considered.

Class V

When caries affects the gingival third of the facial or lingual surfaces of teeth, a glass ionomer cement restoration (for posterior teeth class V cavities) and composite resin (for anterior teeth class V cavities) are best suited. Hypoplastic areas as well as decalcified cavitated lesions located in the cervical one third of the teeth can also be restored using GIC, Resin modified GICs, composite resin or compomers [6] (Fig. **4**). The carious lesion is removed using spoon excavators and rotary instruments taking care to place the axial wall on sound dentine. The cavosurface margins on the enamel surface are bevelled in case of composite resin restorations. In instances where adequate isolation is not possible, GIC or resin modified GIC is preferred for class V restorations.

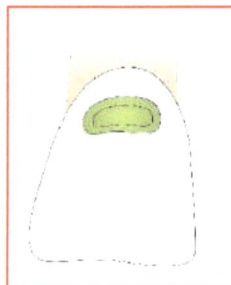

Fig. (4). Class V cavity preparation.

Matrices and Wedging

A matrix system provides a temporary wall for the proximal tooth surface in order to achieve a good restoration of proximal contours and contact points to their normal shape and function. The primary function of a matrix band is to compensate for missing walls of the tooth and thus provide containment for the filling material. Matrix bands are also indispensable for preventing iatrogenic damage to the adjacent tooth during placement of a restoration [7]. Traditionally, matrix bands were manufactured from thin, flexible, flat pieces of metal and were placed circumferentially around the affected tooth. If necessary, the matrix bands can be contoured using the contouring pliers or ball and socket pliers for an accurate reproduction of the approximal surface. Use of a well contoured matrix band along with wedges is crucial to prevent an overhanging restoration [8].

Matrix bands are positioned with the help of various types of retainers. Ivory no. 1 and Ivory no. 9 matrix retainers have been in use for silver amalgam restorations for long (Fig. **5**). Newer matrix systems have been introduced which help in holding the matrix band in a proper position. They consist of "retainer less" matrix systems, incorporating attributes of preformed, spring-loaded, circular bands and novel tightening wrenches. *E.g.*, sectional matrix and smart view matrix system which can be used for class II amalgam and composite restorations [9].

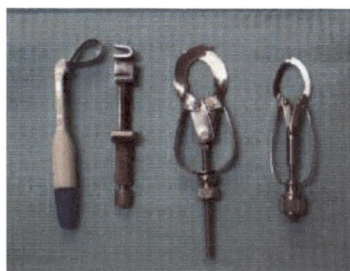

Fig. (5). Matrix band retainers – Disposable (Plastic, adjustable) retainer with matrix band.

Wedges

Wedges are small, tapering, triangular pieces of wood or plastic about ½ inch in length. They are used to adapt the matrix band closely to the tooth, beneath the point of contact to prevent overhang of the restorative material. Wedges are available in plastic, wood, metal, and celluloid (Fig. **6**).

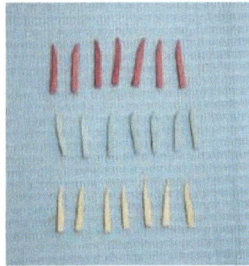

Fig. (6). Colour coded wooden wedges.

Types of wedges:

- According to material used: -
  - Plastic
  - Wood
- According to colour: -
  - Coloured
  - Light reflecting
- According to anatomy: -
  - Anatomical

(Plastic, adjustable) retainer with matrix band

Function of Wedges

Close adaptation of matrix band to tooth, stabilization of band, and to provide a slight degree of tooth separation to enable proper placement and finishing of a proximal restoration.

Clinical Implications

Treatment of caries should meet the needs of each particular patient, based on their individual caries risk. Restorative decisions for the primary dentitions are taken based on different objectives and expectations than those for permanent dentition. Picking the 'right' restoration involves understanding the limitations of the primary dentition to hold certain types of restorations over time and the durability of the restorative options available. The factors to be considered prior to restoring a cavity are enlisted in Table **4**.

Table 4. Factors for consideration prior to restoration of a cavity.

Factors to be Considered Prior to Restoration of Primary Teeth
☐ Extent of caries
☐ Pulpal involvement
☐ Radiographic evaluation
☐ Possibility of adequate isolation ☐ Length of time remaining prior to tooth exfoliation
☐ Limitations of restorative material to be used
☐ Patient's caries risk
☐ Ability of the child to cooperate during treatment
☐ Esthetics considerations
☐ Operator skill

Based on these considerations, the American Academy of Pediatric Dentistry (AAPD) guidelines 2019 recommends [10]:

1. For small occlusal lesions, a conservative preventive resin restoration, using composite or compomer in conjunction with the sealant, would be more appropriate than the classic Class I amalgam preparation. Care should be taken to achieve a good isolation of the tooth for the preventive resin restoration and/or sealant placement.
2. There is strong evidence that dental amalgam is efficacious in the restoration of Class I and Class II cavity restorations in primary and permanent teeth. However, the use of amalgam has declined over the past decade, due to the controversy surrounding the perceived health effects of mercury vapour, environmental concerns from its mercury content, and increased demand for esthetics alternatives.
3. For Class I cavities in primary teeth, conventional Glass ionomer cement, composites, compomers and resin modified GICs can be used (Fig. **7**). All of the above mentioned except conventional GIC are recommended for class II cavity in primary teeth (Fig. **8**).
4. If the carious lesion is extensive and/or involving more than 2 tooth surfaces, full coverage restoration – stainless steel crowns or Hall technique is recommended. Use of stainless-steel crowns is the preferred restorative option in case of children with a high caries risk exhibiting multi-surface cavitated or non-cavitated lesions on primary molars.
5. For Class III and class V restorations in primary anterior teeth, composites offer greater esthetics and longevity than glass ionomer cements; provided

adequate isolation can be obtained (Fig. **9**).

6. For extensive caries involving anterior teeth, or teeth with class IV cavities, pulp therapy followed by full coverage restoration using strip crowns, open face stainless steel crowns, pre-veneered stainless-steel crowns or zirconia crowns are indicated.

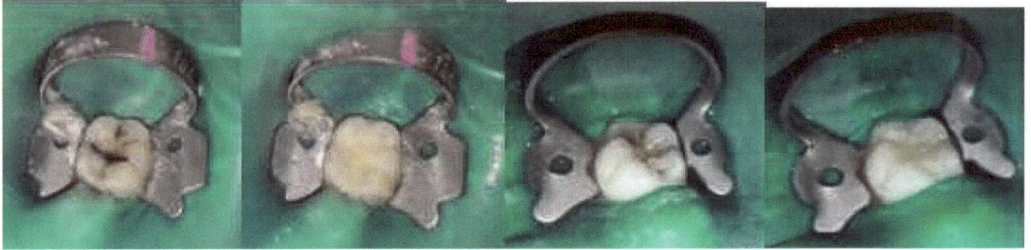

Fig. (7). Class I restoration using resin modified GIC.

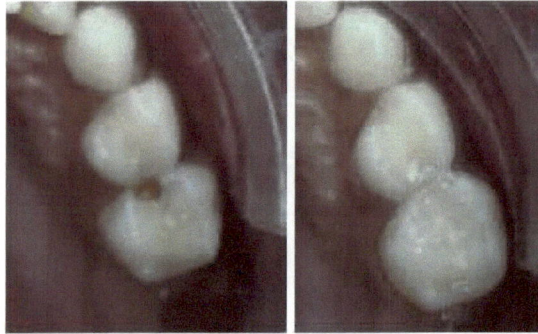

Fig. (8). Class II cavity restored with composite resin.

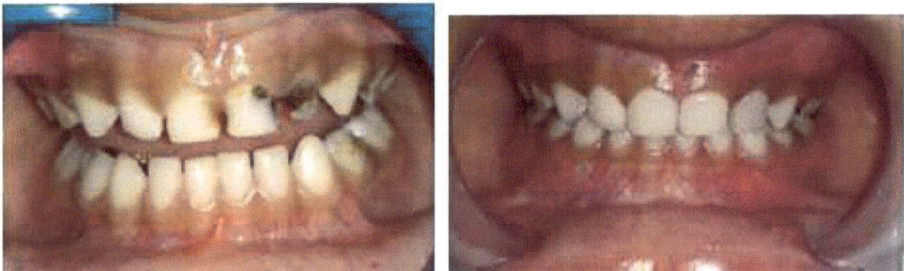

Fig. (9). Class III & V cavities restored using composite resin.

It is imperative to note that the objective of cavity preparation is to prepare the tooth as conservatively as possible and maintaining as much sound tooth structure as possible [11]. Failing to achieve this objective can lead to a reduction in the longevity of the tooth due to:

- Increased susceptibility to fracture
- Restoration of fracture
- Recurrent dental caries
- Pulp exposure during caries excavation
- Iatrogenic damage to adjacent teeth

With a greater emphasis currently being laid upon conservative cavity preparations and minimal intervention modalities, the following clinical alternatives must be considered wherever possible:

Enameloplasty

Enameloplasty is the removal and reshaping of enamel pits and developmental fissures using rotary instruments to create a smooth, saucer-shaped surface that is self-cleansing. Bodecker (1929) suggested that deep occlusal fissures can be reshaped by reducing the cuspal inclines so that the occlusal surface is more easily cleaned. It is intended to be a prophylactic procedure to prevent dental caries in deep pits, fissures, and supplemental grooves. Though the application of pit and fissure sealants does not mandate tooth preparation, enameloplasty is sometimes performed prior to sealant application. As an alternative to using rotary instruments for reshaping of the pits and fissures, air abrasion can also be used. For those pits and fissures already affected by dental caries, the tooth is prepared in an ultra-conservative manner and filled using preventive resin restoration [12].

Resin Infiltration

Resin infiltration is a micro invasive treatment procedure for enamel white spot lesions. The porosities present within the enamel lesion act as diffusion pathways for acids and dissolved minerals. The infiltration of these pores with a low viscosity resin can cause an arrest of the early stages of demineralization. Resin infiltration is especially recommended for smooth surface and proximal surface decalcified lesions. The lesion surface is prepared by application of 15% hydrochloric acid for 2 minutes. This is followed by desiccation using 99% ethanol for 30 sec followed by air drying. Ethanol wet bonding facilitates the penetration of hydrophobic resin into the etched enamel surface giving rise to a well-defined, resin-infiltration layer. Low viscosity resin is applied and allowed to penetrate the prepared lesion surface for 3 mins followed by light curing. Re application of another coat of the resin is recommended to compensate for the possible polymerization shrinkage [13].

Current ADA clinical practice guidelines for non-restorative treatment for non –cavitated interproximal caries lesions conditionally recommends resin infiltration for treatment of these lesions. An additional use of resin infiltration has been suggested to restore white spot lesions formed during orthodontic treatment. Resin infiltration can possibly eliminate or postpone the need for restoration of such incipient lesions.

CONCLUSION

The management of cavitated and non cavitated carious lesions differ significantly. Innovative developments in the field of dental materials enable the pediatric dentist to prioritize conservative and non-invasive treatment approach for dental caries. With this in mind, cavity preparation should maximize retention of healthy tooth tissue, preserve damaged tissues which have the potential to repair and selectively removes weakened tooth tissue that is liable to fracture. Despite best practices, restorations do fail, leaving the tooth vulnerable to recurrent caries or a greater tooth structure loss due to replacement of restoration. Mere restoration of cavities without a comprehensive management of dental caries is futile because recurrent or secondary caries may propel the tooth towards a 'death spiral' or 'tooth countdown' that ultimately results in tooth loss [11]. Therefore, the importance of preventive aspects of dental caries cannot be overemphasized and prevention should go hand in hand with restorative management of tooth decay.

CONSENT FOR PUBLICATION

Not applicable.

CONFLICT OF INTEREST

The authors declare no conflict of interest, financial or otherwise.

ACKNOWLEDGEMENT

Declared none.

REFERENCES

[1]   BaniHani A, Duggal M, Toumba J, Deery C. Outcomes of the conventional and biological treatment approaches for the management of caries in the primary dentition. Int J Paediatr Dent 2018; 28(1): 12-22.
[http://dx.doi.org/10.1111/ipd.12314] [PMID: 28691235]

[2]   Bailey O, Vernazza CR, Stone S, Ternent L, Roche AG, Lynch C. Amalgam phase-down part 1: uk-based posterior restorative material and technique use. JDR Clin Trans Res 2020; 2380084420978653.
[PMID: 33300416]

[3]   Riccio C, Piccirillo P, Belnome G, Serpico R. [Class II cavity for amalgam. Proposed new modifications related to material characteristics]. Arch Stomatol (Napoli) 1990; 31(4): 683-91.
[PMID: 2100480]

[4]   Khandelwal D, Nihalani S, Priyank H, Verma A, Chaudhary E, Nihalani S. *In vitro* Comparative

Evaluation of Various Restorative Materials used for restoring Class III Cavities in Deciduous Anterior Teeth: A Clinical Study. J Contemp Dent Pract 2016; 17(12): 1022-6.
[http://dx.doi.org/10.5005/jp-journals-10024-1975] [PMID: 27965491]

[5]   Piyapinyo S, White GE. Class III cavity preparation in primary anterior teeth: *in vitro* retention comparison of conventional and modified forms. J Clin Pediatr Dent 1998; 22(2): 107-12.
[PMID: 9643182]

[6]   el-Kalla IH. Marginal adaptation of compomers in Class I and V cavities in primary molars. Am J Dent 1999; 12(1): 37-43.
[PMID: 10477997]

[7]   Milic T, George R, Walsh LJ. Evaluation and prevention of enamel surface damage during dental restorative procedures. Aust Dent J 2015; 60(3): 301-8.
[http://dx.doi.org/10.1111/adj.12230] [PMID: 25283817]

[8]   El-Shamy H, Sonbul H, Alturkestani N, *et al.* Proximal contact tightness of class II bulk-fill composite resin restorations: An *in vitro* study. Dent Mater J 2019; 38(1): 96-100.
[http://dx.doi.org/10.4012/dmj.2017-279] [PMID: 30381630]

[9]   de la Peña VA, García RP, García RP. Sectional matrix: Step-by-step directions for their clinical use. Br Dent J 2016; 220(1): 11-4.
[http://dx.doi.org/10.1038/sj.bdj.2016.18] [PMID: 26768458]

[10]   The Reference Manual of Pediatric Dentistry. Chicago, Ill.: American Academy of Pediatric Dentistry 2020; pp. 371-83.

[11]   Mackenzie L, Banerjee A. Minimally invasive direct restorations: a practical guide. Br Dent J 2017; 223(3): 163-71.
[http://dx.doi.org/10.1038/sj.bdj.2017.661] [PMID: 28798466]

[12]   Konark , Singh A, Patil V, Juyal M, Raj R, Rangari P. Comparative evaluation of occlusal pits and fissures morphology modification techniques before application of sealants: An *In vitro* study. Indian J Dent Res 2020; 31(2): 247-51.
[http://dx.doi.org/10.4103/ijdr.IJDR_956_19] [PMID: 32436905]

[13]   Anand V, Arumugam SB, Manoharan V, Kumar SA, Methippara JJ, Methippara JJ. Is Resin Infiltration a Microinvasive Approach to White Lesions of Calcified Tooth Structures?: A Systemic Review. Int J Clin Pediatr Dent 2019; 12(1): 53-8.
[http://dx.doi.org/10.5005/jp-journals-10005-1579] [PMID: 31496574]

SUBJECT INDEX

A

Acids 183, 323, 324, 325, 326, 329, 335, 342, 357, 363, 392
  freeze-dried 326
  hydrochloric 357, 392
  iticonic 324
  maleic 324
  orthophosphoric 329
  phosphoric 335, 357
  polyacrylic 323, 324, 363
  polymeric 325
  stearic 342
  tartaric 324, 326
  tricarballylic 324
Acute disseminated histiocytosis 9
Addison's disease 43
Age, gestational 302
Agents 66, 152, 279, 285, 310, 313, 314, 358, 365, 377
  ant-cholinergic 152
  antifungal 285
  chemo-mechanical 365
  chemotherapeutic 310
  immunosuppressive 279
Amalgam 319, 320, 323, 321, 322, 366
  restorations 319, 320, 321, 322, 366
  scrap 323
Ameloblastoma 16, 20
  hemangiomatous 16
Amelogenesis 371, 373
Anaerobic bacteria 54
Anaesthesia 356
Anemia 2, 7, 37, 38, 42
  hemolytic 37
Ankylosis 43, 187
Antibiotic(s) 8, 54, 273, 283, 293, 296
  cephalosporin 54
  therapy 273, 283
Antimicrobial 276, 367
  mouth rinse 276
  properties 367

Antiviral drug therapy 283

B

Bacteria 125, 269, 281, 297, 304, 310, 333, 359
  heterotrophic water 125
Barr virus 289
Bioactive glass (BAG) 346
Biodegradable waste management 107
Bio dentine application 349
Biological toxins 128
Biomedical waste management 127, 128
Bone marrow transplantation 2
Bony resorption 12
Brushing technique 38, 301, 313
Burkitt's Lymphoma 25

C

Caffey's disease 7
Candida albicans 285
Capnocytophaga sputigena 292
Cardiac arrhythmias 280
Cavitated lesions 318, 356, 363
CBCT 79
  images 79
  machine 79
Cephalometric 74, 85, 86, 105
  imaging 74
  radiography 85, 86
  roentgenography 105
Chicken pox 47, 373
Christian disease 283
Chronic 43, 209
  lymphadenitis 43
  nasal respiratory distress 209
Cognitive skills 309
Collagen 5, 7, 295
  fibers 5
  maturation 7

www.ingramcontent.com/pod-product-compliance
Lightning Source LLC
Chambersburg PA
CBHW050759220326
41598CB00006B/65